Advocacy in Neurology

Advocacy in Neurology

Edited by

Wolfgang Grisold
Neurologist
Ludwig Boltzmann Institute for Experimental and Clinical Traumatology
Vienna, Austria

Walter Struhal
Neurologist and Chair of the Department of Neurology
University Clinic Tulln
Karl Landsteiner University of Health Sciences
Tulln, Austria

Thomas Grisold
Research and Teaching Associate
Vienna University of Economics and Business
Vienna, Austria

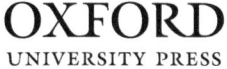

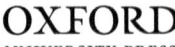
UNIVERSITY PRESS

Great Clarendon Street, Oxford, OX2 6DP,
United Kingdom

Oxford University Press is a department of the University of Oxford.
It furthers the University's objective of excellence in research, scholarship,
and education by publishing worldwide. Oxford is a registered trade mark of
Oxford University Press in the UK and in certain other countries

© Oxford University Press 2019

The moral rights of the authors have been asserted

First Edition published in 2019

All rights reserved. No part of this publication may be reproduced, stored in
a retrieval system, or transmitted, in any form or by any means, without the
prior permission in writing of Oxford University Press, or as expressly permitted
by law, by licence or under terms agreed with the appropriate reprographics
rights organization. Enquiries concerning reproduction outside the scope of the
above should be sent to the Rights Department, Oxford University Press, at the
address above

You must not circulate this work in any other form
and you must impose this same condition on any acquirer

Published in the United States of America by Oxford University Press
198 Madison Avenue, New York, NY 10016, United States of America

British Library Cataloguing in Publication Data

Data available

Library of Congress Control Number: 2018956188

ISBN 978–0–19–879603–9

Oxford University Press makes no representation, express or implied, that the
drug dosages in this book are correct. Readers must therefore always check
the product information and clinical procedures with the most up-to-date
published product information and data sheets provided by the manufacturers
and the most recent codes of conduct and safety regulations. The authors and
the publishers do not accept responsibility or legal liability for any errors in the
text or for the misuse or misapplication of material in this work. Except where
otherwise stated, drug dosages and recommendations are for the non-pregnant
adult who is not breast-feeding

Links to third party websites are provided by Oxford in good faith and
for information only. Oxford disclaims any responsibility for the materials
contained in any third party website referenced in this work.

Contents

Contributors *ix*

Section 1 **What is advocacy?**

1 **What is advocacy?** *3*
   Wolfgang Grisold, Walter Struhal, and Thomas Grisold

2 **Taking an epistemological perspective on advocacy** *21*
   Thomas Grisold and Oliver Lukitsch

3 **Advocacy in history and culture** *33*
   Wolfgang Maderthaner and Wolfgang Grisold

4 **Ethical issues in neurology** *41*
   Jan J. Heimans

5 **Physician autonomy and the pharmaceutical industry** *53*
   Tissa Wijeratne, Essie Low, and Christopher Neil

6 **Advocacy, campaigning, lobbying: Good or bad?** *61*
   Mohammad Wasay

Section 2 **Why is advocacy needed?**

7 **Knowledge and science are not enough** *69*
   Wolfgang Grisold

8 **Perspectives on advocacy of medical doctors** *83*
   Mohammad Wasay

9 **Advocacy and the perspective of (neurology) nursing** *89*
   Hanneke Zwinkels

10 **Patient and caregiver advocacy** *97*
    Helen Bulbeck

11 **Patient involvement in European cancer societies: The example of ECCO—the European CanCer Organization** *113*
    Françoise Van Hemelryck

12 **Advocacy for neurology in migrants** *123*
    Mustapha El Alaoui Faris

13 **Advocacy for neurology: Local, regional, and national** *135*
    Apoorva Pauranik

14 Advocacy in the international arena *153*
   Raad Shakir

15 Working with others, the lesson of the European Brain Council *159*
   Jes Olesen and Frédéric Destrebecq

16 SOS Children's Villages: Rediscovering advocacy to increase relevance and impact. A high-level case study *167*
   Richard Pichler

Section 3 What tools can be used for advocacy?

17 Project management techniques for advocates *179*
   Walter Struhal and Thomas Grisold

18 International advocacy: Case studies and lessons learnt *193*
   Wolfgang Grisold, Anna Klicpera, and Thomas Grisold

19 Using PR tools for advocacy *205*
   Birgit Kofler

Section 4 Advocacy in different neurological diseases

20 Advocacy for stroke *219*
   Tissa Wijeratne, Sheila Crewther, and David Crewther

21 Two decades of patient advocacy in multiple sclerosis: The success story of the European Multiple Sclerosis Platform *229*
   Christoph Thalheim

22 Advocacy in amyotrophic lateral sclerosis *243*
   Albert C. Ludolph

23 Neuromuscular disorders and advocacy *253*
   Elaine C. Jones and John D. England

24 Advocacy for movement disorders *265*
   Francesca Mancini and Carlo Colosimo

25 Advocacy for brain tumours *281*
   Riccardo Soffietti, Christine Marosi, Roberta Rudà, and Wolfgang Grisold

26 Advocacy in dementia *291*
   Gorazd B. Stokin

27 Advocating for orphan diseases in neurology *303*
   Fritz Zimprich

28 Palliative care *315*
   David Oliver

29 **Advocacy for epilepsy: From the shadows to centre stage: Stand up for epilepsy** *327*
   Jules C. Beal and Solomon L. Moshé

30 **Advocacy for patients with headache** *339*
   Timothy J. Steiner and Jes Olesen

31 **Advocacy for patients with neuropathic pain** *347*
   Ligia Onofrei and A. Gordon Smith

Section 5 Outlook, follow-up, results, ending, conclusion, and debriefing

32 **Continuation or ending and 'debriefing'** *363*
   Wolfgang Grisold and Thomas Grisold

33 **Results, outlook, and goals of this book** *369*
   Wolfgang Grisold, Walter Struhal, and Thomas Grisold

Index *375*

Contributors

Jules C. Beal
Saul R. Korey Department of Neurology, Albert Einstein College of Medicine and Montefiore Medical Center, Bronx, NY, USA

Helen Bulbeck
Brainstrust, Cowes, Isle of Wight, UK

Carlo Colosimo
Department of Neurology, Santa Maria University Hospital, Terni, Italy

David Crewther
Centre for Human Psychopharmacology, Swinburne University of Technology, Melbourne, VIC, Australia

Sheila Crewther
Department of Psychology and Counselling, La Trobe University, Melbourne, VIC, Australia

Frédéric Destrebecq
European Brain Council, Brussels, Belgium

Mustapha El Alaoui Faris
Department of Neurology and Neuropsychology, Mohamed-V University, Rabat, Morocco

John D. England
Department of Neurology, Louisiana State University Health Sciences Center, School of Medicine, New Orleans, LA, USA

Thomas Grisold
Vienna University of Economics and Business, Vienna, Austria

Wolfgang Grisold
Ludwig Boltzmann Institute for Experimental and Clinical Traumatology, Vienna, Austria

Jan J. Heimans
Department of Neurology, VU University Medical Centre, Amsterdam, the Netherlands

Elaine C. Jones
Department of Neurology, Specialists On Call, Reston, VA

Anna Klicpera
Paracelsus Private Medical University, Salzburg, Austria

Birgit Kofler
Bettschart & Kofler Kommunikationsberatung, Vienna, Austria

Essie Low
Department of Psychology and Counselling, La Trobe University, Melbourne, VIC, Australia

Albert C. Ludolph
Department of Neurology, University of Ulm, Germany

Oliver Lukitsch
Department of Philosophy, University of Vienna, Vienna, Austria

Wolfgang Maderthaner
Austrian State Archives, Vienna, Austria

Francesca Mancini
Department of Neurology Stroke Unit and Laboratory of Neuroscience, Istituto Auxologico Italiano IRCCS, Milan, Italy

Christine Marosi
Department of Internal Medicine I,
Clinical Division of Medical Oncology,
Comprehensive Cancer Centre Vienna,
Medical University, Vienna, Austria

Solomon L. Moshé
Saul R. Korey Department of Neurology,
and Dominick P. Purpura Department
of Neuroscience, Albert Einstein College
of Medicine and Montefiore Medical
Center, Bronx, NY, USA

Christopher Neil
Department of Neurology, Western
Health, St Albans, VIC, Australia

Jes Olesen
Department of Neurology, University of
Copenhagen, Copenhagen, Denmark

David Oliver
Tizard Centre, University of Kent,
Canterbury, UK

Ligia Onofrei
University of Utah School of Medicine,
Salt Lake City, UT, USA

Apoorva Pauranik
Director, Pauranik Academy of
Medical Education;
Ex Professor of Neurology M.G.M.
Medical college, Indore, India

Richard Pichler
Special Representative for External
Affairs and Resources, SOS Children's
Villages International, Vienna, Austria

Roberta Rudà
Department of Neuro-Oncology,
University and City of Health and
Science Hospital, Turin, Italy

Raad Shakir
Division of Brain Health, Imperial
College London, Charing Cross
Hospital, London, UK

A. Gordon Smith
Division of Neuromuscular Medicine,
University of Utah School of Medicine,
Department of Neurology, Salt Lake
City, UT, USA

Riccardo Soffietti
Department of Neuro-Oncology,
University and City of Health and
Science Hospital, Turin, Italy

Timothy J. Steiner
Department of Neuroscience,
Norwegian University of Science and
Technology, Trondheim, Norway;
Division of Brain Sciences, Imperial
College London, UK

Gorazd B. Stokin
International Clinical Research Centre,
St. Anne's University Hospital, Brno,
Czech Republic

Walter Struhal
University Clinic Tulln, Karl Landsteiner
University of Health Sciences, Tulln,
Austria

Christoph Thalheim
European Multiple Sclerosis Platform,
Brussels, Belgium

Françoise Van Hemelryck
European CanCer Organisation,
Brussels, Belgium

Mohammad Wasay
Department of Neurology, the Aga Khan
University, Karachi, Pakistan

Tissa Wijeratne
Department of Neurology, Western
Health, St Albans, VIC, Australia

Fritz Zimprich
Department of Neurology, Medical
University of Vienna, Austria

Hanneke Zwinkels
Department of Neurology, Haaglanden
Medical Center, the Hague, the
Netherlands

Section 1
What is advocacy?

Chapter 1

What is advocacy?

Wolfgang Grisold, Walter Struhal, and Thomas Grisold

Introduction

Neurological diseases affect the brain, spinal cord, and neuromuscular system or can affect many other organ systems. Neurological diseases can be acute, or chronic and residual. Progressive disease often results in disability and handicap leaving the patient and carer in permanent need of assistance. Neurological diseases have many causes and the group of neurological diseases caused by non-communicable diseases is increasingly becoming the predominant group worldwide.

Advocacy can be aimed at individuals and groups, or have goals that do not address individuals directly but concern indirect patient-related questions. These include research, health system aspects, education in medicine, public access to treatment and care, and legislative issues dedicated to serving patients' best interests.

While modern science provides various opportunities to extend and develop scientific knowledge and management of neurological diseases, we often overlook the fact that patient well-being also depends on factors beyond the clinical context. This can imply that society acknowledges and responds to special needs of patients, or patients are provided with an opportunity to exchange experiences with equally affected individuals. Activities that go beyond the sphere of medical care in neurology can be subsumed under the term 'advocacy', although the spectrum is wider. Activities can be local, national, and international and will be classified at the micro, meso, and macro levels in this book.

Advocacy has become an essential part of medicine in general. However, there is no coherent working definition for advocacy, either in medicine or in the field of neurology. This book seeks to close this gap and to explore how neurologists and related health groups see and advocate for patients with neurological diseases. By related health groups, we mean other stakeholders who serve as advocates in neurology (e.g. doctors from other fields, nurses, physiotherapists, occupational therapists, and others). Patients and carers are increasingly involved in advocacy, not only as clients but also by taking an active part in projects and sharing ownership. Education of the public in regard to risk factors or specific diseases is also an issue of advocacy.

As we will see throughout the book, advocacy is a broad term that offers a variety of interpretations and produces different activities. It is important to know the variety of potential for advocacy as contexts differ across diseases, cultures, age groups, and so on. Knowledge of international behaviour is important.[1]

The goal of this book is twofold:

On the one hand, we endeavour to provide a unifying stage for scattered approaches to advocacy in neurology. In a way, we try to capture the state of the art; or rather what is already available. This may help others to see how developed the field is and how future research can build upon existing approaches.

On the other hand, we wish to shed light on how advocacy is and can be deployed in neurology. Throughout this book, the authors present methods, approaches, best and worst practices (Chapter 30), case studies and the like, to explain how effective advocacy can be pursued for different diseases and contexts. By doing so, we hope to empower advocates and people who are interested in the matter to plan and implement advocacy on their own.

This chapter will provide a summary and an outlook synthesizing the different perspectives of the authors involved. The next section summarizes what practitioners mean by advocacy. We will review definitions used in this book and highlight the levels used for advocacy. Finally, we will explain the structure of the book and suggest how the findings and results could be used.

Why do we need advocacy in neurology?

General context of neurological diseases

Stroke is the most frequent neurological disease, the second cause of mortality, and the first cause of disability across the world. Several comprehensive investigations exist on the epidemiology,[2,3] burden, and costs of neurological diseases.[4-6] By way of an example, a detailed review of the activities of the European Brain Council (EBC) can be found in these publications.[7]

In advocacy at the global level, it is also important to consider the local, regional, social, and economic situation, which depends on many factors and contributes to worldwide treatment gaps, as demonstrated by the case of epilepsy.[8,9]

Who needs advocacy?

Potentially, any person can require advocacy for various reasons. The objective of an advocacy campaign can be abstract—as in the case of legislation or the availability of or payment for a drug—or be immaterial and only indirectly related to clients and persons. This more abstract form of indirect advocacy is used at the meso- and macro levels. One example could be the successful relocation of stroke from vascular diseases to neurology in the new ICD-11. This would help to allocate resources towards stroke patients worldwide (Chapter 14).

At the general level, Jes Olesen and the EBC (Chapter 15) may demonstrate that treatment gaps for common diseases exist and need to be tackled. At the other end of the spectrum, Fritz Zimprich (Chapter 27) argues that instruments and advocacy must also be used for rare and orphan diseases.

Who is an advocate?

Any person, or group of persons, irrespective of their profession, can become an advocate. Advocates should have collaboration and communication skills, adopt scholarly practice, have management abilities and professionalism, compassion, empathy, and perseverance. Some of the attributes are summarized in the CanMED,[10] and some additions have been taken from the references. An attempt to list the essential attributes of advocates can be found in Chapter 7.

In particular circumstances, persons can advocate for themselves (see Case study 1.1).[11-14] In addition, the term 'non-self-advocacy' has been defined in oncology for a group of patients.[11,15]

Case study 1.1 illustrates the features involved for a patient mastering self-advocacy:

Case study 1.1 Self-advocacy

The example that follows shows that a lay person can efficiently address his/her disease and necessary treatments and can benefit from using their own communicative skills. This vignette is an example of self-advocacy.

Example of a patient: How can patients teach us to be self-advocates?

The patient was 75 years old, active in international tourism, independent, and single. He was diagnosed at the time with hypertension and renal insufficiency, which worsened over the years, eventually forcing him to be included in a dialysis programme. Despite his handicap he continued to travel and to keep his second residency in another European country. He travelled around Europe with American tourists, generally staying in a different city each night. He discovered that dialysis was feasible in several European countries and took advantage of nightly stopovers at hospital to have dialysis. His clients were not aware of this.

Besides his kidney problems and hypertension, he needed a cardiac stent. Severe pain in his feet made it almost impossible for him to walk. He was diagnosed with uremic neuropathy, and the cause was eventually diagnosed as uremic osteoarthropathy. He found a surgeon who could replace his ankle joints with a novel prosthesis, enabling him to walk well again.

He was unexpectedly offered a kidney transplant, which was successfully performed and worked quite well. He was able to manage both the immunosuppression regimens and his increased tendency to infection and continued with his life and work.

In the last months of his life he lost the hearing in one ear (he had been deaf in the other since childhood), rendering him completely deaf. He made several attempts at improvement, trying hearing aids, and exploring the possibility of a cochlear implant. However, the hearing loss did not stop him from travelling and he continued to journey with tourists. Communications were facilitated by writing and the use of laptops and PCs.

Finally, he suffered from severe intermittent thoracic pain, leading to a hospital admission, but it was misdiagnosed as vertebral column-related thoracic pain. A recurrent mediastinal haemorrhage caused by a ruptured aortic aneurysm was the pathologically confirmed cause of death.

This time he had been right to judge the severity of his condition, and unlike the attending physicians, he saw death approaching. He was 75 years old.

The key message from this example is: a person older than 70 years, single, with no medical experience, suffers from several severe medical conditions that make him a candidate for permanent residency at a nursing home. Nevertheless, in his capacity as a lay person, he was able to find out about diseases, treatments, and options, and to successfully manage his life and continue travelling.

He practised self-management, self-efficacy, and problem solving, adopting communication and organizational skills, propelled by natural curiosity.

Can self-advocacy be negative?

Self-advocacy in the negative sense is where a person uses advocacy skills and facilities for the sake of own interest. For example, an individual advocating to obtain a benefit for himself represents a highly subjective rather than an altruistic cause.

Age groups

Advocacy is needed for all age groups: the paediatric population, adults, the ageing population, and the underprivileged of any age.

Children

Paediatricians and obstetricians advocate for children and often siblings, parents, and (social) circumstances. Social aspects and circumstances assume a high value. One particular aspect is the transition from paediatric to adult age.[16]

Productive-age adults

They may need advocacy for other reasons. Health issues, working conditions, and specific disease management may be the content and target of advocacy. A link to the economy and productivity is often made for this age group.

The ageing population

The number of elderly persons is on the rise and they need specific attention.

Increasingly with age, neurological diseases such as stroke, dementia, movement disorders, pain syndromes, or other neurological pathologies associated with systemic disease or cancer begin to appear. The term *ageism* describes the negative and disadvantageous aspects of age.[17,18] In particular, frailty, cognitive impairment, and dementia deserve to be mentioned.

Economic analysis shows that older people cost most in health and social terms in the last years of their life.[19] This is often used as an economic argument but is highly debatable.

The underprivileged at any age

Some groups are underprivileged at any age, including people with mental disorders and the handicapped, who never become part of the productivity cycle at any time during their life. As such they may be rated less apt for advocacy than other vulnerable people and disadvantaged groups.[20]

Migrants and refugees

The topic of migrants and refugees is permanently timely. Migrants have a strong need for advocacy, which decreases from one generation to the next once families become integrated (Chapter 12).

Refugees have emergency status, the circumstances of which often preclude any kind of delay. Both migrants and refugees are in need of advocacy support and communication.[21-24]

Patient empowerment and self-responsibility

Increasingly, patients and carers are involved in advocacy, often in the position of the advocate (patient advocacy ECCO, Chapter 11). This development is also a reflection of the change in relations between medical doctors, health groups, and patient carers (see Chapters 7 and 15).

One example is the involvement of patients in the study design. The issue of patient empowerment,[25] self-responsibility, and patient involvement in studies (PCORI)[26,27] are important developments, which will induce large shifts in responsibility and competence towards self-management (Chapter 7).

As described in Chapter 24, the search for information often starts with what most patients and caregivers do when confronted with a disease, which is to use search engines on the Internet. To understand the advocacy process, it is important to identify the sources and avenues patients and carers use to gather their information.

Who 'owns' an advocacy project?

At times and in complex projects, the borders between advocates and clients disappear or become blurred, grey areas, which can result in procedural issues of various types. Ownership can be of little or all-determining value, once a project undergoes changes, particularly in leadership but even more so in purpose and direction. A transparent definition of ownership and leadership is useful in all advocacy projects.

A good example of shared ownership is provided in the chapter on the creation of the EBC (Chapter 15).

What do/could we mean by advocacy in neurology?

Review of definitions used in this book

There is no uniform model to classify models for advocacy. The term appears not only in medicine but in various unrelated fields, as society, politics, education, research, fundraising, and support and community outreach advocacy, among others. The word advocacy originally comes from law and jurisdiction, and several additional meanings are attached, as adverse advocacy, the issue of dual loyalty,[28] and ethical issues in medicine.[29] More colloquially speaking, advocacy should enable patients and carers to access information and services, promote rights, express concerns and views, explore available options, and finally improve given situations.

In the social context, which is close to medical applications, the role of the advocate is to act according to the ethical principles summarized by Bateman,[30] namely:

- To act in the best interest of clients
- To act in accordance with the wishes of the client
- To keep clients properly informed
- To carry out instructions with competence and diligence
- To act impartially and offer frank and independent advice
- To maintain the client's confidentiality

These principles come from the context of social work advocacy but contain all elements that can be used for advocacy projects in neurology.

Other definitions of advocacy can be distinguished descriptively, according to the action involved: partisan[31] and guerrilla advocacy[32]; 'grassroot' and 'grasstop' advocacy[33]; top-down or bottom-up advocacy; and advocacy by coalition. Advocacy can aim at community-based groups[34] or at media, legislative, and regulatory targets, among others. Advocacy ranges widely from informal to formal domains, embracing all levels from local to regional, from state to federal to global.

Legislative advocacy can, for example, be needed to change laws for the purpose of advocacy goals. These laws may deal with discrimination or tackle other issues in conjunction with advocacy. The Neurology on the Hill event exemplifies a successful approach to political advocacy where direct political contacts are used for advocacy.[35]

Distinguishing between advocacy and lobbying is often cause for debate and not always straightforward. In the definition of advocacy and lobbying, a distinction can be made in regard to legal issues. Generally speaking, (ageing) advocacy is the process of making voices (or a voice) heard at the required level (micro-, meso-, macro) and of finding solutions. Lobbying, be it directly or indirectly, is the exertion of direct influence on legislation.

Advocacy needs to be heard. Tools used in public relations are often useful. Chapter 19 discusses this aspect.

An overview on the chapters and their content

Table 1.1 provides an overview of the individual book chapters, and in addition to the working definition, captures general considerations, level of advocacy, and context. The table is meant to be a helpful tool for viewing the book contents.

Review of advocacy levels considered in this book

For clarification purposes, the scope of advocacy will be divided into three levels:

Micro level: meaning advocacy in a local environment. This refers to advocacy for a person or a group of persons and, in a more abstract sense, for a small or regional project.

Meso level: exceeds the local boundaries of a micro project. In regional terms, this could include projects intended for a town, region, or even a state. The goal could concern patients, diseases, and also changes in policy and legislation, in addition to treatment availability.

Table 1.1 Overview of the individual book chapters capturing general considerations, level of advocacy, and context

Chapter no.	Author(s)	Working definition	General considerations or specific case	Level (Micro/meso/macro)	Context
1	Wolfgang Grisold, Walter Struhal, and Thomas Grisold	Review of definitions	General outlook; case vignettes	All levels	Introduction to this book
2	Thomas Grisold and Oliver Lukitsch	Taking the voice of the patient	General considerations	Micro	Philosophical context
3	Wolfgang Maderthaner and Wolfgang Grisold	Advocacy to overcome societal issues	General considerations	Micro/macro	Historical perspective
4	Jan J. Heimans	Acting in the best interest of the patient	Specific case	Macro	Coma Patients, patients unable to speak for themselves
5	Tissa Wijeratne, Essie Low, and Christopher Neil	Bringing best and affordable care to patients	General considerations and specific cases	Meso/macro	Autonomy, relations with the industry, and pharmaceutical interests
6	Mohammad Wasay	Structured advocacy as a powerful force to create changes in societies and other systems	General considerations	All levels	Use and abuse of advocacy. Potential sources of problems and danger
7	Wolfgang Grisold	Advocacy as caring and taking responsibility beyond the medical treatment	General considerations	All levels	View on the spectrum of advocacy; attributes and abilities of advocates
8	Mohammad Wasay	Perspectives on advocacy of medical doctors	General considerations	Meso and macro	Advocacy in the context of health system
9	Hanneke Zwinkels	Advocacy as an activity to act in the best interest and in accordance with the wishes of the patient	Specific case	Micro/meso level	Perspective of/for neurology nurses; potential problems in advocacy

(continued)

Table 1.1 Continued

Chapter no.	Author(s)	Working definition	General considerations or specific case	Level (Micro/meso/macro)	Context
10	Helen Bulbeck	Advocacy promoting the development of patients' capabilities to minimize the impact of the disease; caregivers as 'co-pilots'	General considerations	Micro/meso	Patient and carer empowerment in the context of brain tumour
11	Françoise Van Hemelryck	Cancer-targeted advocacy as influencing decisions within political, economic, and social systems and institutions	General considerations	Macro and meso levels, incorporating specific structures	Patient advocacy to represent the interests of patients in decision
12	Mustapha El Alaoui Faris	Advocacy as developing legal rights and applying existing legal provisions for migrants	General issues	Macro	Advocacy for migrants with neurological diseases
13	Apoorva Pauranik	Neurology and advocacy—wide overview with practical examples	General considerations	Micro/meso/macro	Local, regional, and national context for neurology
14	Raad Shakir	Advocacy as influencing decision-making on the international level	Specific case	Macro	Context of international health politics to highest levels
15	Jes Olesen and Frédéric Destrebecq	Advocacy as a 'chain' with multiple elements, including 'the voice of the patient'	Specific and general considerations—formation of a campaign	Macro	Advocacy for neurological diseases in the EU

16	Richard Pichler	Advocacy as a strategy to increase the impact and create multipliers for a cause—how to reach continuous implementation	Specific case from a non-neurology context	Meso/macro	The case of SOS children's villages
17	Walter Struhal and Thomas Grisold	Advocacy as a proactive way of transforming ideas into actions, actions into meaningful reality	General	Micro/meso/macro	Project management techniques for advocacy projects
18	Wolfgang Grisold, Anna Klicpera, and Thomas Grisold	Advocacy as taking the voice of patients to inform, protect and support them; involves raising awareness on behalf of the patient	Specific cases and general considerations	Meso/macro	Best case strategies and lessons learnt in international context
19	Birgit Kofler	Advocacy as presenting issues, what can be learnt from public relations	General considerations	Micro/meso/macro	Public relation tools for advocacy
20	Tissa Wijeratne, Sheila Crewther, and David Crewther	Advocacy as acting on the behalf of stroke patients and families to promote welfare policies	Specific experience and multiple countries	Meso/macro	Advocacy for stroke
21	Christoph Thalheim	Advocacy as satisfying unmet needs of MS patients	Specific context of EU, specific patient aspects	Meso/macro	Advocacy for multiple sclerosis and political implications
22	Albert Ludolph	Advocacy as raising the voice of the patient at different stages of the disease	Specific context of ALS	Micro/meso	Advocacy for amyotrophic lateral sclerosis
23	Elaine C. Jones and John D. England	Advocacy to reduce barriers; support or promote persons, groups, causes for neuromuscular patients	Specific aspect of neuromuscular disease	Micro/meso/macro	Advocacy for neuromuscular disorders

(continued)

Table 1.1 Continued

Chapter no.	Author(s)	Working definition	General considerations or specific case	Level (Micro/meso/macro)	Context
24	Francesca Mancini and Carlo Colosimo	Advocacy to support patients and caregivers and/or promote research	Specific context on movement disorders	Micro/meso	Advocacy for movement disorders and strategic help on the identification of resources
25	Riccardo Soffietti, Christine Marosi, Roberta Rudà, and Wolfgang Grisold	Advocacy as a variety of strategies that are taken in light of specific needs of the patients with brain tumours and cancer related neurological issues	Specific context of neuro-oncology and cancer	Micro/meso/macro	Advocacy for brain tumours and neuro-oncology
26	Gorazd B. Stokin	Advocacy as act or process to influence/support economic and political systems and organizations for dementia	Specific context of dementia	Micro/macro	Advocacy for dementia
27	Fritz Zimprich	Advocacy has many forms and is key to improving the situation of patients disadvantaged by a rare disease	Specific context of orphan diseases	Micro/macro	Advocacy for orphan diseases and possible avenues
28	David Oliver	Advocacy to enable people to be enabled to make decisions and be fully involved in their care	Specific context of palliative care	Micro/meso/macro	Advocacy for palliative care
29	Jules C. Beal and Solomon L. Moshé	Advocacy to raise awareness of epilepsy and fight the associated stigma and discrimination	Specific context of epilepsy	Macro	Advocacy for epilepsy

30	Timothy J. Steiner and Jes Olesen	Advocacy to promote more research and better care for headache	Specific context of headache disorders	Macro	Headache disorders as a large group of diseases
31	Ligia Onofrei and A. Gordon Smith	Advocacy at a patient level, physician level, and a national policy level to align priorities and interests for pain	Specific context of neuropathic pain	Micro/meso/macro	Advocacy for neuropathic pain, pain treatment in general
32	Wolfgang Grisold and Thomas Grisold	Importance of project ending, closing, debriefing	Structural implications	All levels	Important steps and procedures
33	Wolfgang Grisold, Walter Struhal, and Thomas Grisold	Summary of advocacy contexts in this book	General thoughts and goals	All levels	What can we gain from this book?

Macro level: The macro level starts at the state level and extends to continental and global projects. One multinational example is the European CanCer Organisation (ECCO); World Health Organization (WHO) activities are a global case in point.

This classification is artificial but provides a framework for advocacy in terms of the size and volume of projects. The horizontal classification can overlap and potentially transgress boundaries. For instance, a local project can evolve into a national one, requiring different types of tool and support.

Culture and advocates

Advocacy has many aspects and must consider cultural differences at the micro and meso levels (with individuals and groups), as well in the macro level, where the influence of cultural issues on content, negotiation, and decision-making is essential, and often implicit. This is particularly important at the macro level, where unnecessary cultural 'clashes' can negatively influence advocacy projects. This can include the approach to authorities, language, directness, and other aspects.

The term *culture* is also used with a similar meaning to describe behaviour and organizational principles within organizations. These organizational structures may be 'hidden' or invisible to outsiders, and may not even be defined within the organization. It is important for advocates to be aware and have knowledge of these organizational cultures within their own group and with potential partners and adversaries.

Political thinking

One important message from the Palatucci meetings (cf. Chapter 17) was that 'everything is politics', indicating that actions and achievements are often embedded in large, complex 'political' structures and require political thinking.[36] One example of a successful advocacy approach is the creation of the EBC, outlined by Jes Oleson (Chapter 15). This example clearly highlights that excellent ideas and topics not only need appropriate wording but must carefully include all parties involved.

Teamwork and synergy

Teamwork and synergy among the people involved in an advocacy project are important for its success. Communication, transparency, and sharing of information and responsibilities are all needed, and unnecessary competition within an advocacy group should be avoided. Ownership (Chapter 6) should be defined and transparent.

Advocacy can meet resistance

Advocacy not only concerns the advocate and the client, but also the object of the advocacy, which may be an adversary party, structure, or other target.

Advocacy projects may threaten established procedures, induce fear and anxieties, particularly where established procedures are challenged and changed. When engaging in an advocacy project it is important to lay out the ground of the future project. Pros and cons, other interests, and all persons or other bodies that will be involved need to be identified.

Advocacy is rarely executed in linear, foreseeable ways, and flexible adaptations of the advocacy plans must be expected. Curvilinear and 'zig zag' strategies are often needed and may clash with linear structures, especially if current operational systems or procedures are threatened. Resistance, resilience, and commitment are required from advocates, and the failure of projects can be an important source of new advocacy projects (Chapter 18).

Advocacy campaigns need to aim at permanent changes. In the social context, account needs to be taken of the further coexistence of adversaries and opponents in a project.

Case study 1.2 exemplifies a typical situation. A task of routine becomes obsolete, and often fierce resistance is met when implementing changes. Adherence to established rules and structures, as well as unwillingness for unlearning, are the main causes.

Case study 1.2 Meso to macro level: 'The change in institutional procedures'

Vienna once had a large care home for elderly people, which remained open until the early 2000s, housing more than 5,000 people.[37] The example of change outlined next occurred in the mid-1970s, at a time when said institution strictly followed long-observed tradition and procedures.

The institution was founded at the beginning of the twentieth century and was highly advanced at the time of establishment. It would now be considered an historic monument, serving different concepts of patient care. The pavilions were divided into large rooms, inhabited by 30 or 40 patients, deprived of all individual possessions, often bedridden, and without any hope of leaving the place. Their sole possession was a small, sobering bedstead in a large military style room. Personal belongings remained locked away in a remote locker or storeroom. On admission to the home, all their (often meagre) possessions and the contents of rented apartments and rooms were taken by the city running the hospital as symbolic payment, leaving residents no hope of ever returning home, even should their condition improve.

Their income, usually a tiny old-age pension, was also used to cover running costs, and a small percentage was given to patients as pocket money. In some homes, 'favours' (or rather duties) from nursing staff, such as changing clothing, showering, or in some cases changing the bedpans, had to be paid extra or tipped.

Visiting hours were restricted and often handled inflexibly. Visitors were met with the overwhelming, persistent smell of decay. The visits to these helpless people may have brought some hope and joy to the residents, but always left visitors with a sense of sadness, despair, and relief on leaving the home.

Patient care at this time depended almost entirely on the attending physician/nurse, who paternalistically ruled over the patient. Relations with often hopeless, abandoned patients tended to be unilateral.

The admission procedure to the home took the form of a ritual, like many other internal practices at the time. All newly admitted patients were taken to an 'admission' department. Upon arrival they were stripped naked, washed, deprived of all personal belongings, outfitted with new hospital clothes to avoid 'infection', and kept for several weeks in an 'isolation' department before finally being assigned to their future wards. During this time relatives and carers were not permitted to visit.

As many persons did not voluntarily choose to go to a nursing home and even feared the thought, said procedure added to the shock of being institutionalized. Many newly admitted people were heartbroken and humiliated, but there was no way out and no exceptions were made.

A new health director at the city, who was a very committed physician with a great respect for patient issues, inspected the home/hospital and learnt about the admission procedure for himself (Prof Stacher, personal communication). He was informed that the procedure was absolutely essential and could not be changed for hygienic reasons, since it served to avoid infection. There seemed to be no desire on the part of administration office and the staff involved to bring about change.

The health director did instead insist on immediate change and met with fierce resistance. Despite his position he was forced into a short, but intensive struggle to bring about change, and all professionals concerned accused him of making a serious mistake. He was warned that infections would break out and that the change in procedure would violate medical needs and the principles of hygiene. Despite serious resistance and advice, he implemented the change.

The new admissions process had a positive effect on future patients, who were no longer exposed to the humiliation and unnecessary loss of dignity that had been inflicted on several generations of patients before them.

In summary, this vignette exemplifies not only changes in procedure, developments in medical knowledge, human relations, and the Zeitgeist, but also the need to identify, address, and overcome resistance. It shows that health institutions and, on a larger scale, health systems can be rigid and inflexible towards change, often based on regulations. The need to adapt requires the ability not only to learn new issues and content, but also to professionally 'unlearn' old content.

This is an example of a successful advocacy campaign at the meso-macro level producing positive results for future patients, a lost power struggle with a trained, well-established administration, and the courage and insight to recognize and bring about change.[38]

Equity

Many advocacy efforts address health equity, which means that health opportunities and facilities should aim to be equally available to all persons. Awareness and understanding of social determinants of health are essential.[39]

This refers to similar environments and economic conditions. Considering different health systems worldwide and per capita spending in some low-income countries (Chapter 14), this proposal may sound cynical.

The chapter on epilepsy (Chapter 29) very succinctly describes the 'treatment gap', which is a reality among many populations of the world not only as regards epilepsy and neurology but in many other fields, such as cancer.[40]

From success to failure

Despite planning, implementation, and execution, projects can fail at any stage. Advocacy projects may be even more at risk of failure than other projects, as they are often driven by altruism and enthusiasm.

As in other types of project, the details or milestones of advocacy projects are often not all achievable, frequently due to their spontaneous, irregular approach, the involvement of altruistic persons, and the need for persistence and resilience, or quite simply because the goal is not attainable at that particular time.

From an organizational point of view, the failure of an advocacy project is never a loss, as such failures can fuel new projects, which can in turn learn and gather experience from failures.

Closing and ending

Closing, ending, and debriefing is essential in any advocacy project and will be discussed in Chapter 32. This should emphasize that the analysis and evaluation of any advocacy project is just as important as the conception and beginning. This applies to the ending and closing of all advocacy projects, including early closure or termination.

Gains from this book

Advocacy is an increasingly used term. This book attempts to bring more clarity to the meaning and content of the term advocacy. The first chapter gives an overall view, whereas Chapter 7 focuses on additional aspects, particularly the attributes of advocates.

While 'neurology' is a specific medical field, advocacy activities have several aspects, as seen from the standpoint of physicians, other health groups, patients, and carers, and from the overarching viewpoint, as in global neurology.

Advocacy is neither exclusive to medicine, nor to neurology, and it is useful to look at advocacy projects undertaken by other organizations. The pattern of advocacy project management does, however, remain clear and structured; Chapter 17 delineates its basic principles and describes useful approaches.

We have chosen several 'subspecialties' of neurology that have experience in advocacy and use different methods and tools. There is a spectrum of professionalism in advocacy and this book should provide helpful examples and stimulation for new advocacy projects.

We also emphasize that there is much to learn not only from the initiation and maintenance of projects, but also from their ending and closure. Failures are never complete losses but serve as a useful resource for the next project.

References

1. **Meyer, E.** (2014) *The Culture Map: Decoding How People Think, Lead and Get Things Done Across Cultures*. New York: Book Public Affairs.
2. **Hofman, A**, **Mayeux, R.** (2001) *Investigating Neurological Disease Epidemiology for Clinical Neurology*. Cambridge: Cambridge University Press.
3. **WHO**. The top 10 causes of death. Available at: http://www.who.int/mediacentre/factsheets/fs310/en/
4. **Chin, J. H.**, **Vora, N.** (2014) The global burden of neurologic diseases. *Neurology*, **83**(4), 349–51.
5. **Olesen, J.**, **Gustavsson. A.**, **Svensson, M.**, et al. (2012) The economic cost of brain disorders in Europe. *Eur J Neurol*, **19**(1), 155–62.
6. **Gustavsson, A.**, **Svensson, M.**, **Jacobi, F.**, et al. (2011) Cost of disorders of the brain in Europe 2010. *Eur Neuropsychopharmacol*, **21**(10), 718–79.

7. **European Brain Council**. Library. Available at: https://www.braincouncil.eu/library/ebc-studies-and-reports/
8. **Meyer, A. C., Dua, T., Boscardin, W. J., Escarce, J. J., Saxena, S., Birbeck, G. L.** (2012) Critical determinants of the epilepsy treatment gap: a cross-national analysis in resource-limited settings. *Epilepsia*, **53**(12), 2178–85.
9. **Baulac, M., de Boer, H., Elger, C., et al.** (2015) Epilepsy priorities in Europe: a report of the ILAE-IBE Epilepsy Advocacy Europe Task Force. *Epilepsia*, **56**(11), 1687–95.
10. **Flynn, L., Verma, S.** (2008) Fundamental components of a curriculum for residents in health advocacy. *Med Teach*, **30**(7), e178–83.
11. **Hagan, T. L., Donovan, H. S.** (2013) Self-advocacy and cancer: a concept analysis. *J Adv Nurs*, **69**(10), 2348–59.
12. **Test, D. W., Fowler, C. H., Brewer, D. M., Wood, C. H.** (2005) A content and methodological review of self-advocacy intervention studies. *Council for Exceptional Children*, **72**(1), 101–25.
13. **Jonikas, J. A. Grey, D. D., Copeland, M. E., et al.** (2013) Improving propensity for patient self-advocacy through wellness recovery action planning: results of a randomized controlled trial. *Community Ment Health J*, **49**(3), 260–9.
14. **Martin, L. T., Schonlau, M., Haas, A., et al.** (2011) Patient activation and advocacy: which literacy skills matter most? *J Health Commun*, **16**(Suppl 3), 177–90.
15. **Peppercorn, J. M., Smith, T. J., Helft, P. R., et al.** (2011) American Society of Clinical Oncology Statement: toward individualized care for patients with advanced cancer. *J Clin Oncol*, **29**(6), 755–60.
16. **Harris, M. A., Freeman, K. A., Duke, D. C.** (2011) Transitioning from pediatric to adult health care: dropping off the face of the earth. *Am J Lifestyle Med*, **5**, 85–91.
17. **Butler, R. N., Lewis, M. I., Sunderland, T.** (1991) *Aging and Mental Health: Positive Psychosocial and Biomedical Approaches*, 4th edition. New York: Book Merrill/Macmillan Publishing Company, p. 608.
18. **North, M. S., Fiske, S. T.** (2012) An inconvenienced youth? Ageism and its potential intergenerational roots. *Psychol Bull*, **138**(5), 982–97.
19. **Bahler, C., Huber, C. A., Brungger, B., Reich, O.** (2015) Multimorbidity, health care utilization and costs in an elderly community-dwelling population: a claims data based observational study. *BMC Health Serv Res*, **15**, 23.
20. **Hann, K., Pearson, H., Campbell, D., Sesay, D., Eaton, J.** (2015). Factors for success in mental health advocacy. *Glob Health Action*, **8**(10), 3402/gha.v8.28791.
21. **Teunissen, E., Sherally, J., van den Muijsenbergh, M., et al.** (2014) Mental health problems of undocumented migrants (UMs) in the Netherlands: a qualitative exploration of help-seeking behaviour and experiences with primary care. *BMJ Open*, **4**(11), e005738.
22. **Teunissen, E., Tsaparas, A., Saridaki, A., et al.** (2016) Reporting mental health problems of undocumented migrants in Greece: a qualitative exploration. *Eur J Gen Pract*, **22**(2), 119–25.
23. **Priebe, S., Sandhu, S., Dias, S., et al.** (2011) Good practice in health care for migrants: views and experiences of care professionals in 16 European countries. *BMC Public Health*, **11**, 187.
24. **Pottie, K., Greenaway, C., Feightner, J., et al.** (2011) Evidence-based clinical guidelines for immigrants and refugees. *CMAJ*, **183**(12), E824–925.

25. **Raina, R. S., Thawani, V.** (2016). The zest for patient empowerment. *J Clin Diagn Res*, **10**(6), FE01–FE03.
26. **Patient-Centered Outcomes Research Institute**. Available at: http://www.pcori.org
27. **Forsythe, L. P., Alfano, C. M., George, S. M., et al.** (2013) Pain in long-term breast cancer survivors: the role of body mass index, physical activity, and sedentary behavior. *Breast Cancer Res Treat*, **137**(2), 617–30.
28. **Markovits, D.** (2011) *A Modern Legal Ethics: Adversary Advocacy in a Democratic Age*. Princeton, NJ: Princeton University Press
29. **World Medical Association** (2005). *Medical Ethics Manual*. The World Medical Association. Available at: https://www.wma.net/what-we-do/education/medical-ethics-manual/
30. **Bateman, N.** (1972) *Advocacy Skills for Health and Social Care Professionals*. London and Philadelphia, PA: Jessica Kingsley Publishers.
31. **Kim, C.** (2012) Partisan advocates. *Bull Econ Res*, **66**(4), 313–32.
32. **Galer-Unti, R.** (2009) Guerilla advocacy: using aggressive marketing techniques for health policy change. *Health Promotion Practice*, **10**, 325–7.
33. **Grassroots advocacy**. Available at: https://www.ama-assn.org/about/ama-grassroots-advocacy; andhttps://www.thecampaignworkshop.com/grassroots-advocacy-vs-grass-tops-advocacy
34. **Loue, S.** (2006) Community health advocacy. *J Epidemiol Community Health*, **60**, 458–63.
35. **Neurology on the Hill**. Available at: https://www.aan.com/public-policy/neurology-on-the-hill/about-neurology-on-the-hill/
36. **American Academy of Neurology**. Advocacy. Available at: https://www.aan.com/policy-and-guidelines/advocacy/
37. **Wien Geschichte Wiki**. Available at: https://www.wien.gv.at/wiki/index.php/Pflegeheim_Lainz
38. **Foucault, M.** (translated by Knowlton, E., King, W. J., Elden, S.) (2007) Ch. 15: The incorporation of the hospital into modern technology. In: Crampton, J., Elden, S. (eds). *Space, Knowledge and Power: Foucault and Geography*, pp. 141–53. London and New York: Routledge.
39. **Farrer, L., Marinetti, C., Cavaco, Y. P., Costongs, C.** (2015). Advocacy for health equity: a synthesis review. *Milbank Q*, **93**(2), 392–437.
40. **Meyer, A. C., Dua, T., Boscardin, W. J., Escarce, J. J., Saxena, S., Birbeck, G. L.** (2012) Critical determinants of the epilepsy treatment gap: a cross-national analysis in resource-limited settings. *Epilepsia*, **53**(12), 2178–85.

Chapter 2

Taking an epistemological perspective on advocacy

Thomas Grisold and Oliver Lukitsch

Introduction

If done successfully, advocacy activities create and promote awareness for patient groups and/or diseases. This book offers a variety of tools and methods to do so. However, some authors in this edited volume also emphasize that advocacy activities can fail. For example, Chapter 9 presents a case of a nurse that could not reach out to a patient because any attempt was blocked by the patient's husband. Another barrier can be a neurological disease where a patient is unable to speak; Chapter 22 provides interesting accounts for this case. We will argue that there is yet another reason why advocacy activities can fail, namely, when they do not take into account what the patient actually *needs*. We refer to those needs that the patient would understand as his/her own needs. We exclude cases where one might deny having a specific need while someone else claims that the person has it. While most of the chapters focus on *why* advocacy is needed (relevance) and *how* it is done (practical implications), we will shed light on *what* advocacy should be about (content of advocacy).

Whatever is done on behalf of the patient should take into account what the patient needs *in his/her view, as opposed to someone else's view*. As many definitions in this book show, in-depth knowledge is the basis for advocacy. It is about 'acting in the best interest of the patient' (Chapters 4 and 9), being 'the voice of the patient' (Chapters 15 and 22), or planning activities in the light of a patient's 'specific needs' (Chapter 21). At the same time, attention is not brought to the difficulties in getting to know the needs in the first place. Some would reply that needs are universal constructs that are shared among all human beings, regardless of culture and religion (as propagated by Maslow's popular theory about needs).[1] Following this logic, we would only have to see what has helped other patients with a specific disease and advocate for those needs. However, we follow more recent approaches to the concept of need and stress the *subjective* dimension of needs.[2-4] What a person *needs* to thrive and flourish depends on his/her history and personal context, and for planning advocacy activities, it is necessary to take these dimensions into account.

Then again, one might be tempted to ask; 'What problem can potentially arise when we simply *ask* patients what they need?'. The problem here is that most of these needs are hidden underneath the threshold of conscious awareness. Oftentimes, when we say that we need something we do not refer to the need as such, but rather to the object that satisfies our needs.[5] The underlying need remains itself unknown. As we will argue in this chapter, some of the knowledge about our needs is not *explicit* but *tacit*, that is, non-articulable. When we are planning advocacy activities, we have to consider that patients 'know more than they can tell'.[6] This poses a serious challenge to anyone who is doing advocacy.

Imagine the case of patient X, a 75-year-old male who was diagnosed with renal failure and required dialysis on a 2-day basis (see also Case study 1.1). Usually, such cases follow similar procedures; the patient is encouraged to choose a hospital that is in easy reach and provides the infrastructure needed for regular treatments. In the case of patient X, however, the physician noticed that this prospect seemed unsettling for the patient. Willing to provide support, the physician interrogated the patient and by getting to know his background, the physician made an intriguing discovery. It was not the dialysis per se that unsettled the patient. Rather, the patient was worried about giving up his job as a tour guide travelling all around the world and losing his independence. Working jointly on ideas on how to solve this problem, the physician understood that the patient spoke many languages fluently and that he had remarkable organizational skills. Finally, contrary to any of the patient's expectations, the physician suggested that the patient could identify and contact suitable hospitals in the countries he was touring. This way, the patient could receive required treatment but he could still travel and guide tours; this solution was consistent with the patient's notion of a happy and fulfilling life.

For the purpose of this chapter, this case is illustrative in two respects. On the one hand, it shows that the needs of a patient might not be obvious; they are, at times, tacit in the way that the patient cannot articulate them off-handedly. With the support of the physician, the patient's knowledge about his/her needs crystallized over time. On the other hand, it also shows that advocacy starts when the common clinical work ends. The physician could have stopped upon presenting a list of hospitals in reach of the patient's home. However, the physician was willing to go beyond the regular procedures to provide suitable solutions.

Advocacy consists of three cornerstones. It is (1) *about* something, that is, in the most general sense, the well-being of the patient, (2) done *by* an advocate, and (3) *on behalf* of the patient. Focusing on the third aspect, we show that only certain ways of empathic engagement allow the physician to access the patient's tacit knowledge. On that account, it can be avoided that information is neglected that can otherwise serve as a means for successful advocacy. Central to our argument is that advocacy activities must build on the *uniqueness, or individuality* of the patient considering how she/he experiences the disease and its consequences.[5]

This chapter contributes to this edited volume in two respects. On the one hand, we stress that advocacy starts with getting to know the patient on a fundamental level because only when we know what the patient really needs can we plan and implement effective activities. On the other hand, we will offer concrete strategies and tools that physicians, nurses, and any other advocates can use to gain access to the patient's knowledge and acquire relevant knowledge about his/her needs.

In the next section, we will further elaborate on the notion of 'tacit knowledge'. In the subsequent section, we will present tools and methods that can grant access to the patient's tacit knowledge. We will propose that this can be done on three levels. The advocate can leave behind at least *some* assumptions and expectations in given situations, the patient can provide documentation of his/her daily life, and that this can be achieved if advocate and patient work together. Finally, we present the 'Theory U', which is as a framework that is used in innovation research and that can guide advocates through the process of realizing projects.

Theoretical background

In this chapter, we approach advocacy from an *epistemological* perspective. As a branch of philosophy, epistemology refers to the study of knowledge and justified true belief. Epistemology enquires how we gain knowledge, investigates its conditions, and how it is constructed and spread. It is also concerned with different types of knowledge. For instance, we can have knowledge about how to drive, we can know a person, or a country, and we can also have conceptual knowledge, like knowledge about scientific propositions.

In this chapter, we focus on so-called *tacit knowledge* and explain how it is important for advocacy. Tacit knowledge is a type of knowledge that can be, in its simplest form, described as knowledge that cannot be put into words. One example would be our knowledge about how to ride a bike. It is fairly difficult to convey to someone exactly how to do this. Yet, we have tacit knowledge about how to go about this activity. Sometimes we can even learn to put into words, that is, to express tacit knowledge. This is exactly when tacit knowledge is translated into explicit knowledge, where 'explicit knowledge' simply refers to knowledge that can be put into words.

Tacit knowledge of one's needs

Here, we are concerned with tacit knowledge about oneself[i] and, in particular, of one's needs. For the purpose of getting to know what the patient needs, we need to consider what the patient has experienced and what he/she knows about his/herself. Sometimes the patient has explicit knowledge at his or her disposal, meaning that he/she can convey his/her needs by way of simply talking to the physician, nurse, or other advocate. This is only possible, however, if the patient has *explicit* knowledge of his/her needs. For instance, I know that I am x old, that I suffer from y or I know that I require some medication, and I can put this knowledge into words. But I might also have knowledge about myself that I cannot put into words easily or even not at all; viz. *tacit knowledge about oneself*.

We sometimes *experience* how we feel or what we need but we cannot *say* it. Let us elaborate on this. By way of an example, one might not be happy in being stuck in a particular situation, but does not realize that this is so. For instance, one might be

---

[i] Tacit knowledge of oneself is not to be confused with what is called 'self-knowledge' in philosophy of mind. As opposed to knowledge of oneself, *self-knowledge* is the kind of knowledge we have about our mental states or events. When I currently (and also consciously) believe that p, then I also *know* that I believe p. Self-knowledge is thus one type of knowledge that one can have about oneself.

caught in an unhappy relationship and only after the breakup one would acknowledge that one was unhappy before. This is not to say, that one did *not* know that one was unhappy. In such a situation, one usually experiences oneself as being unhappy, but often not in a way that allows one to talk about it yet. One's unhappiness is not simply isolated from one's conscious life. It is expressed in all our shared activities with the partner, and we know about it tacitly.

The inability to put one's unhappiness into words is often exacerbated by the fact that we do not want to know about our unhappiness. Psychoanalysis refers to this as a repressive mechanism that inhibits one's unconscious beliefs to turn into conscious beliefs. Based on these profound psychoanalytic insights, the phenomenologist Merleau-Ponty[7] has argued that the above-mentioned repressed mental events still infuse with our *experiences*, however, in such a way that we cannot express these experiences propositionally—that is, we might not be able to articulate them. How shall we conceive of these experiences then? One way to make sense of them is to describe them as *bodily knowledge* of the kind that also comes to bear when we ride a bike, for example. It is the kind of knowledge we cannot express but on which we still retain an experiential grasp. This is precisely what we intend to show with our example: we can experience our unhappiness without knowing that we are unhappy *explicitly*. Yet, to know one's unhappiness can be expressed in a prelinguistic, bodily way.

Let us now turn to our prime goal; the patient. Consider a patient that has a certain need that ought to be considered by the advocate. Imagine the patient has the need x, but is unable to express this need. The patient, however, is not fully *unaware* of his/her need. That is, the need is not merely a non-conscious mental state or event. Suppose the patient would know about his/her need *tacitly*. The patient cannot put it into words, but he/she experiences his/her need, and, by the same token, knows about it. If we assume that this is a possibility, then the question arises as to how the advocate and the patient can access the patient's need in order to make it explicit. In other words, how can we access the patient's tacit knowledge? We shall pursue this question in the following section.

Getting to know the patient's tacit needs: Tools and strategies

The notion that one's knowledge does not merely depend on conscious and explicit thoughts has been acknowledged in fields other than philosophy, such as psychotherapy, innovation, and management; in particular, we draw on design thinking, which is a 'human-centred' approach in management that focuses on identifying and utilizing the latent needs of those who are involved in a business process (e.g. consumers when a new product is created).[8,9] These fields share the belief that tacit knowledge, which can be found in patients, peers, and social systems more generally, can be employed to meet, for instance, therapeutic or consolatory goals. Since advocacy should also make use of the patient's tacit knowledge, the above-mentioned resources might as well be of use for advocacy, or so we argue.

In the following, we develop a framework that allows for accessing the patient's tacit knowledge for advocacy. We suggest that this framework consists of three pillars: the physician, the patient, but also the physician–patient as dual system. Accordingly, we introduce three strategies.

Our framework is built on the premise that the most important situation in this process is the advocate–patient interaction. We believe that situations when physicians, nurses, and other advocates speak to patients, provide the highest potential for accessing the tacit knowledge of the patient. In the following, we will explain each of these strategies. Furthermore, we will suggest tools to illustrate how these strategies can be applied to practice.

Physician-centred strategy

The clinical environment is characterized by complex decisions that have to be taken in a limited time.[10] Undoubtedly, relying on intuitions and snap judgements is crucial for anyone who is working in such an environment. As experience grows, analysis gets 'frozen into habit',[11] which is, in many cases, both time- and cost-efficient. At the same time, such 'mental short-cuts' can lead to negative outcomes, such as making wrong decisions because environmental cues have not been taken into account sufficiently.[12] Furthermore, practising advocacy based on a patient's needs requires us to take an opposite approach, as we should appreciate that patients and their situations are individual after all. Of course, that is not to say that the physician must not rely on his/her experiences as a clinician, but rather that one's experience should be applied against the backdrop of appreciating the case's individuality. To do so, physicians have to be able to attune to the patient, listen to him/her and, most importantly, understand what he/she means beyond the words she/he says. Listening in that regard may be best understood as a process of data gathering which *precedes* understanding.[13] Grasping signs of tacit knowledge may involve recognizing subtle signs. In the following, we will present mindfulness as a technique to train and foster the ability to communicate with the patient.

Example: Mindful communicating—'Mindfulness'[ii] is a technique[iii] that can support advocates to attend to the patient more *openly* so as to avoid biases that ensue due to the physician's former experience. The goal of this technique is, essentially, to gain a heightened awareness of what is happening in the situation at large.[14] It calls for maintaining focus to perceive the world as it appears to us *here and now*, and thereby provides a less biased view of events.[15]

By interacting with patients with the aid of this technique, we can direct our attention to them in ways that help us to attend to aspects of the situation that might have otherwise been disregarded by the physician. As discussed earlier in 'Theoretical background', tacit knowledge often figures implicitly in what the patient says but also

---

[ii] Several studies investigate the positive effects of mindfulness on cognitive function and performance.[15] Significant effects can be noticed even within a short period of time (e.g. daily practice of 20 minutes over a few weeks).

[iii] We acknowledge that many authors would insist that mindfulness is more than a technique (e.g. meditation). However, for the purpose of this paper and the application-wise description, we refer to it here as a technique.

in his/her bodily behaviour more generally. This is important, since if one tries to understand others one usually tends to hold on to what we assume and expect in the first place.[16] Meanwhile, some of the patient's utterances can be straightforwardly taken at face value, regardless of whether the physician has certain expectations with respect to the case. However, tacit knowledge might, as we showed, remain unnoticed all the more if the physician loses hold of his/her clinical biases. Tacit knowledge can be made more salient by bracketing one's expectations, routines, and prejudices.

An important aspect of patient interaction is to acknowledge what the patient says but also what lies beyond spoken words.[13,17] Around 60–65% of communication is non-verbal but transmitted via cues, such as body language; in their everyday work, physicians must attend to these cues in order to understand what a patient needs.[18] However, since non-verbal cues highly depend on a patient's context (e.g. culture), it is impossible to give general rules on how to interpret them. Following Shea,[19] we have to attend to certain aspects, such as 'kinesics' and 'paralanguage' to understand non-verbal cues. *Kinesics* refers to bodily cues, such as body language, facial expressions, and gestures. *Paralanguage* includes other signs of mental states, such as volume and pitch of speech. While kinesics and paralanguage can match the patient's actual utterances, and therefore the content of his/her speech, they can also convey information that exceeds the content of the patient's utterances. That is not to say that this additional non-verbal cue indicates the existence of tacit knowledge. Paralanguage and kinesics are nevertheless the locus of manifestation of the patient's tacit knowledge about his/her needs. As we showed earlier, tacit knowledge expresses itself non-verbally as a *bodily knowledge*. Non-verbal kinesic and paralinguistic cues are also bodily in nature and are therefore poised to express the patient's tacit knowledge about his/her inexplicable needs.

Being mindful during physician-patient conversations may facilitate to detect and understand such cues as it increases attentiveness and the physician's focus on the here and now.[18,20]

Patient-centred strategy

Our chapter is based on the idea that effective advocacy activities align with the needs of a patient, which are oftentimes *tacit*. Accordingly, when following a patient-centred strategy, we aim at designing situations where a patient's needs come to light *for the patient his-/herself*. When do such situations arise? Chapter 1 of this book shows that advocacy activities are necessary because a patient has difficulties and issues that have not been addressed or resolved so far. The need for advocacy arises in situations where she struggles and experiences barriers that are caused by a disease—thus, when approaching advocacy from the view of the patient, we have to immerse ourselves into the role of the patient to fully understand how he/she experiences the world ('Lebenswelt'). In some cases, the needs may be fairly obvious for an experienced physician or nurse. Consider a patient who reports on pain in the back; by telling the advocate about the kind of pain, how it feels like, and so on, the advocate may be able to identify situations in which there is a need for advocacy (say, because the patient suffers from back pain and the advocate appoints someone to help him/her doing grocery shopping). In other cases, however, needs may be subtler and identifying them can even be counterintuitive. For example, Chapter 9 reports about a patient whose treatment was obstructed by a family member. How can we become aware of such needs? This will be explored in the following.

Example: Self-documentation of the patient
Originally developed in the field of design thinking, 'self-documenting' is a method to develop or refine products for customers by getting a better understanding of how, when, and why a customer uses or might use a product.[9] For the context of advocacy, it seems promising too, since it helps the patient to explore his/her needs so as to get to know where they might depend on, and profit from advocacy.

The idea is, in essence, that patients get to document their everyday lives with an emphasis on challenges, struggles, but also on aspects of their lives that facilitated their well-being up to now. The documentation is construed as an open, creative engagement, carried out with different tools such as photography, filming, but also drawings, among other things. The material is then used for identifying underlying patterns, which enable the advocate to better understand the broadly ecological profile of the patient's needs. The search for the patient's profile will be carried out jointly (with the advocate and the patient participating) and is understood as an inductive process with the goal to account for the patterns that ensue from the data.[21] The process is repetitious in the sense that after each iteration the finding of a pattern is imposed onto the data, such that it is eventually possible to account for the entire data set. As we already noted in the previous section, it is important here as well to keep an open mind and to be aware of biases that could avert important findings.

Collaborative strategy

While the first strategy addressed the advocate's ability to engage with the patient and the second strategy explored how we can help the patient to make tacit knowledge explicit, the third strategy represents an interplay of the two. A collaborative strategy focuses on the interaction between advocate and patient to jointly identify needs and work on possible advocacy projects. This approach is based on ideas in design thinking and innovation research where authors highlight collective creativity as a means to develop new ideas, products, and services. Following this, we emphasize that a participatory process works best when the people involved (in our case, the advocate and the patient) work on eye level, that is, the advocate should not take the role of an expert; rather, he/she should act as a facilitator who asks the right questions and provides the right environment.[22,23]

The strength of this approach is that both advocates and patients can jointly learn from each other. Such an approach can make sense in cases where an advocate cannot identify what the patient really needs; as argued before, every patient can have unique needs which the advocate has no reference for. Furthermore, one need can lead to different solutions to satisfy this need. A collaborative strategy can support the process of developing methods that can help the patient on the one hand and that can be realized by the advocate on the other hand.

Example: Appreciative inquiry
Appreciative inquiry (AI) is a collaborative method that provides a solution to this problem. Originally designed for the field of organizational management and change,[24]

it has found its way into educational and therapeutic contexts.[25] AI is an interviewing technique where both the interviewer (the advocate) and the interviewee (the patient) cooperate to 'sustain momentum for ongoing positive change'.[24] It can be done in one-on-one settings, but it is also suitable for groups (e.g. a group of patients with the same disease), and is participatory by nature.[26] Just like in design thinking,[8] AI aims at establishing unfulfilled needs, yet, aspects and states of affairs that already contribute to the patient's well-being are taken to be the point of departure for any future changes. Hence, the focus lies on inquiring the conditions of the patient's well-being (a more detailed description can be found in[27]).

The first step in AI consists in finding a positive subject of inquiry concerning, primarily, aspects of the patient's life that contribute to their well-being. Secondly, patients should report moments in which they deemed themselves happy and in which they felt supported. In this way, patients 'envision' their well-being in order to enable the physician to access non-explicit (yet crucial) conditions for the patient's well-being. Thirdly, the advocate draws upon the implicit knowledge to which he/she gains access in step 3. The patient's tacit self-knowledge is thereby transferred into explicit knowledge and can be put into words.

In collaboration with the patient, the fourth step comprises the development of a potential scenario for successful advocacy in which the patient is poised to feel appreciated and supported. This fourth step can then serve as a feasible blueprint for taking action in advocacy.

Throughout this chapter, we argued that knowledge about the patient's needs can inform effective advocacy activities. This section pointed to strategies and tools to access the tacit knowledge of a patient. However, what happens *after* we found out what the patient needs? After all, it might be the case that the resulting need is unknown to the advocate and/or may seem impossible to realize. We will now turn to the challenge of bringing advocacy activities to life in order to respond to a patient's need.

Turning tacit knowledge into advocacy projects: The Theory U

So far, we focused on tacit knowledge, its potential to inform advocacy activities and how we can get access to it. The question we are asking now is: how can we turn this knowledge into a working project? To answer this question, we draw upon the *Theory U* as a guiding framework.[28] The Theory U aims at creating *profound* innovations, that is, innovations that go beyond the further development of already existing ideas and solutions. By taking a closer look at the underlying systematics, we can draw parallels to what we proposed in the preceding sections. Thus, it can serve advocates by providing a systematic guideline to access tacit knowledge, to make it explicit, and to realize concrete projects. Fig. 2.1 depicts the Theory U and the respective steps.

The left side as well as the bottom of the U-process entails the steps 'suspending', 'redirecting', 'letting go', and 'presencing'. The general idea behind these steps is that one has to go through different phases to gain a new perspective on a problem.[28,29] By *suspending* our familiar solutions and proven approaches to a problem, we get into a state of 'pure receptiveness'.[30] *Redirecting* involves directing attention to one's inner

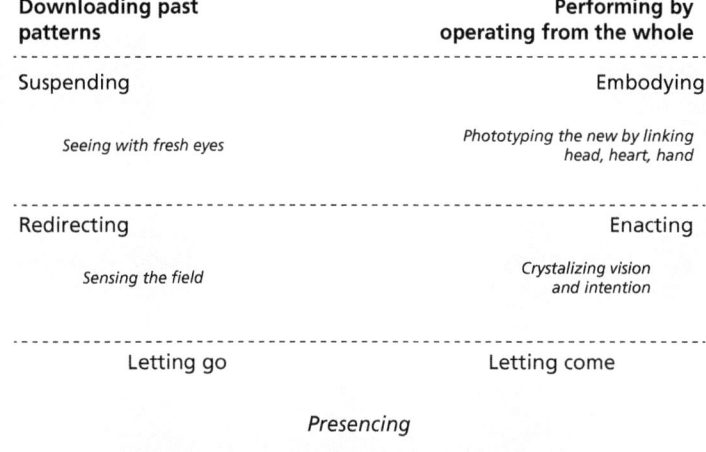

Fig. 2.1 The Theory-U entails different steps; suspending, redirecting, letting go (left side); presencing (bottom); letting come, enacting, embodying (right side).
Adapted from Scharmer CO, Theory U: Leading from the future as it emerges. The social technology of presencing, Copyright (2007), with permission from Society for Organizational Learning.

assumptions and premises and to see why one has attained a certain viewpoint on a problem or matter. *Letting go* is about setting these established mental models aside, and *presencing* requires one to keep a state of heightened awareness, to attune to the environment and get into a mode of 'deep or primary knowing'.[30] In essence, these steps capture what we have proposed so far; at the core of any advocacy process should be a deep understanding of the patient to get a full grasp of the uniqueness of their need. Thus, the advocate must ensure that his/her own ideas, assumptions, and beliefs are not projected on the patient. The Theory U can facilitate this process by providing concrete steps that the advocate can follow through this phase.

The right side, that is, the upward movement of the U focuses on the steps that concern the emergence of new knowledge; 'letting come', 'enacting', and 'embodying'. The following steps can guide an advocate in the process of planning and realizing concrete activities that are based on an identified need.[28-30]

'Letting come' and 'enacting' is all about making sense of what the advocate has perceived so far. It is about articulating the patient's need, or in other words, it is the point where tacit knowledge is made explicit. This step can entail dialogues and other forms of interaction between advocate and patient to ensure that the advocate has found a need that the patient can identify with.

Since the identified need might not correspond to what the advocate has expected or which he has experienced so far, it might be difficult at first to successfully develop and implement an appropriate advocacy project. 'Embodying' requires the advocate to experiment with ideas and develop different possible realizations. Here, it is important that prototypes are being verified, discussed with others, and feedback is provided. There can be a tension between 'what should be done' and 'what can be done'. This tension can be resolved during this step.

'Performing' is the last step in the Theory U. Now, the advocate brings the prototype to life. Depending on the level on which advocacy should take place, this can imply the implementation in practices, decision-making routines, policies, laws, and so on.

To summarize, the Theory U enables profound innovation by emphasizing an unbiased look at problems for the purpose of providing unique solutions. In that regard, this approach is similar to what we propose in this chapter. Only when we connect with the patient in a deep and meaningful way, we might be able to access his tacit knowledge and understand what he/she needs. The Theory U offers a systematic structure which can be used in advocacy projects because it can guide an advocate through different steps during planning and realizing (for additional tools and materials, see [31]).

Outlook

In this chapter, we provided an epistemological perspective on advocacy. We argued that definitions of advocacy presuppose that the advocate understands the needs of the patient from the patient's perspective. In many cases, it is obvious what patients need (for example, Chapter 14 presents advocacy activities to provide adequate medical attention to a disease). As we showed in the first part, however, identifying the needs of a patient can also be challenging because most knowledge is tacit. It is hidden in the patient's unconsciousness and patients cannot put it into words. To access this knowledge, we proposed a framework that entails three strategies; (1) the physician can use techniques to get a clear understanding of what the patient says, what he is trying to say and what he means; (2) the patient can provide detailed knowledge about his/her everyday experiences that can inform concrete activities; and (3), both advocate and patient can collaborate and jointly identify needs. We suggested tools that come from psychotherapy, design thinking, and innovation research to realize these strategies. Furthermore, we introduced the Theory U as a systematic process to realize advocacy projects.

We are aware that the strategies and tools might not be easily implemented in the clinical environment on an everyday basis since they can require a lot of time and effort. At the same time, we argue that a profound understanding of a patient's need might ensure efficient and sustainable advocacy activities. This understanding can only be provided by accessing the patient's tacit knowledge.

References

1. **Maslow, A.** (1943) A theory of human motivation. *Psychol Rev*, **50**(4), 370–96.
2. **Gasper, D.** (2007) Conceptualising human needs and wellbeing. In: Gough, I., McGregor, J. (eds). *Wellbeing in Developing Countries*. Cambridge: Cambridge University Press, pp. 47–70.
3. **Kenrick, D. T., Griskevicius, V., Neuberg, S. L., Schaller, M.** (2010) Renovating the pyramid of needs: contemporary extensions built upon ancient foundations. *Perspect Psychol Sci J Assoc Psychol Sci*, **5**(3), 292–314.

4. **Kesebir, S., Graham, J., Oishi, S.** (2010) A theory of human needs should be human-centered, not animal-centered: commentary on Kenrick et al. *Perspect Psychol Sci J Assoc Psychol Sci*, **5**(3), 315–9.
5. **McLeod, S. K.** (2011) Knowledge of need. *Int J Philos Stud*, **19**, 211–30.
6. **Polanyi, M.** (1966) *The Tacit Dimension*. Chicago: The University of Chicago Press.
7. **Merleau-Ponty, M.** (1962) *Phenomenology of Perception*, 1st edition. London: Routledge.
8. **Mootee, I.** (2013) *Design Thinking for Strategic Innovation*. Hoboken, NJ: Wiley & Sons.
9. **Roberts, J. P., Fisher, T. R., Trowbridge, M. J., Bent, C.** (2016) A design thinking framework for healthcare management and innovation. *Healthcare*, **4**(1), 11–4.
10. **Bornstein, B. H., Emler, A. C.** (2001) Rationality in medical decision making: a review of the literature on doctors' decision-making biases. *J Eval Clin Pract*, **7**(2), 97–107.
11. **Simon, H. A.** (1987) Making management decisions: the role of intuition and emotion. *Acad Manag Exec (1987-1989)*, **1**(1), 57–64.
12. **Klein, J. G.** (2005) Five pitfalls in decisions about diagnosis and prescribing. *BMJ*, **330**(7494), 781–3.
13. **Makari, G., Shapiro, T.** (1993) On psychoanalytic listening: language and unconscious communication. *J Am Psychoanal Assoc*, **41**(4), 991–1020.
14. **Bishop, S. R.** (2004) Mindfulness: a proposed operational definition. *Clin Psychol Sci Pract*, **11**(3), 230–41.
15. **Kabat-Zinn, J.** (2003) Mindfulness-based interventions in context: past, present, and future. *Clin Psychol Sci Pract*, **10**(2), 144–56.
16. **McWilliams, S. A.** (2010) Inherent self, invented self, empty self: constructivism, buddhism, and psychotherapy. *Couns Values*, **55**(1), 79–100.
17. **Philippot, P., Feldman, R., Coats, E.** (2003) *Nonverbal Behavior in Clinical Settings*. New York: Oxford University Press.
18. **Foley, G. N., Gentile, J. P.** (2010) Nonverbal communication in psychotherapy. *Psychiatry Edgmont*, **7**(6), 38–44.
19. **Shea, S. C.** (1998) *Psychiatric Interviewing: The Art of Understanding*, 2nd edition. Philadelphia, PA: Sanders.
20. **Burgoon, J. K., Berger, C. R., Waldron, V. R.** (2000) Mindfulness and interpersonal communication. *J Soc Issues*, **56**(1), 105–27.
21. **Strauss, A., Corbin, J.** (1997) *Grounded Theory in Practice*. Thousand Oaks, CA: Sage Publications.
22. **Björgvinsson, E., Ehn, P., Hillgren, P.-A.** (2012) Design things and design thinking: contemporary participatory design challenges. *Des Issues*, **28**(3), 101–16.
23. **Sanders, E. B.-N., Stappers, P. J.** (2008) Co-creation and the new landscapes of design. *CoDesign*, **4**(1), 5–18.
24. **Cooperrider, D., Whitney, D. D.** (2005) *Appreciative Inquiry: A Positive Revolution in Change*. Oakland, CA: Berrett-Koehler Publishers, p. 77.
25. **Rubin, R., Kerrell, R., Roberts, G.** (2011) Appreciative inquiry in occupational therapy education. *Br J Occup Ther*, **74**(5), 233–40.
26. **Aldred, R.** (2011) From community participation to organizational therapy? World cafe and appreciative inquiry as research methods. *Community Dev J*, **46**(1), 57–71.
27. **Center for Appreciative Inquiry** (2016) Generic Processes of Appreciative Inquiry. Available at: https://www.centerforappreciativeinquiry.net/more-on-ai/the-generic-processes-of-appreciative-inquiry/

28. **Scharmer, C. O.** (2007) Theory U. *Leading from the Future as It Emerges: The Social Technology of Presencing.* Cambridge, MA: Society for Organizational Learning.
29. **Scharmer, C. O.** (2001) Self-transcending knowledge. Sensing and organizing around emerging opportunities. *J Knowl Manag*, **5**(2), 137–50.
30. **Peschl, M. F.** (2007) Triple-loop learning as foundation for profound change, individual cultivation, and radical innovation. Construction processes beyond scientific and rational knowledge. *Constr Found*, **2**(2–3), 136–45.
31. **Scharmer, O.** (2018) Tools. Available at: http://www.ottoscharmer.com/tools

Chapter 3

Advocacy in history and culture

Wolfgang Maderthaner and Wolfgang Grisold

Introduction

The cultural proliferation of fin-de-siècle and interwar Vienna provided for the emergence of a world-renowned medical school whose concerns in many aspects exceeded the more limited purposes of traditional medicine. An integral part of the contemporary *Late Enlightenment* project, it conceived of methods and concepts advocating for a self-determined individual fully aware of his or her potentials and prospects—be it as a highly complex mechanism of the interplay of the conscious and the unconscious, or as an insoluble part of a social collective. Resulting from both a unique flourishing of Jewish creativity during the final years of the Habsburg Empire, as well as from the traumatic social and cultural consequences of that empire's disintegration in the immediate aftermath of World War I, these concepts, though unfolding from a specific intellectual context they had in common, differed widely in methods and outlook. They may be best represented by the achievements of two of the most outstanding proponents of the *Vienna Modern*: depth psychologist Sigmund Freud, the founder of psychoanalysis, and anatomist and social welfare politician Julius Tandler.

Vienna as the locus for emerging advocacy: The historical context

The Vienna of 1900, or *fin-de-siècle Vienna* as it is often addressed, was a peculiar and somehow solitary conglomerate of some of the most divergent, yet mutually dependent, social, political, and cultural developments of the time—simultaneously a laboratory of the Apocalypse and the birthplace of epoch-making modern trends and achievements. In many respects, it is what we nowadays would label a global city, and was the place of the last of the Habsburgs as well as that of young Adolf Hitler, and of Theodor Herzl, the founder of modern Zionism. It was the city of the patriarchal mayor Karl Lueger, who shaped modern anti-Semitism into a political mass movement, and the home of one of the pioneers of democratic socialism, the Jewish poor man's doctor, psychiatrist, and social reformer, Victor Adler. It was, by the way, the place where the founding fathers of the Austrian School of Economics conceived of a meta-theory of liberalism—ideas that were finally to become globally dominant, if not hegemonic, from the 1990s onwards.

Vienna was the first metropolis in which organized anti-Semitism was able to seize power, and it was to become, after World War I, the first city with over one million inhabitants under a social-democratic administration. In Robert Musil's words, the Vienna of 1900 resembled a boiling blister of initiations and emergences, one gigantic beat and the eternal dissonance and determent of all rhythms against each other:

> No one knew exactly what was in the making; nobody could have said whether it was to be a new art, a new humanity, a new morality, or perhaps a reshuffling of society. These were certainly opposing and widely varying cries, but uttered in the same breath.[1]

In the city's coffeehouses and salons, writers, artists, and scientists searched for a common denominator to all these contradictions and seemed to detect it in psychophysics, expressionism, an aesthetically sophisticated nervousness, and, above all, psychoanalysis. Fin-de-siècle Vienna then is probably best known for its cultural innovations: Arnold Schönberg's 12-tone compositions; Karl Kraus's linguistic criticism; Arthur Schnitzler's fictional psychology; Ludwig Wittgenstein's dismantling of metaphysics; Ernst Mach's empirical criticism; and, of course, Sigmund Freud's reshaping of psychology.

Freud and Adler were to become outstanding proponents of a Late Enlightenment, the cultural revolt of their generation heightened their awareness of the value of psychological investigation, of the basic psychic dispositions of the individual. This background led them towards a diagnosis of what was the *other*, the unfathomable, the secret. And when one of them, by profession a 'doctor of nervous diseases', extended the individual body to a social body, which was to be healed by the means of mass psychology and mass politics, the other, theoretical anthropologist and neurologist, deliberately kept his distance from vis-à-vis politics to devise his revolutionary system of a depth psychology of the individual.

Advocacy for the individual: The case of Sigmund Freud

In his *revolutionary dream* that has become legendary, written down in *The Interpretation of Dreams*, Freud recalled a fierce dispute with Adler at the Reading Club of German Students of Vienna ('*Leseverein der deutschen Studenten Wiens*'):

> There was a debate in a German student's club about the relation of philosophy to the general sciences. Being a green youth, full of materialistic doctrines, I thrust myself forward in order to defend an extremely one-sided position. Thereupon a sagacious older fellow-student, who has since then shown his capacity for leading men and organizing the masses, and who, moreover, bears a name belonging to the animal kingdom, rose and gave us a thorough dressing-down; he too, he said, had herded swine in his youth, and had then returned repentant to his father's house. I jumped up (as in the dream), became piggishly rude, and retorted that since I knew he had herded swine, I was not surprised at the tone of his discourse. (In the dream, I am surprised at my German Nationalistic feelings.) There was a great commotion, and an almost general demand that I should retract my words, but I stood my ground. The insulted student was too sensible to take the advice which was offered him, that he should send me a challenge, and let the matter drop.[2]

The anecdote appeared in one of the most important, influential, and probably most widely read books of the twentieth century. Though it was published on

14 November 1899, the year of publication is given as the programmatic 1900, due to a little publicity trick of the editor Franz Deuticke (Leipzig and Vienna). It is, in fact, a book of the century. The atheist, enlightener, and positivist Freud derived his method from religious hermeneutics and thus demystified a universal psychic phenomenon, to open a key path, a *via regia*, leading to a realm so far considered beyond elucidation—the human unconscious. Freud's radically progressive perspective was to bring the negated, suppressed unconscious to awareness, to make it understandable and explainable and therefore accessible to objective analysis and diagnosis.[3]

Now Freud—not least because of his training with Theodor Meynert and the influence of Josef Breuer, later for the most part to be denied—stood in the strictly empirical, rationalistic tradition of the more recent Vienna School of Medicine. Positive sciences had conquered the last bastion and subjected even the human psyche to a rational model of interpretation and explication. It has comprehensibly been argued that this model is derived from the world of thought of liberal economics, and that the human individual is being conceptualized as a psychological small enterprise. Psychoanalysis has decoded the complex libidinal economy, the psychic apparatus of this enterprise as a multilayered dynamism of the unconscious and the conscious, of Id, Ego, and Superego. The social supervisory body of the Superego, in contestation with the Ego, keeps the libidinal instincts within the boundaries of self-preservation. Thus, in spite of the inevitable formation of neuroses, a more or less liberal interplay of subjects is made possible, which is the basic prerequisite of free market economy.[4] Even though this retrospective dependence of Freud's theories and procedures on his ideological and intellectual culture of origin is brilliant, his method points far beyond this.

The great anti-metaphysician, the materialist, sceptic, and relativist, who regarded *Reason* to be his exclusive and only authority, did create a deterministic psychology of freedom.[5] With his *Interpretation of Dreams* Freud, however, has also established psychoanalysis above all as a technique of interpretation.[6] In this the *Jew without God*, as Renate Schlesinger convincingly pointed out, makes use of the hermeneutic tradition of Talmudic research—a *deconstructive* method of association, of dialogic reflection, the creation of manifold inner relations, and latent signification. His method of interpretation pertains to the latent dream content, not to the manifest dream. The dream, without being real itself, refers to reality, and this quality of reference makes it require interpretation. The truth of the dream is founded in the human psyche itself; it finds its ways of expression in complex ways leading from the unconscious to the conscious. Freud has thus introduced a new model of the psychic structure; he has comprehensively addressed its uncivilized, irrational, forbidden, libidinal aspects, its erotic, egoistic, destructive impulses, and opened a revolutionary anthropological perspective. Freud describes and analyses the more or less unlimited capacities of the unconscious, while at the same time determining those limits which are set to his objective and subjective awareness.

Freud's influence on twentieth-century thought was in fact enormous, overarching civilizations via the detour of his Anglo-American reception. He was certain of several of his epoch-making discoveries: understanding the basic order of the psychic structure; the dynamic unconscious; the dualistic theory of libidinal impulses; the universality of the Oedipus complex; the interaction of conflict, defence, repression; the sexual aetiology of neuroses. With the concepts of taboo, censorship, and regression, he set psycho-political and emancipatory milestones: 'Where there was Id shall be Ego.'

He also made use of the historical method—and this was perhaps hardly possible otherwise in a metropolis which derived its identity from the imagination of its historic importance and made its architectural redesign draw upon the historic model of the *Gründerzeit* era. In Freud's view, what is known does not result from new experience but from what is remembered, what has already happened. What counts is the *milieu intérieur*, the substratum of psychic instincts which determine the outer behaviour. Knowing the past is the key to the future; it develops out of decoding, deciphering those hidden forces of the unconscious, which underlie social action and the libidinal structure of the Ego.[7]

Advocacy for the Collective: The case of Julius Tandler

This very specific conception of *time* Freud shared with the so-called *Austromarxists* in the immediate succession of Victor Adler. They on their part had secularized essential moments of the Jewish-Christian millenarian tradition, placing them within a historic process. Freud, however, would not accept their fundamentally optimistic concept of humanity. And while Freud's outlook and methods increasingly gained global significance, the Austromarxists had to act within the rather restricted bounds of a city acquiring a markedly different status. In the immediate post–World War I period the transnational, if not global position of Vienna changed dramatically, as the city was transformed from a formerly highly celebrated and praised imperial metropolis to the somewhat isolated capital of a newly formed and unwanted small state in the very centre of Europe.

According to a political concept that was derived from what Victor Adler had introduced as the key moment of social-democratic politics, only a well-schooled and disciplined workforce that had attained intellectual and cultural hegemony over a majority of the population could guarantee the victory of democracy. This attributed prime significance to the field of education. The workforce needed to be placed in a position to develop within itself those intellectual and moral qualities without which democracy could not be realized.[8] The will to achieve power and cultural hegemony (*Machtwille* and *Kulturwille*) could be synthesized; and from a condition of being without culture at all there could be developed an intellectually active working class striving for ever greater cultural acquisition. The transformation of society was thereby linked to the reshaping of the individual and to the anticipation of what was melodramatically hailed as der *Neue Mensch* (the New Man) in the context of setting free the elements of the new society within existing conditions.[9]

For a decade and a half in the Vienna of the interwar years, this conception was put into practice in an astonishingly faithful manner. Local politics concentrated above all on the area of reproduction and were predicated on a complete reorganization of the administrative and technical functions of the city. The three main pillars were municipal housing, school reform, and social welfare policy.[10] The achievement of an ambitious and (on an international scale) unique programme of social housing proved to be both a symbolic and pragmatic keystone of Viennese municipal experiment. As a recognizable, indeed unmistakable *urban signature*, communal housing had the most direct and most significant effect. The building programme made political control over the urban fabric available to the organized working class as the new buildings across the whole of Vienna opened up a discursive space between those very buildings and the historical city. For the first time, the working population became the subject of its direct environmental milieu.[11]

The socio-political project operated similarly. It conceptualized the city principally as an example of social technology and offered a virtually paradigmatic illustration of the rational and emancipatory character of municipal reform. When the Social Democrats assumed control of the city's administration in the summer of 1919, the areas of devastation left behind by the war were clearly and tangibly evident across the whole city. The collapse of the city's sanitation systems, a population virtually under siege from hunger, malnutrition, and rampant Spanish influenza, a dramatic rise in instances of tuberculosis and sexually transmitted infections (which matched an equally dramatic growth in the numbers of homeless people and those without any means of support), a general lack of all kinds of necessities for living, public and private destitution, the constant threat of epidemics—all this reinforced the omnipresent scenario of a 'dying city'.[12]

On 22 November 1920 Professor Julius Tandler, who until then had been the Deputy Secretary of State responsible for health in the new Republic, was appointed City Councillor for Welfare Services. He was a highly regarded clinical anatomist and one of the ever-dwindling number of Jewish professors at the Faculty of Medicine (of which he had been Dean from 1914 to 1917), and with his strongly social-Darwinist, eugenicist, and neo-Lamarckian tendencies represented the scientific mainstream of the age. Tandler combined these traits with a civilizing ethos, as was manifested in his reorganization of the city's welfare and social care systems, making use of the latest technological and bureaucratic developments in the field.[13]

In conducting this reorganization Tandler referred to decisive stages in enlightened bourgeois developments in social reform, particularly in the Anglo-Saxon world; concepts that were principally concerned with the social stabilization of the urban and industrial working class. The *Vienna System*, which emerged pragmatically from the exigencies of dealing with actual problems, soon concentrated on the area of preventive measures, on the care of juveniles, and the establishment of optimal socialization conditions for future generations.

> For the more we take care of the young, the less we shall have to take care of the old. What we spend on facilities for young people we shall save on prisons. What we deploy for the care of pregnant women and new-born infants we shall save on institutions for the mentally ill.[14]

In a deliberate reversal of the traditional principles of charity, Tandler took as his basis the social obligation to provide welfare and the individual's right to it. The organic capital of a society, according to him, lay in the community of living human beings, and there was just as strong a duty to manage this capital as there was to manage other social assets, regardless of whether they were cultural or material.

Thus, in a system of social welfare based on generative ethics, welfare workers were holding society's mandate, and those they cared for stood in a relationship of mutual rights and duties.[15]

The successes of the Vienna System were impressive. The overall mortality rate fell by a quarter compared with the period before World War I, and infant mortality fell by half. The number of kindergartens rose more than fivefold; by 1931 they were caring for some 10,000 children and their educational methods were based on principles of developmental psychology in the tradition of Froebel and Montessori. In 1932 prophylactic medical examinations encompassed more than 132,000 children and adults. Open-air pools for children were put into parks and into the courtyards of the newly built communal blocks, and the city was dotted with public swimming baths. By 1927 there were children's pools, public showers, a steam bathhouse, a bathing beach, two outdoor swimming pools with extensive grounds, and the luxurious *Amalienbad*, or 'Workers' Palace' as it was generally called. In district youth offices and in many communal blocks, centres were set up offering marriage counselling or advice to mothers, and from 1927 on all mothers, regardless of circumstances, were given a large box containing a complete infant layette. These boxes bore the slogan *Kein Wiener Kind darf auf Zeitungspapier geboren werden* ('No Viennese child should be born on newspaper sheets anymore') and a picture of Anton Hanak's statue *Die große Mutter* (The Great Mother), which topped the fountain in front of the municipal Children's Reception Centre (Kinderübernahmestelle). This was a monumental figure of a caring mother with her arm placed protectively around a group of children threatened by snakes spouting water, which were intended to symbolize the dangers of the big city.

The majority of measures taken and institutions established were strictly related to families, aiming at an increase in the birth rate, a rise in reproductive health overall and in general hygiene, and at improvements in parental care. Tandler's social reforms and his new, socially and technically inspired conception of the fabric of urban life, proved to be a profoundly enlightened project, a project to cleanse the body of the city and establish the conditions for the emancipation of the individual via social intervention. It combined the provision of social and welfare services with the promotion of family life and an element of social supervision.[10]

As did Freud's project, Tandler's conception of a new urban fabric met with furious opposition, generating wild storms of anti-Semitism. As, in the course of the Great Depression, Nazi-terrorism intensified with Tandler's Vienna University as one of the major objects, he increasingly lost faith in the perspectives of his welfare-based reform endeavours. The crash of civilizations following the Great Depression of the early 1930s-induced cultural barriers, built up laboriously, to break, setting free a crazed and untamed instinct on a large scale, mobilizing what is dark, abysmal, and hidden in civilization. It was the release of anger, of the urge to destroy of the pauperized individual, deprived of hope and perspectives. The anti-Semites, as Theodor Adorno described in his *Dialectic of Enlightenment*, had started to convert the world into the hell they had always seen in it. It was at the same time the end of those emancipatory concepts of *advocacy*, as they had been formulated (though not yet labelled as such) by prominent members of the Vienna School of Medicine—whether with reference to the individual and their psychic condition, or with reference to their potentials of development and design as a member of a specific community, that is, with reference to the more collective aspects of advocacy.

Freud stayed in Vienna until 1938, when he, advanced in years and gravely ill, was driven into exile by the Nazis. Tandler in 1933 accepted an invitation from the Chinese government to the University of Shanghai, but when he heard of the bloody civil war in February 1934, he returned to Vienna where he was immediately arrested. After his release, he went back to China and from there to the Soviet Union, where he was to undertake the reorganization of important areas of the rather inefficient health system. He died on 26 August 1936 in Moscow, and is nowadays, very much in contrast to Freud, hardly remembered at all.

Conclusion

The Vienna School of Medicine, being constituted in the late nineteenth century and acquiring worldwide fame later on, was one of the institutions to explore new avenues in a variety of ways: brilliant in diagnosis, nihilistic in therapy (not least because of a lack of suitable therapeutic means and instruments). Some of its leading representatives followed concepts which we today would probably subsume under the term *advocacy*. This chapter has testified two very specific ways of interpreting this originally rather vaguely defined concept: Sigmund Freud's exploration of the unconscious to promote the individual's status and self-perception, and Julius Tandler's endeavour to improve decisively collective living conditions by means of social technology. As exemplary enterprises of *Late Enlightenment*, both projects, in their radically progressive stance, can with good reason be seen as parallel actions—in so far, as they were, each in their ways, trying to transform mass objects into self-assertive individuals.

References

1. **Musil, R.** (1995) *The Man Without Qualities*. New York: Alfred A. Knopf, p. 53.
2. **Freud, S.** (1913) *The Interpretation of Dreams* (translated by Abraham A. Brill). New York: Macmillan, p. 122.
3. **Schlesier, R.** (2002) Hermeneutik auf dem Königsweg zum Unbewussten. Freuds Traumdeutung. In: W. Erhard, H. Jaumann (eds). *Jahrhundertbücher. Große Theorien von Freud bis Luhmann*. München: C. H. Beck, pp. 22ff.
4. **Horkheimer, M., Adorno, T. W.** (1988) *Dialektik der Aufklärung. Philosophische Fragmente*. Frankfurt/Main: S. Fischer, p. 212.
5. **Gay, P.** (1999) *Ein gottloser Jude*. Frankfurt: Fischer, p. 59.
6. **Schorske, C. E.** (1980) *Fin de Siècle Vienna. Politics and Culture*. New York: Random House, pp. 169ff.
7. **Alt, P.-A.** (2016) *Sigmund Freud: Der Arzt der Moderne*. München: C. H. Beck.
8. **Maderthaner, W.** (2006) Austro-Marxism: Mass Culture and Anticipatory Socialism. *Austrian Studies*, **14**, 21.
9. **Rabinbach, A.** (1983) *The Crisis of Austrian Socialism. From Red Vienna to Civil War*. Chicago: Chicago University Press, pp. 44ff.
10. **Gruber, H.** (1991) *Red Vienna: Experiment in Working-Class Culture, 1919–1934*. New York/Oxford: Oxford University Press.

11. **Blau, E.** (1999) *The Architecture of Red Vienna 1919–1934*. Cambridge, MA/London: Harvard University Press.
12. **Maderthaner, W.** (2005) *Kultur Macht Geschichte. Studien zur Wiener Stadtkultur im 19. und 20. Jahrhundert*. Wien: LIT Verlag, pp. 198ff.
13. **Sablik, K.** (2005) Tandler, Julius. In: W. E. Gerabek, B. D. Haage, G. Keil, W. Wegner (eds). *Enzyklopädie Medizingeschichte*. Berlin/New York: De Gruyter, p. 1379.
14. **Tandler, J.** (1925) *Wohltätigkeit oder Fürsorge*. Wien: Volksbuchhandlung, p. 5.
15. **Sablik, K.** (2010) *Julius Tandler, Mediziner und Sozialreformer*. Frankfurt/Main: Peter Lang.

Chapter 4

Ethical issues in neurology

Jan J. Heimans

Introduction

Ethical issues in neurology are connected with patient care as well as with neuroscience research. Basically, ethics in neurology do not seem to differ very much from ethics in other medical disciplines, such as internal medicine, surgery, or medical oncology, and several issues will be grossly the same. However, some ethical aspects in patient care as well as in research are unique to neurology, and these aspects are not the least important.

Neurology concerns diseases of the brain, the spinal cord, the peripheral nerves, and the muscles. This implicates that patients who are struck by a neurological disorder may not only be severely handicapped by loss of physical functions (such as motor, sensory, or visual function), but will often not be able to make their own decisions due to cognitive function impairment or impairment of consciousness.

Problems concerning medical decision-making in various disorders of consciousness and in patients with dementia or other cortical function disorders (stroke, brain injury, brain tumours) frequently occur in the care for neurologic patients. Further, the decision-making process is also crucial in items such as brain death and organ donation. Research in comatose patients and in patients with dementia or other cerebral function disorders leading to impaired or lost consent capacity is characterized by comparable dilemmas that are more or less unique to brain disease.

If we consider these ethical issues in the context of advocacy, as highlighted in Chapter 1 with reference to Bateman,[1] several ethical principles come up for discussion. One of the leading principles in advocacy is that we act in the best interests of our patients and that we do so in accordance with the wishes of the patients. But in patients with severe brain damage, the question of what is in the best interest of the patient is sometimes not easy to answer. And we often grope in the dark about the wishes of a patient, because there is no written advance directive and the patients' proxies are not aware of any wishes because they never discussed these issues with their beloved ones.

In this chapter, only a selection of ethical issues in neurology will be discussed and the main focus will be on the decision-making process in patients with brain disease.

Disorders of consciousness and the decision-making process

Persons with chronically impaired consciousness are extremely vulnerable, as they are not able to express themselves.[2] Medical decision-making in these patients who are not able to express their wishes with regard to any therapeutic measure, like respiratory support or treatment with antibiotics, is a problem that neurologists are frequently confronted with. Especially in the intensive care department, family members of neurologically devastated patients often must act as representatives. In some instances, these relatives do not have the disposal of an advanced directive of the patient and in most instances, relatives will only have a very limited experience with medical decision-making. This may lead to disconcerting situations in which relatives do not accept a dismal prognosis and insist on medical interventions that are not indicated in the eyes of the medical team. But also, the reverse may happen: family members raise objections against proposed interventions which by the physicians are thought to be in the best interest of the patient.

Disorders of consciousness may be transient or permanent. This seems to be a self-evident remark but the first and major question that we are confronted with is when we are allowed to speak of a permanent state.

Various grades of disturbed consciousness

Coma may be defined as a state of loss of spontaneous or stimulus-induced arousal. This comatose state is self-limiting: either the patient regains consciousness or there is (after approximately two weeks) a transition into a vegetative state or a minimally conscious state.[3] In a vegetative state, there are no purposeful responses to visual, auditory, tactile, or noxious stimuli and there is no evidence of any form of communication. The distinction with coma, however, is that there is spontaneous eye-opening. This latter phenomenon may be very confusing for proxies who tend to think that opening of the eyes is an indication of recovery of cerebral functioning. It is one of the major tasks of neurologists to explain phenomena like this and to guide proxies of patients with long-lasting disturbances of consciousness during the course of the disease. Advocacy in this respect not only concerns the patient but also extends to the patients' relatives who see themselves confronted with confusing and frightening signs of a severely injured brain in their beloved one.

When the vegetative state is still present after one month the term 'persistent vegetative state' is applied, and this persistent state may become a 'permanent vegetative state' after 3–12 months, depending on the aetiology. This wide time range was the reason that the Aspen Neurobehavioral Conference Workgroup suggested to abandon the term 'persistent vegetative state' and to use the term vegetative state only in association with the aetiology and the length of time since the onset of the condition.[4] Because of the (unintended) denigrating association with a 'vegetable-like condition', the European Task Force on Disorders of Consciousness proposed the term 'unresponsive wakefulness syndrome', which reflects the major quality of the condition: a state of wakeful unconsciousness.[5] This renaming of a pathophysiologic condition only out of respect for patients as well as their relatives should also be interpreted as an act of advocacy.

Coma may also be followed by a so-called 'minimally conscious state'. A patient who has been diagnosed with this condition shows minimal evidence of awareness. This condition usually reflects a transition to regain of consciousness after coma (or after a vegetative state) or is part of a gradually progressive decline. It may be difficult to distinguish a persistent vegetative state from a minimally conscious state purely on the basis of clinical signs and symptoms. A meta-analysis from the literature by Bender and co-workers showed that modern diagnostic techniques can contribute significantly to the diagnostic assessment of this minimally conscious state.[2]

Communication with proxies and decision-making

Within the emergency department, where almost all patients with severe brain injury stay during the first days or weeks after the injury, the neurologist is an indispensable member of the medical team which usually also consists of specialists in emergency medicine, anaesthesia, neurosurgery, pharmacy, and nursing. During the various stages of diminished consciousness of a patient, the medical team has several tasks. Providing information to the proxies on the diagnosis, on the various aspects of the actual medical condition, and especially on prognostic aspects and uncertainties, is one of the main tasks. An excellent review by Rubin and co-workers[6] provides a 'code of professional conduct for the Neurocritical Care Society' for those who work with these patients in an intensive care department. Aspects like personal behaviour, relationships with other team members, expert testimony, conflicts of interest, and ethics of research are covered in this paper.

In case of a devastating brain injury, management during the first days after the injury requires special management skills and knowledge of guidelines. A position statement for the management of these patients during the first 72 hours after the injury has been given by the Neurocritical Care Society, and this paper contains a number of recommendations that are worthy of consideration.[7] Devastating brain injury has been defined as 'neurological injury where there is an immediate threat to life from a neurologic cause'. The authors state that in case of such a severe neurological insult, it can be necessary to consider early limitation of therapy, which is defined as treatment of disease, 'in favour of an emphasis on care, e.g., the provision of comfort measures'.

This means that the proxies of these patients must be informed on the medical situation from the very beginning and that the proxies will also be involved in the decision-making process. This so-called 'surrogate decision-making' in patients who are not able to express their wishes is an ethical item that frequently arises, both in neurological patient care as well as in neuroscience research.

A prerequisite for optimal communication with proxies is that clinicians acknowledge the almost continuous need for information and emotional support during this first phase of a devastating brain injury in a beloved one. Only then, family members who are in a state of emotional shock will be able to participate adequately in the decision-making process. In the communication with family members, prognostic uncertainty, especially during the first 72 hours after a serious brain injury, should be expressed clearly[7,8]: usually proxies appreciate an honest approach more than a reassuring attitude that is not based on evidence, although cultural factors may affect this appreciation.

One major question during the first days after a devastating brain injury is whether the patient should be resuscitated. It should be recognized that prognostic uncertainty makes it very difficult to formulate clear guidelines in this delicate matter. If there is no known objection to resuscitation, it is important to realize that restoration and optimization of physiologic homeostasis are pivotal to the neurological outcome in serious brain injury. Apart from that, optimization of the physiologic condition is required when organ donation may be an option. Especially during the first hours and days after a devastating brain injury, these items should be explained and discussed with family members in such a way that relatives are able to understand the extreme complicated decision-making process.

Rubin describes this decision-making process with surrogate decision-makers extensively and points to the major problem arising from the fact that surrogates often do not know what the patient might have wished in a situation like this.[9] For that reason, they tend to express what they themselves would prefer. In the same article, the author pays attention to the decision-making process and the importance of a shared decision-making model. He illustrates this by first describing the two most extreme methods of communication that are used by physicians who lack experience with the shared decision-making process. The first extreme is characterized by an attitude of paternalism, where the physician decides on the basis of what she/he thinks is in the patient's best interest without giving attention to what the patient has previously expressed as his wish or what the surrogate thinks. Before 1980, the paternalistic approach of patients was the prevalent approach in the Western world. The second extreme approach is called by Rubin 'isolated autonomy': the patient—or his surrogate—has to make a decision without being able to weigh and discuss a doctor's advice. The first extreme approach disregards the principle of patient's (or surrogate's) autonomy, whereas the second extreme approach leaves the unexperienced patient (or surrogate) without the doctor's guidance. Patient autonomy is nowadays a widely accepted principle in Western medicine, but it is important to emphasize that physicians always have the moral obligation to make their patients and the representatives of their patients aware of any ill-conceived decisions which could result in actual harm.[10] In this respect, it is important to realize that nowadays people have easy access to many sources of information, and that they will use this often confusing and overwhelming amount of information in their discussion with healthcare professionals.

It may be clear that both extreme approaches should be avoided as much as possible. In a shared decision-making model, physicians carefully and repeatedly formulate their advice and continuously check whether the patient or proxy understands which decisions are under discussion and what the reach of these decisions is. This is one of the most ultimate aspects of advocacy. In the case of devastating brain injury, either by a traumatic or by a non-traumatic (e.g. a massive subarachnoid haemorrhage) cause, hard decisions should be made during the first hours and days. And in almost all cases the patient himself will be unconscious, so a proxy should act as surrogate decision-maker. It is important that the guidelines on communication during the decision-making process, as described by Rubin,[10] are observed as much as possible. Devastating brain injury is almost always an acute event and there is only a short time for decisions, which implies that the surrogate will hardly be able to reflect on what she/he has heard, or to discuss the proposed strategy with other proxies.

Life-sustaining treatment: Yes or no?

The first decision to be taken, and to be discussed with the proxies, is on life-sustaining treatment. Often this treatment will have been started during the transport of the patient to the hospital. In the recommendations of the Neurocritical Care Society, a 72-hour observation period is advised. During this period, the decision on withdrawal of life-sustaining treatment should be postponed, if possible.[7] Another item that should be discussed with family members as soon as possible is whether the patient should be resuscitated. Not resuscitating a patient with a devastating brain injury will limit both the opportunity for optimal recovery as well as the opportunity for organ donation. The only exception to this rule would be that there is a pre-existing objection to resuscitation attempts. It is important to stress that the decision to resuscitate a patient should not depend on the organ donor status.

Equally important is that patients with a severe cerebral injury should receive sedative and analgesic medication, if appropriate. Also, this decision should not depend on the organ donor status. The Neurocritical Care Society even recommends that palliative sedation does not exclude the possibility of organ donation.

In every patient who receives life-sustaining treatment (including mechanical ventilation) after a devastating brain injury, the decision on either continuing or stopping this treatment will have to be taken. If the patient will be physiologically stable after stopping artificial respiration, the question is not relevant any more, but if the patient appears to be dependent on measures like artificial respiration, the question arises for how long these should be continued.

Several papers have been written on withdrawal of life-sustaining treatment. A recent systematic review[11] provides an overview on the variability concerning life-sustaining treatment in various countries in North America, Europe, Asia, the Middle East, and Australia. The first striking finding from this review is the wide variability among countries but also the variability among ICU units within one country. This underlines that there are virtually no uniform rules or guidelines for physicians to tackle this problem. The authors point to the fact that withdrawal of life-sustaining treatment differs ethically from withholding life-sustaining treatment, in the respect that withdrawal is an active process whereas withholding is the absence of action. That will likely also be the reason that withholding life-sustaining measures is less consistently documented in the files of terminally ill patients, especially in those cases where advance directives fail.

Stroke is an important cause of devastating brain injury. Although the incidence of stroke is decreasing due to improved vascular risk factor control, care for stroke patients is a large part of neurological practice. Notwithstanding positive developments in the treatment of stroke in the acute phase, many stroke patients will be confronted with serious and persisting disabling symptoms and still a considerable number of them will die. This makes palliative care in stroke patients an important responsibility of the neurologist.[12] Also, with these severe stroke patients important decisions have to be made in the initial phase of the disease: intubation and mechanical ventilation, but also brain surgery should be considered. Furthermore, in this category of patients these decisions often have to be made in close collaboration with family members, because the patients themselves will be unable to communicate. Neurologists and other healthcare workers are familiar with a large degree of uncertainty concerning the prognosis of stroke patients, and they know that significant functional improvement during the weeks and months after the incident is one possibility, but they also realize that severe physical and cognitive limitations may persist. It is extremely difficult to communicate this uncertainty with family members who are involved in the decision-making process and to avoid that they experience an almost unbearable sense of responsibility.

Brain death and organ donation

Nowadays, we are more or less used to the concept of 'brain death', but this has not always been the case. In an overview on the definition and criterion of death, which contains several interesting historical landmarks, Bernat[13] refers to the report of the ad hoc committee of the Harvard medical school.[14] This was the first paper that made the medical community, as well as the general public, aware of the use of the absence of brain functions as a method to define death, and their opinions had a profound influence on the discussions that followed during the next decades. The term *brain death* has given rise to a lot of confusion and discussion, because it suggested that brain death was a special form of death, to be distinguished from ordinary death, but in the end the term has survived and is now commonly used. Also in the world's major religions, brain death is an accepted concept. In Bernat's aforementioned article,[13] the view of various religions (Roman Catholic, Protestant, Jewish, Islamic, Hinduism, Buddhism) on the concept is described conscientiously and it is interesting to see that conclusions are largely the same.

Although the concept of brain death apparently does not give rise to seriously diverting opinions, the technical aspects are complicated and it requires an expert to make the diagnosis. Brain death results from an unrelenting acute brain injury which usually starts as a hemispheric lesion and progresses to a brain stem lesion: the brainstem injury advances caudally, starting in the mesencephalon and progressing to the medulla oblongata.[15] When the medulla oblongata ceases functioning, pontine reflexes will have disappeared and the cough response will stop. In this stage, spontaneous breathing will have stopped and ventilation will only be possible by means of artificial respiration. A thorough neurologic examination at this stage usually will show that the patient fulfils the criteria of brain death. The neurologic examination should be carried out by an experienced expert who is able to identify any reflex motor responses as spinal reflexes, who is able to test pupillary, cornea, and oculocephalic reflexes in an appropriate way and who is able to judge the absence of oculovestibular responses, gag, and cough reflexes. Also, the performance of the apnoea test is part of this complex procedure. For the proxies of a patient, it may be very difficult to understand that spinal motor responses may persist in a person who is declared to be brain dead. A very important task for the neurologist is to explain this phenomenon to family members as well as to medical, paramedical, and nursing staff who are closely involved with the patient.

Notwithstanding intensive efforts to optimize communication with family members, in some instances there may be opposition to the declaration of brain death and this may particularly be the case when the patient is a child or young adult. Relatives simply cannot accept the fact that a person with a continuous heart beat and persisting (spinal) motor responses is declared dead, and there have been sporadic cases in which the family maintained in refusing to accept the death of a beloved one for a longer time.

As soon as a person is declared brain dead, and there is consent for tissue and organ donation, the care of the patient shifts to the protection of organ viability.[15] This shift should be explained clearly to the relatives of the patient. In the United States the topic of organ donation is usually not mentioned by the medical and nursing staff who take care of the patient before brain death is determined. Consent should preferably be obtained by a specially trained person who was not involved in the care of the patient. However, this is not the case in all countries. Within the context of this chapter, it would be too much to go into detail with respect to various aspects of organ donation, but it should be emphasized that in the very complex process preceding this procedure, it is again the neurologist that has an extremely important role.

Decision-making and giving consent in patients with cognitive impairment

As with unconscious patients, in patients with various disturbances of cortical functions medical decisions often have to be discussed with relatives. Various types of dementia, but also Parkinson's disease, brain tumours, stroke, post-traumatic encephalopathy, and post-ischaemic encephalopathy are examples of brain disorders that may interfere severely with cognitive functioning leading to impaired decision-making capacity. One of the most severe and most dramatic consequences of many brain disorders is that patients may undergo a change of personality during the course of their illness. This is particularly the case in advanced Alzheimer's disease and other forms of dementia, but also in patients with brain tumours, multiple sclerosis, or Parkinson's disease, emotional and cognitive changes may be part of the clinical picture. This makes it that many people fear brain diseases more than any other disease: not only their lives, but also their identities are threatened.[16] Not recognizing one's own children any more is often considered as the utmost terror. But also in milder forms of disturbed brain functioning, patients may not be capable of understanding problems which are connected with medical decision-making. As long as the problem is relatively simple (e.g. the question of whether or not a flu vaccination is indicated), surrogate decision-makers can easily assist, but in more complex situations the burden for these relatives will often be heavy.

If someone has made written advance directives, the problem for the family members seems less difficult, but the major question the family members are confronted with is whether the patient is still the same person as the one who wrote these directives.

This problem is well illustrated by Chiong, who addresses this as the 'someone else problem', by an actual (modified) case which has been discussed extensively in the literature.[17] The patient is an independent and intellectual woman, who has expressed the wish at various occasions not to be treated for a potentially treatable infection if she was living in a demented state. Then, unfortunately, she develops Alzheimer's disease: during the advancing disease process, she does not repeat her former wishes and seems to be content with simple pleasures. What should be done in case she would develop pneumonia? When her formerly expressed wishes would be respected, no antibiotics should be prescribed. But if we recognize that the disease has changed her and that—in fact—she now is a different person, there would be no reason to withhold antibiotics. In fact, we may observe this shift also in people who are functioning normally and without any cognitive limitations: as long as they are in good health, they may express the wish not to live any longer if they would be met with a serious and crippling disease; but if they are actually struck with that fate, they can change their view and prove to be able to live with a severe limitation.

Chiong[16] further explores the implications of the decision-making process and personal identity in dementia and states that dementing illnesses strike at cognitive capacities that are pivotal to personal identity, thus raising important philosophical but also major practical problems. One of the most crucial practical questions is how to handle advance directives. Here also, just as in those cases in which the patient is unconscious due to catastrophic brain injury, the opinion of relatives in the role of surrogate decision-maker is important. There is, however, one big difference: catastrophic brain injury is an acute event, whereas dementia is a gradually progressing condition. In the first case, relatives are all of a sudden confronted with a dramatic and highly threatening situation and they have to participate in the decision-making process when they are still in a state of emotional shock, or at least in a more or less confused state of mind. In the case of a developing dementia syndrome, relatives witness gradually decreasing cognitive abilities in a beloved person. Although this may have a severe emotional impact, it also enables relatives to discuss eventual decisions with the patient during a stage of the disease where such is still possible. Moreover, relatives have the time for reflection and exchange of thoughts with others.

Earlier in this chapter we have pointed to the importance of the shared decision-making model in acute situations in the intensive care department. Physicians should avoid both the 'paternalistic' approach, as well as the 'isolated autonomy' approach. These rules also apply to the guidance of dementing patients and their beloved ones. Doctors should be able to guide patients and their relatives and to provide them with as much relevant and objective information as possible. The decision on whether or not to treat a case of pneumonia during an advanced stage of dementia will be easier when all aspects and prospects have been discussed thoroughly in an earlier phase.

Driving ability

The decision on treatment of life-threatening complications in an end stage of dementia is one end of the spectrum. In earlier stages of dementia, other decisions may be under discussion. One of these is the problem of driving fitness. This problem seems trivial in comparison with end-of-life decisions such as withholding of antibiotic treatment, but being able to drive a car, especially in older people, contributes strongly to social participation and independency.

Driving in modern traffic, however, requires several complex skills and these depend on a certain level of cognitive functioning, especially in the domains of attention, memory, and visuo-spatial orientation.[18] A physician who is confronted with a patient suffering from dementia or any other brain disease that leads (or may lead) to cognitive impairment, should raise the subject of driving ability. This is not as simple as it seems, because often the relatives of the patient insist on a prohibition to drive, but the patient is not willing to acknowledge his or her limitation. The warning of a physician may help, but will not always be obeyed. In some countries (e.g. the Netherlands) professional confidence does not allow a physician to report the driving inability to the authorities, whereas in other countries (e.g. Sweden) physicians should report patients who are unfit to drive to the licensing authority.[18] This is an interesting and rather striking legal difference, but considered in more detail is maybe less striking than it seems, because Swedish doctors may also reach an agreement with their patients to abstain from driving. Lovas and co-workers performed a cross-sectional study in which they included over 15,000 patients suffering from dementia. Only 9% of these patients were reported to the authorities, whereas in the large majority an agreement was made. However, in 16% of patients who were demented and had a driving licence, no action was taken by the physician. This means that with these patients, either the proxies had the task to persuade them to refrain from driving, or the patients had to take this decision on their own. Generally speaking, the ideal situation would be that the physician, together with family members of the patient, which will usually be the partner or the children, explains to the patient that driving a car is no longer an option. Also in these cases a paternalistic approach should be avoided as long as possible, although here not only the safety of the individual but also the safety of others is at stake, which eventually could lead to a more constrained approach. Advocacy in these cases is not restricted to the patient and his proxies but also extends to society in general when the safety of other road users is an issue.

Participation in research

Another item that deserves attention is the participation of people with cognitive impairment in research projects. Dementia affects millions of people worldwide and there is urgent need for research into causes and treatment of various types of dementia. This implicates that patients participate in clinical trials and give informed consent. Patients with mild cognitive impairment will be able to give this consent but patients who suffer from more advanced stages of dementia often will have lost consent capacity; in those cases, it could be considered that surrogate decision-makers give consent. The process of decision-making for participation in research has been studied by Black et al.[19] They found that the decision on whether or not to join a study usually was a complex and dynamic collaborative process between the patient and the relative, but in most cases the patient ultimately made the decision. The surrogates usually played a greater role when subjects were more impaired.

The question arises whether the use of advance research directives should be encouraged. Dementia is a gradually progressive disorder and giving advance directives with regard to future participation in research projects will usually be possible in the early stages of the disease. Jongsma and van de Vathorst argue that advance directives are a morally defensible basis for the inclusion of persons with impaired consent capacity in research projects and they raised some questions with regard to the use of proxy consent.[20] Proxies are supposed to act on the basis of the persons' presumed will, but often, especially in unusual situations (such as research projects), this has never been a subject of discussion. Apart from that, proxies may have problems with the responsibility of making decisions and may experience guilt and stress. Despite these considerations, the authors recognize that legal representatives remain to play a role also when an advance research directive exists. But it is obvious that such an advance directive will make the decision-making process easier: both authorization and protection are served.

Treatment restrictions in patients with neurologic disease

Motor neuron disease (amyotrophic lateral sclerosis), various forms of dementia, Parkinson's disease, multiple sclerosis, and glioma are examples of incurable and progressive neurologic disorders. Although in some of these diseases (i.e. glioma, multiple sclerosis, Parkinson's disease) various forms of treatment will be given during initial stages, what these disorders have in common is that definitive cure is not an option. When the disease advances and therapeutic options become limited, the emphasis will gradually shift to palliative and symptomatic care. Especially in brain tumours this shift can be illustrated by the fact that 'tumour-directed treatment'—in terms of surgery, irradiation, and chemotherapy—will be replaced by symptomatic treatment (i.e. corticosteroids and analgesics), when the tumour progresses. With regard to an inevitable end-of-life stage, other restrictions such as resuscitation and treatment of potentially treatable infectious complications should be discussed, preferably in an earlier stage.

In a literature search for empirical studies about restricting treatment in the course of chronic neurologic conditions, only a few studies about decision-making practices were found. The authors identified three scenarios: (1) acute devastating disease (severe stroke); (2) stable severe neurologic deficit with complications (brain damage after stroke); (3) progressive disease with complications.[21]

Decision-making, including the role of relatives, in acute, catastrophic brain injury (scenario 1) has extensively been discussed in former paragraphs. In patients with chronic severe brain damage after stroke (scenario 2), the problem of communication with the patients and consequently the role of surrogate decision-makers arises and this issue also received attention in previous paragraphs. But in a disease like amyotrophic lateral sclerosis, or ALS (scenario 3), which has a predictable fatal course with preservation of cognitive functions (and as such can be considered as a classical model for advance care planning), the patient himself can give directives with respect to therapeutic restrictions and end-of-life decisions. Invasive as well as non-invasive mechanical ventilation, artificial nutrition, artificial hydration, and treatment of complicating infections are items that can be discussed in a relatively early stage of the disease. In the review by Seeber and colleagues, attention is paid to several studies on advance care planning in ALS patients and one of these studies[22] has shown that patients with ALS wanted to get detailed information on their present state of health, but almost half of them refused to consider end-of-life palliative treatment possibilities, and only 20% of the population were willing to give explicit advance directives.

Decision-making in the end-of-life phase of high-grade glioma patients has aspects in common with decision-making in other forms of cancer (i.e. the shift from 'aggressive' tumour directed treatment to symptomatic, palliative treatment), but has also aspects in common with end-of-life treatment in other types of progressive brain disease (i.e. impaired decision-making capacity and the more important role of surrogate decision-makers). This combination makes that advance care planning at an early stage in patients with brain tumours should be encouraged because the ability to express wishes will decrease with tumour progression. Sizoo et al., in a retrospective descriptive study, found that as many as 40% of patients' physicians were unaware of their patients' end-of-life preferences.[23] This finding illustrates that communication on end-of-life issues between physicians and brain tumour patients can be optimized. End-of-life preferences were less often discussed with brain tumour patients than with other cancer patients, probably because such discussions are often postponed until the last weeks of life, and in that stage brain tumour patients will usually not be able to express their will any more. This again stresses the importance of early discussion of end-of-life preferences between physicians, brain tumour patients, and their relatives.

Conclusion

The care for neurologic patients and the execution of research protocols in neurologic patients are both strongly connected with cognitive functioning and the ability of patients to participate in the process of decision-making. This ability will be impaired or even completely lost in a considerable number of patients with any form of brain disease. Making decisions for further care in these patients makes high demands upon neurologists and patients' relatives who have to act as surrogate decision-makers, especially when decisions on the withdrawal or withholding of life-sustaining treatment are concerned, or when participation in research protocols is considered. All competences connected with these processes can be regarded as parts of advocacy where neurologists commit themselves to acquire maximal and current knowledge on all major aspects of brain disease and treatment protocols, as well as to train their skills in communication, especially in the context of decision-making.

References

1. **Bateman, N.** (2000) *Advocacy Skills for Health and Social Care Professionals.* London and Philadelphia, PA: Jessica Kingsley Publishers.
2. **Bender, A., Jox, R. J., Grill, E., Straube, A., Lulé, D.** (2015) Persistent vegetative state and minimally conscious state—a systemic review and meta-analysis of diagnostic procedures. *Dtsch Artztebl Int*, **112**, 235–42.

3. **Giacino, J. T., Fins, J. J., Laureys, S., Schiff, N. D.** (2014) Disorders of consciousness after acquired brain injury: the state of the science. *Nat Rev Neurol*, **10**, 99–114.
4. **Giacino, J. T., Kalmar, K.** (2005) Diagnostic and prognostic guidelines for the vegetative and minimally conscious states. *Neuropsychol Rehabil*, **15**, 166–74.
5. **Laureys, S., Celesia, G. G., Cohadon, F., et al.** (2010) Unresponsive wakefulness syndrome: a new name for the vegetative state or apallic syndrome. *BMC Medicine*, **8**, 68.
6. **Rubin, M., Bonomo, J., Bar, B., et al.** (2015) The code of professional conduct for the Neurocritical Care Society. *Neurocrit Care*, **23**, 145–8.
7. **Souter, M. J., Blissitt, P. A., Blosser, S., et al.** (2015) Recommendations for the critical care management of devastating brain injury: prognostication, psychosocial, and ethical management. *Neurocrit Care*, **23**, 4–13.
8. **Payne, S., Burton, C., Addington-Hall, J., Jones, A.** (2010) End-of-life issues in acute stroke care: a qualitative study of the experiences and preferences of patients and families. *Palliat Med*, **24**, 146–53.
9. **Rubin, M. A.** (2014) The collaborative autonomy model of medical decision-making. *Neurocrit Care*, **20**, 311–18.
10. **Pellegrino, E. D., Thomasma, D.** (1988) *For the Patient's Good: The Restoration of Beneficence in Medical Ethics*. New York: Oxford University Press.
11. **Mark, N. M., Rayner, S. G., Lee, N. J., Curtis, J. R.** (2015) Global variability in withholding and withdrawal of life-sustaining treatment in the intensive care unit: a systematic review. *Intensive Care Med*, **41**, 1572–85.
12. **Creutzfeldt, C. J., Holloway, R. G., Curtis, J. R.** (2015) Palliative care. A core competency for stroke neurologists. *Stroke*, **9**, 2714–19.
13. **Bernat, J. L.** (2013) The definition and criterion of death. In: Bernat, J. L., Beresford, R. (eds). *Handbook of Clinical Neurology*. Vol 118 (3rd series). *Ethical and Legal Issues in Neurology*. Edinburgh: Elsevier BV, pp. 419–35.
14. **Ad Hoc Committee** (1968) A definition of irreversible coma. A report of the Ad Hoc Committee of the Harvard Medical School to examine the definition of brain death. *JAMA*, **205**, 337–40.
15. **Wijdicks, E. F. M.** (2015) Determining brain death. *Continuum*, **21**, 1411–24.
16. **Chiong, W.** (2013) Dementia and personal identity: implications for decision-making. In: Bernat, J. L., Beresford, R. (eds). *Handbook of Clinical Neurology*. Vol 118 (3rd series). *Ethical and Legal Issues in Neurology*. Edinburgh: Elsevier BV, pp. 409–18.
17. **Firlik, A. D.** (1991) A piece of my mind. Margo's logo. *JAMA*, **265**, 201.
18. **Lovas, J., Fereshtehnejad, S., Cermakova, P., et al.** (2016) Assessment and reporting of driving fitness in patients with dementia in clinical practice: data from SveDem, the Swedish dementia registry. *J Alzheimer's Dis*, **53**, 631–8.
19. **Black, B. S., Wechsler, M., Fogarty, L.** (2013) Decision making for participation in dementia research. *Am J Geriatr Psychiatry*, **21**, 355–63.
20. **Jongsma, K. R., Van de Vathorst, S.** (2015) Beyond competence: advance directives in dementia research. *Monash Bioeth Rev*, **33**, 167–80.
21. **Seeber, A. A., Hijdra, A., Vermeulen, M., Willems, D. L.** (2012) Discussions about treatment restrictions in chronic neurologic diseases. *Neurology*, **78**, 590–7.
22. **Albert, S. M., Murphy, P. L., Del Bene, M. L., Rowland, L. P.** (1999) A prospective study of preferences and actual treatment choices in ALS. *Neurology*, **53**, 278–83.
23. **Sizoo, E. L., Pasman, H. R. W., Buttolo, J., et al.** (2012) Decision-making in the end-of-life phase of high-grade glioma patients. *Eur J Cancer*, **48**, 226–32.

Chapter 5

Physician autonomy and the pharmaceutical industry

Tissa Wijeratne, Essie Low, and Christopher Neil

Introduction

There are not many topics, other than that of the 'physician and pharmaceutical industry', which is capable of generating heated debate among physicians.[1] The relationship between the medical community and pharmaceutical industry is necessary despite the existence of negative beliefs in the contemporary world. It has certainly evolved into one where both parties acknowledge the differences in interests and opinions. The complexity that comes with differences in interests and opinions itself makes it mandatory for us to address this issue with a view to continue the dialogue of bringing the best, affordable care to our patients.

Worldwide, the primary duty of a neurologist is to act in the best interest of patients. In doing so, neurologists must maintain their professional autonomy, integrity, and independence. The relationship between the profession and the pharmaceutical industry must not cross boundaries, must not compromise, or be perceived to be compromised by the society and patients; it must have the capacity to serve patients in their best interests and to establish trust by virtue of the physician's professional judgement.

The history of healthcare delivery worldwide includes interactions between doctors and pharmaceutical industries with extension to continuous medical education and medical research. Neurologists understand that they have a responsibility to ensure that participation in collaborative efforts in neuroscience research, and engagement in medical education across clinical and experimental neurology, is in keeping with their primary responsibility for their patients. To an extent, it is imperative to avoid any conflict of interest when interacting with pharmaceutical industries by way of practising a high level of professionalism and by adhering to ethical and moral standards.

Pharmaceutically driven clinical trials and clinical research studies in hospitals do indeed facilitate clinical translational research in the neurosciences globally. Specifically, the output generated from such clinical trials help to generate new evidence and therapeutic armamentarium for a variety of neurological disorders, including multiple sclerosis, Parkinson's disease, stroke, and migraine, among many others.

It has been known that patients who participate in clinical trials and research studies in hospitals have better outcomes and lower mortality.[2] In this context, it would be possible for pharmaceutical industry-sponsored clinical trials and research to influence neurologists' clinical practice and prescription pattern. It is important for neurologists and the hospital's respective research governance directorate to manage this risk through strict adherence to national research governance policies (and procedures and guidelines), as well as the institution's standard operating procedures. Those countries that are not regulated by national research governance policies and procedures would imminently face significant risk of undue influence from pharmaceutical industries, even in the context of clinical trials and clinical research.

In a qualitative study involving semi-structured interviews by Prosser and Walley (2003), the authors investigated the reasons behind physicians' willingness to receive visits by pharmaceutical representatives.[3] One hundred and seven general practitioners (GPs) across practices from two health authorities in the North West of England participated in this study. Based on the interviews, findings revealed that physicians received such visits due to the following reasons:

1. Pharmaceutical industry representatives were able to introduce new drug information in a speedy manner.
2. The visits were convenient.
3. The visits were accessible.
4. The visits were time-saving and effortless, which is to the benefit of GPs.
5. Many GPs felt that they had the skills to critically appraise the evidence regarding trials.

In addition, this study demonstrated that pharmaceutical industry representatives could exert a significant impact on the decision-making of the GPs through personal selling techniques, gift giving, and through their personal and social interaction skills.

Interactions between physicians and industry

One of this chapter's authors (TW) recalled initial interactions with pharmaceutical industries as early on as the second year of medical training. Specifically, TW recalled attending medical meetings as a medical student, where he would often correspond with pharmaceutical representatives and subsequently receive printed material regarding pharmaceutical products. This is indeed a common experience for the many physicians practising medicine today. As physician training continues to progress, the degree of interaction with pharmaceutical industries increases as a function. Weekly clinical case conferences, local and regional clinical meetings, and international clinical and scientific meetings further foster these interactions.

Ashley Wazana reviewed the issue of physicians and pharmaceutical industry in 2000.[4] The author's aim was to identify the extent and attitudes towards the link between physicians, industry, and pharmaceutical representatives, and the impact of this relationship on physician's behaviour, knowledge, and attitude.

The predominant findings from Wazana's review[5] mostly indicate negative outcomes associated with these interactions. The inability to identify incorrect facts and claims about the medications that were marketed, a friendly attitude towards the pharmaceutical representative, early prescription of the marketed product, and irrational prescriber behaviour were among these negative outcomes.

Clinical trials

Many landmark trials were funded by pharmaceutical industries (at times exclusively, at times partly) for several decades now. In fact, almost all acute stroke trials involving new generation anti-coagulants and thrombectomy-related trials would not have been successfully executed without funding support from pharmaceutical industries. These clinical trials are critical to promote better therapeutics for patients with neurological disorders such as migraine, stroke, multiple sclerosis, Alzheimer's disease, Guillian–Barré syndrome, and Parkinson's disease. Given that the pursuit for research funding through government agencies is highly competitive, this has encouraged researchers and clinicians to find matched funding through non-governmental organizations, including the pharmaceutical industry.

Potential relationships between physicians and pharmaceutical industry

Physicians may own shares or similar options in the pharmaceutical industry. It is not uncommon for some of the leading physicians to provide a service to the pharmaceutical companies as to be an advisory board member, consultant, director, or even as an employee at times. Physicians often attend meetings that are supported or sponsored by these companies, including continuing professional development, educational and scientific meetings, both locally and internationally. In fact, it is possible for travel and accommodation expenses to be covered by pharmaceutical sponsors at times, as this paves the way for countries to continue to take part in continuous medical education activities among physicians.

What are the disadvantages of commercial pharmaceutical promotion via pharmaceutical industry representatives and physician interactions?

There is a significant risk for pharmaceutical industry representatives to have an impact on prescriber behaviour through undue influence. For example, it is highly likely that the information provided by pharmaceutical industry representatives is significantly biased towards the benefit of their respective company.[6-9] Furthermore, the Prosser study, alongside some others, have suggested that doctors tended to be passive recipients of information.[3,6] Therefore, it is crucial for physicians to practice the habit of critically appraising information provided by pharmaceutical industry representatives, and to strive towards appropriate prescribing.

How does pharmaceutical industry influence physicians?

Pharmaceutical industry representatives (PIR) may be genuinely friendly, but it is important to note that they are preselected for their outgoing nature, as well as their presentation and personality.[10] PIR are trained to study physicians very much like car salesman are trained to sell cars to their customers. Friendly physicians are likely to make life quite easy for reps. Reps study physicians carefully and collect information about the physicians and use their personal information to strengthen their relationship (personal communication with a senior product manager, pharmaceutical industry, Sri Lanka). Once the friendship is well-established, it is easier for the reps to ask for favours, for example, 'please prescribe my product . . . Don't forget my product . . .' can be commonly heard during the conversation at times.

In an article by Fugh-Berman and Ahari (2007), the authors revealed a series of strategies that were used by a sales representative to exert influence on the physician's decision-making (regarding trial-related activities).[10] These tactics include framing discussions and conversations; offering free samples, meals, and office lunches as a gesture of friendship, rather than the part of the job of the pharmaceutical representative for the friendly and outgoing physicians. Making an appointment to visit physicians with journal articles that would specifically counter the physician's perceptions on a product that the representative market, playing the dumb role while physician does the explaining of the journal articles for physicians who are sceptical of a product.

If a physician prefers a competing product, representatives will seek to understand the reasons underlying the physician's decision. They may then attempt to lavish the physician with his/her product and try to win the physician over. While it is very likely that the product shows no difference in efficacy compared with a similar product from a competitive company, the PIR, in this situation, will attempt to advocate for superiority of their product.

The pharmaceutical industry is often interested in opinionated leaders among physicians. Representatives will therefore specifically target such individuals to determine if these physicians would cooperate with the company's public relations department. Representatives would also often observe lectures given by physicians, to establish physicians' prescription pattern and handling of questions from the audience, with a view to target the speaker more than the audience.[10]

Understanding of the pharmaceutical industry by physician trainees

The pharmaceutical industry spends nearly $60 billion per year on marketing of clinical trials to physicians,[11] the largest share of this expenditure being fed into interactions with physicians that includes medical students, junior residents, senior residents, and consultants. Austad and colleagues from Harvard Medical School surveyed a nationally representative sample of first and fourth year medical students and third year residents (via a series of multiple choice questions) to determine students' knowledge on the appropriate treatment for hypothetical patients with diabetes, hypertension, difficulty sleeping, and hyperlipidaemia. Some 1,601 students (49.5% response rate) and 735 residents (42.9% response rate) reported use of resources such as Google (74.2–88.9%) and Wikipedia (45.2–84.5%), which are unfiltered sources of information on drugs.[12] Furthermore, a 10-point higher industry relations index was associated with 15% lower odds of selecting an evidence-based prescribing choice, with an odds ratio of 1.08:95% CI,1.00–1.16). Data from this paper indicates that pharmaceutical marketing is more strongly linked with a lack of evidence-based prescribing decisions, and a higher tendency towards expensive brand names at the expense of generic products that may have equal or, in fact, better efficacy.

The story of essential drug policy in Sri Lanka

Essential drug policy may not provide a solution to the above-mentioned issues in the current era of practice of medicine. None the less, this remarkable story from Sri Lanka is still worth discussing and reflecting upon.

Sri Lanka went on to made major policy reforms in national pharmaceutical policy in 1971 which was a world's first to address some of these issues.[13-15] In 1971, at least 75% of the domestic market was dominated by multinational corporations. In Sri Lanka, there was a landslide election in 1970 for the inauguration of a strong coalition government between the Sri Lanka Freedom Party (SLFP) and two Marxist parties. There followed a transformation of the Sri Lankan economy with a significant shift towards nationalization and growth of the corporate public sector. The new prime minister established a two-member committee, including the late Professor Senaka Bibile, professor of Pharmacology, and a member of parliament, the late Dr S. A. Wickramasinghe, to prepare a report on measures to rationalize the pharmaceutical industry in Sri Lanka. The late Professor Bibile was regarded as a visionary, a high-level academic, and a humanitarian of very high calibre. The duo came up with the national drug policy, an 'essential drug policy' which was presented to the prime minister of Sri Lanka on 23 March 1971.

Introduction of the new essential drug policy was not smooth sailing in Sri Lanka at the time. Drug manufacturing multinationals were operating in multiple fronts, including strong protest from US-based multinational pharmaceutical industries. Eventually, essential drug policy took off the ground and the State Pharmaceutical Cooperation (SPC) was born. Bibile became the first managing director. SPC began manufacturing high-quality essential drugs for Sri Lanka, which the public could easily afford. The country was able to save lot of foreign exchange by limiting drug imports. Many world leaders invited Professor Bibile to their countries with the view of developing similar policies. On 22 September 1977, Professor Bibile passed away in Guyana, Caribbean, while he was assisting the development of essential drug policy in that country.

The new government that came to power in 1977 in Sri Lanka reversed the crucial elements of essential drug policy with free market economy. At present, the undue influence of pharmaceutical industry is significant, with government policies that are vital to regulate such issues being absent. Pharmaceutical industries have direct access to the number of scripts produced by each physician, and the industry also support 'continuous medical education' to physicians almost exclusively. There is no mandatory reporting to the regulatory authorities in Sri Lanka.

Increasingly, the pharmaceutical industry gifts to physicians are under attack and regularly subject to bans and restrictions globally.[16] Brody (2005) argued the case for why physicians should refuse to see the PIR.[17] The author believed that the reason for the willingness of medical practitioners to accept offers of gifts is due to long-standing habits rather than a conscious choice. Brody argued that consultations with representatives are time-consuming and not in the best interest of patients. According to Brody, it is better to care about professional integrity as well as one's commitment to the well-being of patients.[17]

There have been significant improvements in the quality and integrity of industry conferences globally. There are almost no purely commercial medical conferences today.

The complexities in the dynamics of the relationship between such industries and physicians are here to stay. Physicians should display professional principles in maintaining a positive relationship with pharmaceutical organizations, with the clear aim that patient care trumps pharmaceutical agendas. We should encourage the industry to support our educational initiatives without having undue influence on the content. We should encourage the industry to support our initiatives in clinical and experimental research with complete independence on the research process and academic work.

It is important to understand the real and potential conflicts of interests and manage these appropriately. As defined by the Medical Board of Australia,[i] a conflict of interest arises when a doctor, entrusted with acting in the best interests of patients, also has financial, professional, personal interests, or relationships which may affect their care of the patient. Doctors may also be influenced by interests that extend to other persons connected to the provider.[ii]

Neurologists may also have conflicts of interests with the pharmaceutical industry. These must be secondary to the primary duty of serving their patient's interests. If the community or patients perceive that a neurologist is placing his or her personal interests above patient's interest, this is likely to undermine professional trust.

The best way to manage real or perceived conflicts of interest is to maintain openness and transparency. In Australia, every relationship between the industry and physicians are openly disclosed in the public space.

Doctors who participate in medical research involving human participants must ensure that they have a duty to protect the life, health, dignity, integrity, right to self-determination, privacy, and confidentiality of the research participants in accordance with the Helsinki declaration. The well-being and health of research participants take the highest priority over other interests. They should only participate in industry-sponsored research if these studies are scientifically sound, ethically approved, and genuinely worthy of doing.

---

[i] Medical Board of Australia. Good Medical Practice. A Code of Conduct for Doctors in Australia.

[ii] The Royal Australasian College of Physicians' *Guidelines for Ethical Relationship Between Physician and Industry*, 3rd edition (2006) defines 'interest' as follows:

- An 'interest' is a commitment, goal or value arising out of a social relationship or practice;
- A duality of interest arises when two more interests coexist. These interests may or may not conflict, depending on the specific circumstances; and
- A duality may become a conflict of interest when a particular relationship or practice gives rise to two or more contradictory interests.

Industry-sponsored financial and other material support are hugely important in clinical and scientific meetings today. These should be openly disclosed and easily accessible for public scrutiny. Ideally the contents of the meeting should be independent of the industry. This can be achieved through an independent organizing committee with full power to make decisions on the selection of speakers and topics.

Industry advocacy and the need to avoid dependency

Hidden dangers of pharmaceutical industry sponsorship and dependence must be considered. Pharmaceutical industry may fund projects that appear to promote better patient care, translational research, and additional support to the workforce (e.g. fellowship positions, nurse support positions) with the hidden agenda of getting their products prescribed through this 'dependency'. One may argue the overall benefit of such funding towards better patient care. The physician must be cautious and vigilant to ensure the hidden danger is addressed and be very careful to be professional all times.

Gifts should generally be rejected. The Royal Australasian College of Physicians (RACP), Australia recommendations provide a solid framework in dealing with industry advocacy.[18]

Conclusion

The relationship between physicians and industry is here to stay. While there may be potential for conflicts of interests between parties, there are overall benefits to society through professional, ethical relationships between these two groups. Proper management of these conflicts of interests, transparency, and open disclosure should minimize further risks. Ongoing dialogue, discussion, and collaboration will help to facilitate the current and future needs of our patients and the society.

The pharmaceutical industry will be a strong advocate for the medical profession. PIR will continue to focus on getting their products promoted through sponsorship, scientific meetings, and educational meetings, despite their agenda being hidden in most cases. Physicians must adhere to strict professional standards and strong ethical principles. Our priority is delivering the best possible care for the patient, while we use the resources that come our way through pharmaceutical industry partnership for patient benefit. One must never cross the boundaries in this complex interaction. We should continue to be the best advocates for our patients, not the pharmaceutical industry.

References

1. **Erola, J. A.** (1994) We need dialogue and discussion, not a new Berlin Wall. *CMAJ*, **150**(6), 955–6.
2. **Majumdar, S. R., Roe, M. T., Peterson, E. D., Chen, A. Y., Gibler, W. B., Armstrong, P. W.** (2008) Better outcomes for patients treated at hospitals that participate in clinical trials. *Arch Intern Med*, **168**(6), 657–62.

3. **Prosser, H., Walley, T.** (2003) Understanding why GPs see pharmaceutical representatives: a qualitative interview study. *Br J Gen Pract*, **53**(489), 305–11.
4. **Wazana, A.** (2000) Physicians and the pharmaceutical industry: is a gift ever just a gift? *JAMA*, **283**(3), 373–80.
5. **Wazana, A.** (2000) Gifts to physicians from the pharmaceutical industry. *JAMA*, **283**(20), 2655–8.
6. **Ziegler, M. G., Lew, P., Singer, B. C.** (1995) The accuracy of drug information from pharmaceutical sales representatives. *JAMA*, **273**(16), 1296–8.
7. **Spurling, G. K., Mansfield, P. R., Montgomery, B. D., et al.** (2010) Information from pharmaceutical companies and the quality, quantity, and cost of physicians' prescribing: a systematic review. *PLoS Med*, **7**(10), e1000352.
8. **Lexchin, J.** (1989) Doctors and detailers: therapeutic education or pharmaceutical promotion? *Int J Health Services*, **19**(4), 663–79.
9. **Lexchin, J.** (1993) Interactions between physicians and the pharmaceutical industry: what does the literature say? *CMAJ*, **149**(10), 1401–7.
10. **Fugh-Berman, A., Ahari, S.** (2007) Following the script: how drug reps make friends and influence doctors. *PLoS Med*, **4**(4), e150.
11. **Gagnon, M. A., Lexchin, J.** (2008) The cost of pushing pills: a new estimate of pharmaceutical promotion expenditures in the United States. *PLoS Med*, **5**(1), e1.
12. **Austad, K. E., Avorn, J., Franklin, J. M., Campbell, E. G., Kesselheim, A. S.** (2014) Association of marketing interactions with medical trainees' knowledge about evidence-based prescribing: results from a national survey. *JAMA Intern Med*, **174**(8), 1283–90.
13. **Wickremasinghe, S. A., Bibile, S.** (1971) Pharmaceuticals management in Ceylon. *BMJ*, **3**(5777), 757–8.
14. **Lall, S., Bibile, S.** (1978) The political economy of controlling transnationals: the pharmaceutical industry in Sri Lanka, 1972–1976. *Int J Health Services*, **8**(2), 299–328.
15. **Reich, M. R.** (1995) The politics of health sector reform in developing countries: three cases of pharmaceutical policy. *Health Policy*, **32**(1–3), 47–77.
16. **Steinbrook, R.** (2009) Physician-industry relations—will fewer gifts make a difference? *N Engl J Med*, **360**(6), 557–9.
17. **Brody, H.** (2005) The company we keep: why physicians should refuse to see pharmaceutical representatives. *Ann Fam Med*, **3**(1), 82–5.
18. **The Royal Australasian College of Physicians** (2006) Guidelines for Ethical Relationships Between Physicians and Industry. Available at: https://www.racp.edu.au/docs/default-source/advocacy-library/guidelines-for-ethical-relationships-between-physicians-and-industry.pdf

Chapter 6

Advocacy, campaigning, lobbying: Good or bad?

Mohammad Wasay

Introduction

'Advocacy—a human behaviour'

Structured advocacy is a relatively new concept in healthcare. Basic concepts of advocacy including identification and evaluation of better options, discussion, and opinion-making, convincing or lobbying, and making joint efforts for a cause have existed since the early days of humankind. We can consider advocacy an important part of human behaviour.

Advocacy is a special ability of humankind largely utilized in politics, sociology, law-making and legal affairs, and administration for centuries. Advocacy for healthcare started more recently. The term *healthcare advocacy* is relatively new, and advocacy in some forms was always available. Important advocacy landmarks may include patients' rights, physician's responsibilities, and the role of society and governments in healthcare.

Health is a basic human right as per the United Nations declaration,[1] but it took years of advocacy to make health part of this declaration. In reality, most people living in the world do not have access to this right. Large-scale, long-term, sustainable advocacy efforts are needed at global level for provision of this right for all human beings.

Advocacy as a tool

Structured advocacy is a tool that converts human behaviour into a strong, useful force to bring forth changes in society, system, and infrastructure for the sake of patients. However, advocacy skills and tools could be used in ways that are both good or bad. This important distinction needs to be kept in mind, as usually advocacy is considered in a positive sense. There may be exceptions and there is also the danger of misuse. This chapter will be devoted to explaining and discuss this issue. The objective is not to discourage advocates, but to make them aware of the strong tool they have.

A whole country or nation could be directed towards war and destruction by using advocacy tools. World Wars I and II and the invasion on Iraq are recent examples of these negative advocacy campaign outcomes. On the other hand, eradication of chickenpox and almost complete eradication of polio from the world map are prime examples of positive advocacy outcomes.

Advocacy as a tool has been applied for centuries for development and growth of societies and countries. Law-making is an outcome of extensive advocacy practices. The same is true for formation of all democracies, civil society organizations, and function of governments. However, this tool could be used effectively for both good and bad purposes.

'Good' and 'bad' are relative terms. When used in advocacy, good usually means something beneficial for society in general or a group in society. Good versus bad advocacy could be identified by analysing objectives and outcomes of advocacy. Prospective analysis of advocacy objectives is essential for estimated outcome. Review of outcome of an advocacy project or activity may lead to identification of good or bad outcome.

Purpose of neurology advocacy

The burden of neurological diseases is probably one of the highest in the world but awareness among public and healthcare authorities is probably one of the lowest. The purpose of neurology advocacy is to improve patient care related to neurological diseases. Improved patient care is an outcome which needs improvement in many domains across all regions of world. These domains may include awareness, financing, perceptions, training of healthcare personnel, regulations, and so on. Neurology advocacy is a structured effort in all these domains.[2,3]

Advocacy and conflicting interests

Society is a collection of various groups with conflicting interests and demands. It is possible that an advocacy activity may be good or useful for one group but bad or detrimental to another. It is important for an advocate or groups of advocates to carefully review if their advocacy interests and activities match or differ from the interests of other groups, or do not hurt the society at large. It is inevitable to avoid such conflicts while advocating for any purpose. When advocating for any cause, there will be a question of whether this advocacy effort is good or bad for society at large or a component of society. This is a major responsibility of advocacy: to convince all stakeholders with conflicting interests that this advocacy campaign will benefit society. Collaboration with various stakeholders is an integral part of advocacy campaign. This interaction and collaboration is called lobbying; more stakeholders means stronger lobbying. This is essential for success of any advocacy project.[4]

Conflicts of opinion, interests, and demands are common in any society. Advocacy principles in any society follow basic medical ethics principles including no harm, respect, and integrity to stakeholders, especially patients.

Objectives of advocacy: Short term and long term

The outcome of any advocacy project is highly dependent on its objectives. It is essential that objectives are well thought of, well-discussed and well-written, and transparent for all participants. All objectives should be divided into short-term and long-term goals, which are also defined as primary and secondary goals. Advocacy projects could be of short duration and equipped with quickly achievable objectives but their impact lasts much longer. Short-term objectives should outline outcomes at the end of the advocacy project, while long-term objectives should cover expected outcome after one or more years. Why this is important? Sometimes an advocacy project may be good in the short term but may be less beneficial in the long term. The same could be true for the scale of advocacy. An advocacy project could be beneficial at a small scale but at large scale, for example, at national or regional levels, may be complicated and not beneficial.

Advocacy message

The whole advocacy campaign actually relies on a message. It should be positive, explicit, and target oriented. The language must be understandable and target laypeople. A negative or complicated message is one of the most important factors for a failed advocacy campaign. The outcome of an advocacy campaign relies upon the message. As far as possible, help from media and communication experts, marketing, and advertising personnel should be sought before finalizing a message. Methods of message delivery are as important as the message itself.

Types of advocacy campaigns

We can broadly divide advocacy campaigns into two types: *issue-centred advocacy* and *advocate-centred advocacy*.

Issue-centred advocacy

Most of the time, advocacy is targeted towards an issue. The purpose of advocacy is to identify, highlight, and solve an issue. The popularity and uplifting of an advocate's profile is a secondary outcome.

Advocate-centred projects

Popularity and uplifting of an advocate's profile is a primary outcome. Providing a solution to issues or problems is secondary.

Most advocacy projects are issue centred, aiming to find a solution to a specific problem or issue. This requires extensive research in identifying a problem and multilevel efforts in highlighting and solving a problem. All efforts must be directed towards the resolution of the problem. These projects are usually short-term and easier to design. These projects are good for trainees and young advocates.

Advocate-centred advocacy

This is a common approach in conventional politics. This kind of advocacy is centred on the image of the advocate. This approach may be useful for long-term projects where the profile of the advocate is key to solving the problem. Even advocate-centred advocacy requires teamwork and the involvement of many stakeholders. This approach may be useful in image-building and the growth of an advocacy leader. It is not only important for media coverage but also for communicating and dealing with authorities. In these kinds of project, the primary objective is not the solution of the problem but to introduce the advocate to media, public, and authorities as an active stakeholder of society. Once an advocate is known and established as an active society member, then she/he could take on high-impact advocacy projects.

Advocacy leadership training is focused on grooming the advocates' thinking, presenting, and communication skills. Long-term use of these skills for improved healthcare and patient care will transform any person into a celebrated healthcare advocate.

Another chapter considers ownership in this context (see Chapter 1).

Methods: 'Good or bad'

Strategy or methodology is an important aspect of any advocacy project. It must be carefully crafted. Sometimes the wrong methodology could transform a good project into a bad project and outcome.

Example: A group of residents in a training programme started a project to reduce trainee burden and stress and to improve the research expertise of trainees. The objectives were good. However, critical analysis of the current training programme and the faculty involved in training transformed into a conflict between the faculty and trainees. This conflict escalated and ended up in a fight between the faculties and trainees. A project aimed at reducing trainees' burden and stress actually ended up increasing their stress. Any methodology which converts an advocacy project into severe conflict, adversarial relationship, or fighting may create a mishap or totally opposite outcome. Monitoring of methodology and success are one of the most important components of any advocacy campaign. The methodology of an advocacy project has many aspects, including: selection of target audience; data collection; formulation of message; use of media and other communication tools; and negotiations with authorities. Each of these aspects should be evaluated and designed carefully and thoughtfully. Selecting the wrong target audience or improper research data could transform a good project into a bad project. The message and its communication is an extremely important part of the methodology.

Intellectual and financial input

Most projects require intellectual and financial input from various stakeholders. It is important to involve multiple stakeholders, but it should be kept in mind that every stakeholder has an agenda of its own. Collaboration is mandatory for success of any advocacy project, but it should not be at cost of your credibility and the credibility of a project.

Advocacy and financial input are even trickier

One of my colleagues started an anti-tobacco alliance and was able to achieve success in highlighting the issue in the media. He was contacted by tobacco companies with an offer for financial support of this advocacy campaign. He assumed that these funds would be useful to boost the advocacy campaign. He was able to boost his campaign with industry sponsors but as soon as the news came out that he was sponsored by the tobacco industry he and his campaign lost credibility. This led to controversy among team members of this advocacy campaign. Due to these internal credibility issues, the whole campaign failed. Finances may be a key factor for any advocacy campaign. Advocates should be thoughtful and careful in generating and spending finances; issues should be discussed with the team and must remain transparent.

The same is true for intellectual input. All intellectual inputs and feedback from various stakeholders should be carefully reviewed. It is wise to thoroughly discuss and identify collaborators and financial sponsors for advocacy projects, weighing up the pros and cons of each supporter at an early stage. The role of stakeholders should be continuously monitored to ensure they remain an asset for the project and do not become a liability.

Outcome of advocacy

Outcome is highly dependent on objectives. Specific, measurable, assignable, realistic, and time-related (SMART) objectives have a high chance of being successful. There are many secondary objectives in addition to one or two primary objectives. Even if an advocacy project is unable to achieve primary objectives, there is always some success in achieving secondary objectives. There is no failure in an advocacy campaign. In my opinion, there is no bad outcome of an advocacy campaign if the objectives are directed towards the welfare of patients and society. Starting an advocacy campaign or process in itself is great but the positive outcomes of an advocacy project have a huge potential for society. Often it is hard to fully imagine the overall outcome of an advocacy campaign. It is like a small seed which grows slowly and could become a fully grown tree over many years.

Example: We started a tetanus and rabies eradication campaign about 10 years ago in Pakistan. Eradication may still take a decade or more but in recent years, awareness, availability, and utilization of vaccines and post-exposure prophylaxis have increased manyfold. Although our primary objective is not yet achieved, the active running of this advocacy process after 10 years is a huge success in itself.

Counter-advocacy

The impact of advocacy is multidirectional and may affect other stakeholders or persons/groups. One of my colleagues started an advocacy campaign for decreasing the costs of medicines and decreasing co-payment from 20% to 10%. Co-payment is the share of a medication's price paid by an insurer.

Insurance companies perceived this campaign as a threat to their interests. A counter-advocacy campaign was started by companies with involvement of media and other stakeholders. The counter-advocacy campaign message was 'lower co-payment will lead to lower quality medications'. This counter-campaign was strong and effective, and created an impression that advocates for lower co-payment are advocating for lower-quality medications.

As an advocate, one has to be prepared to handle and address these counter-advocacy campaigns. While planning an advocacy campaign it should be decided which stakeholders are going to be affected; and if there is a counter-advocacy campaign, how it will be handled. Most counter-advocacy campaigns represent the interests of a small group, but sometimes can be stronger than advocacy campaign itself.

It may be helpful to discuss issues and plans with other stakeholders, especially if they are going to be directly affected by your advocacy campaign. Your messages and campaign should not be directed towards another stakeholder. Controversy may be helpful for media coverage, but in the end, advocacy goals are hard to achieve amid lots of contention.

Long-term impact

Impact of any advocacy activity, even short-term, could be long-lasting. This should be considered while designing a campaign. Actually, it is the long-term results which will decide the good or bad outcome of an advocacy campaign. A five-year or longer follow-up plan may be helpful in determining the outcome. Whenever starting an advocacy campaign, the long-term (5 or 10 year) outcome should be a part of the discussion, even if your campaign's duration is only 3–6 months.

Conclusion

Advocacy, campaigning, and lobbying are important components of human behaviour and modern civil society. Healthcare advocacy is as important and crucial as any other advocacy. Advocacy is a rather new concept in field of neurology. Many neurologists still question if advocacy is good or bad.

This chapter has tried to answer this question. In addition to basic and clinical sciences, neurology—like any other healthcare specialty—has a strong social scientific component which includes awareness, economics, media, and advocacy. Professional organizations are now putting more and more emphasis on this component. It is now realized that a doctor's job is not just to write prescriptions, but that they are one of the most important stakeholders in society—especially in healthcare. Advocacy is mandatory for the growth and survival of any specialty but it could become a double-edged sword. It has the potential to be detrimental if the objectives, methodology, and outcomes are not evaluated and planned properly.

References

1. **United Nations.** *Universal Declaration of Human Rights.* Available at: http://www.un.org/en/universal-declaration-human-rights/
2. **Wasay, M., Hauth, E.** (2008) Advocacy training in neurology: scope and impact. *Nat Clin Pract Neurol*, **4**(2), 114–5.
3. **Pauranik, A**. (2008) Advocacy in neurology. *Ann Indian Acad Neurol*, **11**(1), 60–5.
4. **Berg, K. T.** (2009) Finding connections between lobbying, public relations and advocacy. *Public Relations Journal*, **3**(3), 1–19.

Section 2

Why is advocacy needed?

Chapter 7

Knowledge and science are not enough

Wolfgang Grisold

Introduction

Medicine is a hybrid among science, skills, narrative, human components, management and, increasingly, resources and economic issues.[1]

The body of knowledge and skills are constantly changing due to ongoing developments in the field. Continuous medical education and continuous professional development are the basis of continuous neurological and professional work.[2]

Growing awareness of doctors' responsibilities and duties has led to implementation of some changes in continuous education and assessment, particularly following serious incidents as the 'Shipman' case, which had a major impact on patient trust in the medical profession.[3,4]

The strength of neurology lies in patient consultation, clinical examination, and the increasing ability to offer effective therapies for neurological diseases. This is, of course, a timely development through which all other fields of medicine must pass, and the change from healer, to physician 'with the lancet', to the present self-image of the neurologist is a contemporary development.

The core competencies of physicians and medical staff are not, however, confined to knowledge, skills, and science, but must include the ability to advocate for patients and carers, as well as promote projects and developments.

This chapter will discuss several important aspects of advocacy in neurology, including its knowledge and science.

Background

The historical context of neurology

Neurology has its origins in the nineteenth century, with Charcot as the 'Übervater' ('supreme father'). In many countries, neurology developed from internal medicine and psychiatry, leaving profound marks on the practice of neurology in many settings.

Neurology soon became known for its precision and 'pinpoint' clinical methods, and deductions were sometimes compared with nineteenth-century 'Sherlockism'.[5]

Neurology has since developed over the decades with medical progress. It has been strongly influenced by contemporary scientific mainstreams such as neuropathology, electrophysiology, neurochemistry, neuroimmunology, neuroimaging, genetics and, more recently, molecular medicine.

Scientific advances have clarified many aspects of the function of the brain and nervous system. This new transparency has helped to demystify neurology,[6] which is an important move forward in terms of patient relations.

Historically, neurologists are trained to base their case on precise history-taking, followed by thorough neurological examination, which can be explicit and useful. Compared to scientific advances, which occur at a logarithmic scale and speed, this basic neurological tool (which highly advanced specialists often contemptuously consider too simple) has remained a basic instrument in clinical practice, partly due to the intensive contact it allows with the patient.

Similarly, there has been a shift in medicine from the profession of healer to that of professional specialist. Medicine, often historically considered 'an art', is becoming more technical. Another important change in practice is the shift from paternalistic medicine towards autonomy, accountability, partnership, and shared responsibility.[7]

Patient autonomy, based on individual values and background needs, respect for patients' decisions, and acceptance of the opinion of competent patients, are the current developments. They are closely linked with consumerism which, among other things, demystifies the 'art of medical care' and treatment, making it a professional exchange of services, mirrored by reimbursement. The trend towards shared decision-making[8] demands greater help with information and public education of patients. A very interesting aspect is patient 'literacy' on health and disease issues, and may be a prerequisite of shared decision-making.[9,10]

Several aspects of the need for individual decision-making and involvement in treatment plans are discussed in the chapters by Zwinkels and Bulbeck (Chapters 9 and 10).

Developments in neurology and the role of science

Recent developments are reducing the role of physician to an expert on demand, with a distinct, increasingly specialized role in a well-defined workflow. This precision 'on demand' view has many advantages, as the person in charge will be well-trained and will ensure high-quality performance and accuracy. Medical institutions' practice and procedures adapt to these developments, which in turn have an effect on treatment practice and patient care.

Patients are exposed to this newly developing situation and their relationship with physicians has also undergone extensive processes of change. Participation in decisions, consent, procedures, and active involvement in therapies have been implemented.[11]

There are some commonalities with consumerism and said new demands will bring about a more subspecialized, often highly specified concept, which can be compared with the term 'Toyotaization', in analogy with the highly logistic and specialized manufacturing techniques used by Toyota Motors.[12] This concept can be advantageous for several processes and has already been very successful in some fields, such as surgery, orthopaedics, and trauma—and, most notably, in the technical and theoretical fields of medicine. It could, however, potentially miss the point of the patient–physician relationship, especially in neurology, where a holistic approach is often needed.

Medicine is always influenced by opinions, beliefs, philosophy, ethical aspects, and so on, and by the current mainstream, which is determined by science and evidence. Yet in these current, increasingly regulated situations, a fair number of patients prefer to use and apply methods that lack sound empirical or scientific evidence.[13] Moreover, other concepts based on psychology, psychosomatics, and the like develop in irrational ways as compared to the structured, scientific, evidence-based pathway of conventional medicine.[14]

Science is the backbone of medicine and neurology and is a highly competitive field, nationally and internationally. Publishing in science and research domains is important as a tool and measurable effect of scientific work. Journals and scientific media are complex structures that screen work to be published, often using a peer-review system. On the subject of topics for publication, editors report that rare, 'interesting', and complicated topics appear to receive more attention, space, and publication pages than do more common themes, which might instead have a greater impact on patient well-being. This seems to be in direct contrast to the purpose of publishing and represents a current publication bias.

Funding for science is important and the source of resources can vary, ranging from governmental institutions to international and national entities, from donors to industry. All sources need to be defined as clearly as possible, and judgement of values or interests for support can lead to highly variable results. The chapter by Olesen and Destrebecq (Chapter 15) describes the procedure for developing a science support concept, and the chapter on orphan diseases (Chapter 27) also alludes to this important connection.

Knowledge and science are not enough

The main target of this book is to describe the purpose of advocacy, how it can be undertaken, and what can be achieved. Nevertheless, we have chosen to include a historic chapter (Chapter 3) describing the activities of two outstanding people whose different achievements can be considered examples of advocacy, even though the term did not exist at the time.

Advocacy is the implicit duty of any physician, in particular of neurologists, and is usually offered by the physician as a token part of treatment and care.

Besides expertise and knowledge, additional 'soft' skills are important, including doctoring, bedside manner, a multitude of personal traits, individual factors, and the human factors associated with patients and carers. The definition of soft or critical skills is difficult and while it is justified to refer to them as 'problem-solving' abilities,[15] this approach does not embrace the whole spectrum.

The process of patient–physician interaction also includes elements that are historically acknowledged and widely known as 'PLACEBO and NOCEBO'.[16,17] These elements go beyond the technical aspects of medicine and are contained in many procedures.[16,18]

Additional features are needed in neurological practice, as practical work with patients, carers, and the multiprofessional and multidisciplinary team within the local environment. In regard to advocacy at the meso and macro levels, expertise and engagement need to go further, require political skills, and can involve national or international bodies.

Advocacy

Advocacy is an important, implicit element of traditional physician relations and the commonly used phrase—'the patient is under my care'[19]—indicates that the physician is not only committed to medical treatment. It implies that importance is also attributed to caring, responsibility, and readiness to advocate for the patient beyond the necessary medical treatment. This all-inclusive concept may nonetheless be considered critical from the point of view of paternalism versus patient autonomy (Chapters 1 and 10).

Many books have been written on what makes a good doctor. The advocacy position of neurologists also depends on their professional role: they may be head of a department, or a neurologist in a large community taking care of many patients, or work in science or healthcare. In addition to their scientific knowledge, all neurologists need to be advocates for their patients, either directly or by fostering and nurturing health issues, resources, or science for their patients.

Attention to and awareness of advocacy is also guided by timely 'mainstream' topics of medicine. Advocacy for some diseases and conditions can also be influenced and driven by industrial interests, thus prompting the need for caution. Industry is not the only concern, as governmental and non-governmental bodies may also influence advocacy work. Historic examples of misguided governmental influence on issues of race, genetics, and disease are numerous and can be disastrous (Chapter 6).

As many topics requiring advocacy are not in the mainstream or are of general interest, advocates must also be prepared to take up less popular topics on behalf of patients, expose themselves to situations that are often unpopular, and meet with resistance and obstacles.

The neurologist as an advocate

Compassion, competence, and autonomy are not exclusive to medicine and include members of other professions, such as psychologists, lawyers and, notably, members of the clergy. Physicians are expected to exemplify these traits to a higher degree than other professions, in accordance with their professional ethos. The word 'clergy' has ancient roots and is usually associated with religious aims and institutions. Wisdom, trustworthiness, and credibility are important characteristics. In both a closer and a more distant sense, these attributes often match the profile of physicians and neurologists. Physician relations with members of the clergy can also be problematic, as highlighted by Kübler-Ross in her milestone publication on death and dying.[20]

Attributes of advocates

Many aspects of the role of advocacy and the importance of advocacy for neurology have been mentioned. Advocates should be knowledgeable in collaboration, have good communication abilities, foster scholarly practice, possess management skills and professionalism, and have compassion, passion, empathy, and resilience. Some of the attributes are summarized in the CanMED[21]; some have been drawn from the contributions of others and from the literature. The list that follows here, given in alphabetical order, is not complete.

Ability to orchestrate

To be able to coordinate and organize various aspects of an advocacy project.[22] This is the ability to organize, understand timely aspects, and identify the best opportunities. Soft management skills, including empathy and elasticity, are needed to orchestrate advocacy.

Acting on behalf of patients

This is one of the main issues in advocacy and can be considered the key theme and purpose of advocacy activities. A good example can be found in Chapter 9.

Authenticity

Both advocate and client need to be authentic and transparent. Conflict of interest and personal interests must be declared and roles in the advocacy process need to be transparent and well defined.

Autonomy

The term autonomy in advocacy can be used in relation to the independence of the advocate in regard to other interests or conflict of interests, or towards patient autonomy.

Patient autonomy is increasingly important and needs to be respected. Autonomy and self-responsibility are essential components of the changing relationship with physicians. Chapter 9 describes the need to respect and safeguard patients' autonomy through their disease trajectory.

Collaboration

Collaboration is an essential feature of advocacy and relies on collaborating with multiple persons in various ways.

Communication

Communication is very important and closely linked to collaboration skills.[23]

Creativity

Any advocacy project requires inspiration, implicit knowledge, and experience, but most of all it needs creativity. Creativity is a term frequently used in the context of art but it can also be successfully applied to health issues (see also Chapters 12 and 21).[24]

Empathy, passion, sympathy

The topics of empathy, passion, and sympathy overlap with each other. Advocacy must encompass all three abilities.

Humility

Humility is an important aspect. Misuse of advocacy leadership for own advantage or self-profiling purposes must be avoided.

Management and professionalism

Management skills and professionalism are also important in advocacy, particularly in project development and maintenance.

Navigating through the healthcare system

Physicians and neurologists have the challenging task not only of diagnosing and treating patients, but also of guiding them through the increasingly complex health system. This gains importance as the complexity of specializations rises. In complicated diseases, a plethora of specialities and different health professions care for patients, and it is the responsibility of the advocate to help focus on achieving the best results.

Neuro-oncology is a good example of a multiprofessional field, as described in Chapter 9.

Passion

Passion is often considered to be an essential part of advocacy. While useful, passion, enthusiasm, and emotion can also be ambiguous and have their own inherent problems.[25]

Perseverance

Perseverance is important in following and maintaining advocacy projects.

Resilience

The word resilience captures several aspects of advocacy; literally it means resistance to deformity and elasticity, which helps to deal with obstacles, lack of success, and frustration. The word is also used in different contexts, such as ecology, and harbours different meanings and interpretations.[26]

Scholarly practice

Scholarly practice is an important skill for successful advocacy.

Whistle-blowing

Whistle-blowing can be helpful in emphasizing patients' rights and needs.[27] Whistle-blowing needs to handled carefully and according to situational needs. It does not play a primary role in advocacy but is considered to be an emergency tool.

Factors and methods

Advocacy projects need to be carefully implemented and handled, often requiring methods that transcend the content of the project. Implementing and positioning advocacy projects is one of the core competencies of advocates.

Methods

Advocacy needs instruments and methods, which can be taught and learnt (Chapter 17). Chapters 17–19 provide a systematic introduction to practical issues. Advocacy can follow a structured concept of development as demonstrated in the chapter on the creation of the European Brain Council (Chapter 15), or can develop over several years in a pre-existing structure (Chapter 16). The chapter on advocacy for epilepsy covers a long-term perspective of advocacy and describes an advocacy pathway across a continuum from low-income situations up to the World Health Organization level (Chapter 14).

The methods used for advocacy projects depend on size, level (micro, meso, and macro) and content. Projects need to be planned, defined, and delivered, and generally require engineering and practical implementation skills. Leadership skills are also needed, in addition to the ability to synchronize and communicate with the team involved. Chapters 17–19 are intended to refer and help to develop these issues.

Stakeholders, as governmental organizations, insurance companies, and professional interest groups, differ in size. Accordingly, advocacy projects and communication tools must be tailored to match the structure being targeted and engage with the respective stakeholders.

It is essential to increase public education to foster the health literacy required for shared decision-making. Building awareness of diseases and their possible dangers, or disseminating the experience of other persons suffering from a given neurological disease can be important. Campaigning for people or patient groups in need can be an important task.

Advocacy for patients or patient-related issues can create conflicts. Changes often meet resistance (see Chapter 1, Case study 1.2). Practically speaking, advocating for patients can create conflicts.

Evaluation of advocacy

It is important to evaluate advocacy projects, the work of advocates, and the results achieved.[28] A range of evaluation models are available, from self-assessment to auditing, depending on the size of the project.[29]

The long-term success of a project is determined by its strategic capacity, as well as the influence it exerts on the desired target as, for example, organizations, institutions, and even legislation.[29]

Immersion as a method for advocacy

Although there is dispute about the concept of historic immersion, immersion is a helpful technique for advocates.[30] Immersion in history means fully entering an appropriate period in history, considering timely contemporary issues, as beliefs, religion, science, ethics, morals, and putting a situation into its historical context.

In analogy in advocacy, it is worthwhile to use this technique to become fully immersed in the situation of the persons involved in the advocacy project, particularly in the role and position of critical or opposing parties and persons.

The experiment can be simply performed, at least psychologically, by changing from the position of neurologist to that of patient or carer (i.e. by 'swapping sides'). This technique can be very effective because understanding or trying to understand specific aspects, points of contention, and adverse situations helps to prevent unnecessary polarization. Blind spots and moral judgement should be avoided.[31]

Disputes and controversies are common and natural in advocacy projects. Bridges of communication need to be maintained despite diverging opinions.

Relations and communication

Communication is an essential skill of advocates and needs to be used abundantly to liaise with everyone concerned. No advocacy activity or campaign can succeed without proper communication, which can range from personal contact to written communications.

Advocates need to be able to connect, communicate, and deliver their message. Ideally an advocacy campaign is prepared in detail, with presentations. Where feasible, graphics, a layout, and professional tools should be used.

'Storytelling' is an excellent way to deliver messages,[32] although this technique has also been criticized.[33] Intriguingly, the 'stories behind', or 'stories about people' can help the advocate to connect with the addressee. In medicine, other people's experience of a disease and the involvement of relatives or friends can help patients to connect with topics. Making the subject more tangible adds life to an otherwise abstract topic. Moreover, stories create mental images which are sometimes more powerful than spoken words.

In other circumstances the opportunity to communicate comes suddenly and unexpectedly. 'Elevator messages' belong to this type of communication. Elevator messages need to be brief and comprehensive and must be delivered in the short time available.

In communications with the press and media, short, comprehensive messages known as 'sound bites' are useful information and communication tools. To focus on the main issue, sound bites need to be precise and to the point, and considerable effort must be devoted to making the 'message' understandable and to hitting the target.

Case study 7.1 illustrates that even within organized medical systems and structures, communication patterns may deviate from the expected pathways.

Case study 7.1 Oncology ward

'At an oncology ward'—a vignette

One of the most memorable lectures I received during my training in haematology was on the communication patterns of and with severely sick patients. As residents, we saw patients during admission, physical examinations, bloodletting, chemotherapy administration, treatment of symptoms, and during numerous ward rounds. We listened to what we were told by patients, which usually centred around the disease, subjective feelings, pain, discomfort, but small talk rarely touched on other needs and desires. Individual patients were discussed and, as residents, we assumed we knew the patients and their medical history well. We knew what type of cancer they had, if they responded to therapy, and if there were any complications. We also knew how patients presented themselves at the patient rounds and how they reported on themselves.

However, there were at least two other communication levels to consider:

1. Nurses and therapists: Nurses and therapists often have a more intimate relationship with patients. The care they provide involves aspects of bodily function and close physical contact, in settings that are less 'glamorous' or structured than formal patient rounds. Communication occurs during times of pain, despair, drowsiness, and nausea, when many

safeguards are lowered and naturally protective mechanisms fail. Accordingly, nurses usually see, experience, and learn a lot more about patients than do physicians. Therapists are exposed to similar communications, being in close contact with the toll taken on patients by physical disability, bodily dysfunction, weakness, and impotence.

2   Cleaning staff

Hospitals have developed along the lines of military organizations and usually have a staff hierarchy. The lowest ranks on patient wards are usually the cleaning staff, who also come into very close contact with patients while doing the rooms, changing the beds, or helping to clean patients' personal belongings. This puts them in a position to communicate with patients and they often know more than the medical staff about them and their specific problems. Patients tend to convey feelings of despair, pain, depression and other symptoms to cleaning staff, rather than talk to the doctor individually or during the daily rounds. There are many reasons for this, such as time constraints, lack of more highly qualified personnel, and worries about voicing complaints or medical problems for fear of exposure to new investigations or new drugs.

The importance of these observations has recently been systematically studied and published.[34]

The lesson to be learnt is that the lower the medical staff qualifications, the stronger the bond created with patients. What this reveals in practical terms is that despite the structured approach to patients in institutions and the many advances in competence, care, and documentation, individual needs for advocacy can be channelled in many different ways.

Can we attach a 'flavour carrier' to our message?

Likewise, 'flavour carriers' are recommended for message transmission. In analogy to culinary techniques, 'flavour carriers' may per se be almost tasteless, but can flavour the recipient.[35] Oil and fat, for example, are often used as food flavour carriers and help to deliver or enhance the development of a flavour. In the advocacy setting, current or timely topics can be included to advocacy-related communications to make them more comprehensible and attractive. Flavour carriers include tools adopted by professional public relations (PR) experts and agencies, which help to wrap and carry the message in a more appealing way. This also involves the electronic media, which can contribute to dissemination and awareness of advocacy issues (see Chapter 19).

Involvement of patients in study design

Studies in neurology have several inherent problems. For example, not all age groups are usually examined, studies tend to be shorter than the duration of the disease, and long-term drug use is often not explored. Results from studies in common diseases are often extrapolated towards rarer diseases. Neuropathic pain is a case in point, where most studies have been carried out in diabetic neuropathy, post-herpetic pain, and trigeminal neuralgia.

One common problem in medicine is that it is easier to publish positive rather than negative results ('Publication bias'[36-38]), despite the fact that negative studies can contain a lot of information.

More patient involvement is needed in study design and practicalities. This is voiced, for example, by the Patient-Centered Outcomes Research Institute (PCORI) group,[39] which seeks to implement patient opinion and patient empowerment in study design.

Several patient perspectives need to be considered and the following list is not exhaustive:

- Patients often expect the development of new drugs to cure their disease, which is understandable.
- Patients want to have a wide safety margin if they participate in studies.
- The time from the development of a new drug to its introduction into clinical practice should be as fast as possible.
- Patients want to be involved in study development and to define the content of studies, with more consideration being taken of their needs.

Patients legitimately wish to find a cure for their disease and increasingly seek to participate in the development and design of advocacy studies.

Open charts and patent access

Patients have usually been given little access to medical records and charts. This is now changing, and patients consider it their right to be able to consult their medical records.

The development of new practices, such as open charts, empowers patients to read and participate in their medical records, which is part of the wider scope of patient advocacy.[40]

Training of advocates

Training is an important part of a neurologist's professional career. Despite the common training basis, considerable differences exist worldwide in terms of textbooks, reference materials, literature, guidelines, and so on. This embraces many aspects such as content, duration, profile, skills, techniques, and the definition of the end of the training period.

Advocacy needs to become part of the training curricula and residents should be introduced to advocacy early on. The American Academy of Neurology (AAN) Palatucci programme clearly covers these aspects.[41] Although these advocacy courses are only available for a comparatively small number of participants, they are well suited to spreading the idea of advocacy and are an excellent multiplicator.

During their instruction, trainees are exposed to many aspects of general medicine and the neurosciences, and may also receive specific training in communication and interdisciplinary and multidisciplinary teamwork. They are likewise invariably exposed to advocacy issues. It is essential to implement a structured approach to the shaping of future neurological training curricula.

Summary and recommendations

This chapter shows that neurology is developing into an increasingly specialized field. Neurology is based on knowledge and science, but neurologists must be aware that advocacy, be it implicit or part of an advocacy initiative, is a key component of their work.

Advocacy is dependent on temporary circumstances and on the advocacy needs that patients present. By definition, being an advocate is implicit in the work of physicians and of neurologists in particular. Besides the attempt to define the large spectrum of advocacy, a list of advocate attributes is provided.

Advocacy uses several methodological approaches, requires evaluation, and is dependent on communication and information. Patients increasingly take part in advocacy issues, as study design, or directly participate in decision-making and shared access to their own medical charts.

Training in neurology is not limited to knowledge and science, but extends to the awareness that advocacy for patients is a key duty of neurologists, and to the awareness that patients, carers, and laypersons increasingly share these responsibilities.

References

1. **Frank, J. R., Danoff, D.** (2007) The CanMEDS initiative: implementing an outcomes-based framework of physician competencies. *Med Teach*, **29**(7), 642–7.
2. **EACCME**. Areas of expertise. Available at: https://www.uems.eu/areas-of-expertise/cme-cpd/eaccme
3. **Smith, J.** (2002) *The Shipman Inquiry. First Report: Death Disguised*. Norwich: The Stationary Office.
4. **Guthrie, B., Love, T., Kaye, R., MacLeod, M., Chalmers, J.** (2002) Routine mortality monitoring for detecting mass murder in UK general practice: test of effectiveness using modelling. *Br J Gen Pract*, **58**(550), 311–7.
5. **Westmoreland, B. F., Key J. D.** (1991) Arthur Conan Doyle, Joseph Bell, and Sherlock Holmes: a neurologic connection. *Arch Neurol*, **48**(3), 325–9.
6. **Menken, M.** (2002) Demystifying neurology. *BMJ*, **324**(7352), 1469–70.
7. **Coulter, A.** (1997) Partnerships with patients: the pros and cons of shared clinical decision-making. *J Health Serv Res Policy*, **2**(2), 112–21.
8. **Barry, M. J., Edgman-Levitan, S.** (2012) Shared decision making—pinnacle of patient-centered care. *N Engl J Med*, **366**(9), 780–1.
9. **Katz, M. G., Jacobson, T. A., Veledar, E., Kripalani, S.** (2007) Patient literacy and question-asking behavior during the medical encounter: a mixed-methods analysis. *J Gen Intern Med*, **22**(6), 782–6.
10. **Cooley, M. E., Moriarty, H., Berger, M. S., Selm-Orr, D., Coyle, B., Short, T.** (1995) Patient literacy and the readability of written cancer educational materials. *Oncol Nurs Forum*, **22**(9), 1345–51.
11. **Ritzer, G.** (2004) *The McDonaldization of Society*. Thousand Oaks, CA: Sage Publications
12. **Liston, D. E., Richards, M. J., Karl, H. W.** (2017) Adapting the Toyota production model to teach systems-based practice to anesthesiology fellows. *J Clin Anesth*, **38**, 87–8.
13. **Ernst, E., Singh, S.** (2009) *Trick or Treatment? Alternative Medicine on Trial*. London: Corgi.

14. **Baskind, R., Birbeck, G.** (2005) Epilepsy care in Zambia: a study of traditional healers. *Epilepsia*, **46**(7), 1121–6.
15. **Dunn, M. C.** (1998) Knowledge helps health care professionals deal with ethical dilemmas. *AORN J*, **67**(3), 658–61.
16. **Carlino, E., Piedimonte, A., Benedetti, F.** (2017) Nature of the placebo and nocebo effect in relation to functional neurologic disorders. *Handb Clin Neurol*, **139**, 597–606.
17. **Bittar, C., Nascimento, O. J.** (2015) Placebo and nocebo effects in the neurological practice. *Arq Neuropsiquiatr*, **73**(1), 58–63.
18. **Carlino, E., Piedimonte, A., Benedetti, F.** (2016) Nature of the placebo and nocebo effect in relation to functional neurologic disorders. *Handb Clin Neurol*, **139**, 597–606.
19. **Peabody, F. W.** (2015) The care of the patient. *JAMA*, **313**(18), 1868.
20. **Kübler-Ross, E.** (2008) *On Death and Dying*. London: Routledge.
21. **Flynn, L., Velma, S.** (2008) Fundamental components of a curriculum for residents in health advocacy. *Med Teach*, **30**(7), e178–83.
22. **Loewy, E. H., Loewy, R. S.** (2002) *The Ethics of Terminal Care: Orchestrating the End of Life*. New York, Boston, Dordrecht, London, Moscow: Kluwer Academic Publishers.
23. **Hanks, R. G.** (2010) The medical-surgical nurse perspective of advocate role. *Nurs Forum*, **45**(2), 97–107.
24. **Madden, C., Bloom, T.** (2004) Creativity, health and arts advocacy. *International Journal of Cultural Policy*, **10**(2), 133–56.
25. **Sprinks, J.** (2011) Drive to find volunteers with a passion for high quality care. *Nurs Manag (Harrow)*, **18**(6), 6–7.
26. **Olsson, L., Jerneck, A., Thoren, H., Persson, J., O'Byrne, D.** (2015) Why resilience is unappealing to social science: theoretical and empirical investigations of the scientific use of resilience. *Sci Adv*, **1**(4), e1400217.
27. **Vaartio, H. L., Leino-Kilpi, H., Salanterä, S., Suominen, T.** (2006) Nursing advocacy: how is it defined by patients and nurses, what does it involve and how is it experienced? *Scand J Caring Sci*, **20**(3), 282–92.
28. **Teles, S., Schmitt, M.** (2011) The Elusive Craft of Evaluating Advocacy. *Stanford Social Innovation Review Summer 2011*. Stanford University.
29. **Kost, R. G., Reider, C., Stephens, J., Schuff, K. G.** (2012) Research subject advocacy: program implementation and evaluation at clinical and translational science award centers. *Acad Med*, **87**(9), 1228–36.
30. **Lipton, P.** (2005) Science and religion: the immersion solution. In: Moore, A., Scott, M. (eds). *Realism and Religion: Philosophical and Theological Perspectives*. Aldershot: Ashgate, pp. 31–46.
31. **Hill, T. E.** (2010) How clinicians make (or avoid) moral judgments of patients: implications of the evidence for relationships and research. *Philos Ethics Humanit Med*, **9**(5), 11.
32. **Sandercock, J., Parmar, M. K., Torri, V., Qian, W.** (2002) First-line treatment for advanced ovarian cancer: paclitaxel, platinum and the evidence. *Br J Cancer*, **87**(8), 815–24.
33. **Koch, T.** (1998) Story telling: is it really research? *J Adv Nurs*, **28**(6), 1182–90.
34. **Jors, K., Tietgen, S., Xander, C., Momm, F., Becker, G.** (2016) Tidying rooms and tending hearts: an explorative, mixed-methods study of hospital cleaning staff's experiences with seriously ill and dying patients. *Palliat Med*, **31**(1) 63–71.
35. **Wolke, R. L.** (2008) *What Einstein Told His Cook: Kitchen Science Explained*. New York: W. W. Norton & Company.

36. **Easterbrook, P. J., Berlin, J. A., Gopalan, R., Matthews, D. R.** (1991) Publication bias in clinical research. *Lancet*, **337**(8746), 867–72.
37. **Malicki, M., Marusic, A., Consortium, O.** (2014) Is there a solution to publication bias? Researchers call for changes in dissemination of clinical research results. *J Clin Epidemiol*, **67**(10), 1103–10.
38. **Begg, C. B., Berlin, J. A.** (1989) Publication bias and dissemination of clinical research. *J Natl Cancer Inst*, **81**(2), 107–15.
39. **PCORI. Patient-Centered Outcomes Research Institute**. Available at: https://www.pcori.org
40. **Yu, M. M., Weathers, A. L., Wu, A. D., Evans, D. A.** (2017) Sharing notes with patients. *Neurol Clin Pract*, **7**(2), 179–85.
41. **American Academy of Neurology.** Palatucci Advocacy Leadership. Available at: https://www.aan.com/conferences-community/leadership-programs/palatucci-advocacy-leadership/

Chapter 8

Perspectives on advocacy of medical doctors

Mohammad Wasay

Traditional and current role of doctors

Doctors are usually considered one of the most needed and respectable components of society. For centuries, their role has largely been limited to providing care to people suffering from diseases. Physicians see patients, evaluate their disease, and prescribe medications or perform procedures. The doctor's role changed to some extent with the evolution of the preventive healthcare model. In this model, doctors help normal children and other people to prevent them from becoming sick. Doctors started providing health screening, vaccines, vector control strategies, and so on; public health became a popular field of medicine. Healthcare used to be a private matter between doctor and patient without any involvement of governments or third parties. However, during the past 50–100 years this has changed, especially in the Western world. We have observed the increasing role of World Health Organization (WHO), governments, non-governmental organizations, and professional organizations in the modification and improvement of healthcare systems around the globe. In recent years, the media, patient support organizations, financial organizations (e.g. insurance companies), lawyers, and economists have also become important stakeholders in healthcare systems and management. Doctors continue to remain at the hub of healthcare provision but as far as the healthcare system is concerned, they were marginalized over the past three to four decades.

About a 100 years ago, healthcare involved a direct pay (fee for service) transaction from patient to doctor. This has changed to a third-party system in a large number of developed countries. It is estimated that more than 70% of doctors are not paid by patients directly but are paid by a third party (government, business organization, non-governmental organization, and so on) in developed countries.

In developing countries, the situation may be different. For example, in Pakistan, more than 70% of healthcare costs are out of pocket. Fees are paid directly by patients to doctors or hospitals in exchange for service. All countries in the world have a health budget, ranging from 1% to 20% of their overall budget being spent on health. Donor agencies including WHO, Gates Foundation, and others are spending billions of dollars through governments and institutions throughout world every year. There are so many stakeholders in managing the healthcare system that doctors or medical communities do not have a clear understanding and knowledge of their roles. Doctors are not taught in depth about healthcare systems at medical colleges. This transformation, which includes multilevel administration and financially driven steering methods, has led to a healthcare system with a very small role for doctors.

Multidisciplinary care model

Another major transformation in health delivery is the concept of specialized and multidisciplinary care. The concept of the primary care physician or general practitioner still exists in large parts of world. Multidisciplinary care means a patient will be seen by many specialists with diverse expertise. These may include nurses, physiotherapists, rehabilitation experts, nutritionists, financial counsellors, and social workers, and so on. There may be multiple doctors involved in the care of a patient. This model has modified the doctor's role to a great extent. In most cases, doctors still have a role in diagnostic and therapeutic planning and execution, but they are not the only one providing care. Care has shifted to a team approach in this model.

This multidisciplinary model has some advantages and disadvantages. The advantages include better quality of care by experts in different dimensions but at the same time it increases cost to great extent. Interaction between various care providers is mandatory. It takes more time and communication on the part of physicians. The number of doctors in the United States and Europe has delegated this responsibility to nurses, nurse practitioners, or physicians' assistants, especially in areas requiring multidimensional care.

Role of doctors in managed care

Managed care is a new and growing healthcare delivery model largely run by business organizations and insurance companies. Managed care is a term which refers to a system largely used in the United States, and is spreading worldwide. Internationally, particularly in Europe, other systems also exist such as publicly funded care, with a wide variation on national level.

Healthcare has become a successful business model in many parts of world, especially in the United States. These healthcare models are run by business and financial experts with doctors playing just a small role. Many governments with huge health budgets are outsourcing part of their delivery to these managed care organizations. These companies may make millions of dollars as revenue or profit.

Both doctors and patients have little say in this model and have to comply with rules and regulations made by these third-party business organizations.[1] The primary objective of these organizations is to maximize profits, with quality of care as second or even third priority. In this model, a large share of healthcare cost is not directly spent on patient care but towards management. This model could be improved by increasing the role of patients and doctors in decision-making processes related to diagnostic workup, therapeutic interventions, and the cost and availability of medication, and so on.

The regulation and monitoring of such healthcare systems by local and national healthcare authorities is of utmost importance.

The social healthcare system and doctors

This is a popular model in European countries, where 10–20% of overall budget is allocated for health, and the government is responsible for providing complete healthcare including prevention, home care, and social support, and even long-term care including rehabilitation. These systems are run by government organizations, like the National Health Service (NHS) in the United Kingdom. Social healthcare systems are largely funded by taxpayers' money and monitored by publicly elected officials. The doctor's role in this system is advisory. Sometimes doctors are part of management in this system and they have a stronger say as compared to managed care models.

Doctors as leaders of the healthcare system

Most of the world's health experts are still doctors. Leadership of healthcare systems is largely provided by business professionals, however. Leadership training, advocacy, financial management, and business solutions are unfamiliar topics at medical schools. Most doctors do not receive training related to understanding and managing businesses. Healthcare technology is another important area where the doctor's role is largely limited to users of these technologies.

These areas, especially economics, regulations, lobbying, and management, are becoming more and more important for doctors, especially if they want to have a leadership role in a future healthcare model. These could be labelled as the 'social science of medicine'. Adding social sciences to a medical school's curriculum will redefine the role of doctors in society.

Doctors as advocates

During the last two to three decades, advocacy has evolved as an important area among healthcare professionals, especially doctors. Doctors have realized that their job is not confined to writing prescriptions or performing procedures only, but they could play an effective role in modification, evolution, and development of the healthcare system. This realization has led to the development of healthcare advocacy as a specialized area for doctors. Many fields, especially paediatrics, have done a great job in training paediatricians to become great doctors and advocates.[2-5] As advocates, doctors become stakeholders of the whole healthcare system. They could be advocating for their patients, other doctors, and other healthcare providers. It is important for doctors to learn advocacy skills early in their course of training.

In this book, several chapters are dedicated to advocacy relating to neurological subspecialties, including stroke, cancer, dementia, and Parkinson's disease, and others.

The role of doctors in patient support groups

Patient support groups are a new dimension in healthcare advocacy. These groups are usually formed by patients and their family members, and could be highly effective and influential in advocacy. Doctors may play an extremely important role in establishing and guiding these groups in an advisory capacity. These groups can play a role in awareness, lobbying, and media management for any advocacy project.

Patients are obviously most important stakeholders in any healthcare system. These groups may define their role in future healthcare models. Patient support groups may be able to lobby and negotiate for better care with managed care authorities or even government authorities.

In future, doctors could team up with patients support groups for many quality care initiatives. Professional societies should have a close communication with patients support groups. The World Stroke Organization (WSO) has adopted a model to have patient support organizations as directors for WSO. Doctors could initiate, motivate, and guide patients to start these groups or become supporters for active groups.

WHO has prepared a database and guide for doctors to assist these support groups.[6]

Professional organizations and healthcare advocacy

Many professional organizations have started advocacy as one of their main activities throughout the year, in addition to scientific teachings and trainings. The American Academy of Neurology (AAN) is a notable example. AAN started advocacy training (Palatucci programme) more than a decade ago and has trained more than 300 neurologists as advocates. AAN started public policy and advocacy fellowship with its 'Neurology on the Hill' programme, when a number of neurologists visit congressmen and senators' offices for lobbying and advocacy on a prespecified day.[7,8]

The World Federation of Neurology (WFN) was effective in publishing its *World Brain Atlas* by WHO. WFN is working with WHO to define stroke as a brain disease. The International League against Epilepsy and International Bureau of Epilepsy have been successful in developing WHO resolutions for epilepsy. Many national societies are actively working with health authorities and governments for improved care for their patients. The World Federation of Neurology also has an effective advocacy programme including World Brain Day and advocacy training workshops at the World Congress of Neurology. Some of professional organizations, especially nurse's organizations, have transformed into strong advocacy groups.

In future, we are going to see stronger roles being played by neurology societies and other professional organizations, especially epilepsy societies and stroke societies, in areas of advocacy and health reform throughout the globe.

Doctors training and advocacy

Advocacy is a skill. These skills can be developed by teaching, training, practice, and mentoring. We have suggested that advocacy training should be a part of residency training programmes, especially neurology residency programmes. An 'Introduction to Healthcare Advocacy' should be taught as a subject in medical schools and universities.

Residency training programmes are more suitable to incorporate advocacy leadership training. All residents should go through a 12–15-hour workshop learning basic concepts and skills. This could also be done through an online course. After the workshop, each trainee should start and accomplish an advocacy project under the mentorship of a trained advocate. This could be added as module or project in a residency programme. The same could be done for young neurologists and junior faculty members.

The AAN Palatucci advocacy leaders' programme is a good model for high-impact short training workshops. Mentoring is extremely important for the long-term growth of these trainees.

Profile of a MD advocate

A doctor with advocacy training and skills can contribute to patient care, health systems, and society more effectively. These doctors are not only involved in direct patient care but are also active in system improvement, patients' rights, economics, and regulations related to healthcare and even local, national, and global health policymaking.

References

1. **Feldman, D. S.**, **Novack, D. H.**, **Gracely, E.** (1998) Effects of managed care on physician-patient relationships, quality of care, and the ethical practice of medicine: a physician survey. *Arch Intern Med*, **158**(15), 1626–32.
2. **Wright, C. J.**, **Moreno, M. A.**, **Katcher, M. L.**, **McIntosh, G. C.**, **Mundt, M. P.**, **Corden, T. E.** (2005) Development of an advocacy curriculum in a pediatric residency program. *Teach Learn Med*, **17**(2), 142–8.
3. **Chamberlain, L. J.**, **Sanders, L. M.**, **Takayama, J. I.** (2005) Child advocacy training: curriculum outcomes and resident satisfaction. *Arch Pediatr Adolesc Med*, **159**(9), 842–7
4. **Wright, C. J.**, **Katcher, M. L.**, **Blatt, S. D.**, **et al.** (2005) Toward the development of advocacy training curricula for pediatric residents: a national delphi study. *Ambul Pediatr*, **5**(3), 165–71.
5. **Shipley, L. J.**, **Stelzner, S. M.**, **Zenni, E. A.**, **et al.** (2005) Teaching community pediatrics to pediatric residents: strategic approaches and successful models for education in community health and child advocacy. *Pediatrics*, **115**(4 Suppl), 1150–7.
6. **Shucart, W. A.** (2003) In memoriam: Donald Moore Palatucci, MD (1940–2002) *Neurology*, **60**, 896–7.
7. **Wasay, M.**, **Hauth, E.** (2008) Advocacy training in neurology: scope and impact. *Nat Clin Pract Neurol*, **4**(2), 114–5.
8. **Pauranik, A.** (2008) Advocacy in neurology. *Ann Indian Acad Neurol*, **11**(1), 60–5.

Chapter 9

Advocacy and the perspective of (neurology) nursing

Hanneke Zwinkels

Introduction

Patient advocacy is recognized as an integral part of nursing; however, a clear understanding of advocacy is needed to address activities that are necessary to deploy nursing advocacy. Within nursing literature during the past decades, several authors have conceptualized the advocate role of the nurse, and identified advocacy activities such as counselling, educating, and empowering the patient while creating an atmosphere which is supportive of patients' decision-making.[1-3] Competences nurses should possess in carrying out their advocacy role include: being sensitive to the patients' needs created by illness[1]; helping the patient discern his own values, and that decisions made by the patient towards treatment should reflect those values[2]; and provide the patient with information adequate to help him make his own decisions.[3] Nevertheless, it still appeared to be difficult to create awareness of the nursing advocacy role, and subsequently, Malliks' research on the perceptions of the nursing advocacy role by nursing healthcare professionals identified the need for professionalization of the role, and the necessity for public recognition and legal support.[4-6] This implicates that patients, as well as the nurse and other healthcare professionals, have to acknowledge the advocacy role of the nurse in order to enable them to be able to fulfil that role. In the 1990s, professional nursing organizations have been adopting advocacy as a required activity, and educational programmes included advocacy as a subject of study, which are aimed at helping nurses exercise their advocacy role.[7,8] Patient advocacy is believed to be a process or strategy consisting of a series of specific actions for preserving, representing, and/or safeguarding patients' rights, best interests, and values in the healthcare system.[9] A process or strategy for acting on behalf of others such as vulnerable patients, with regards towards respect for self-determination, and for help to access healthcare. By their position in the healthcare system, nurses should be able to advocate for patients effectively, however, how to practice advocacy depends on the competences, skills, and autonomy of the neurology nurse. Meanwhile, not only the patient but also the caregiver is affected by illness and disease, and there is more attention given to caregivers' needs in literature and nursing practice. By analysing patients' and caregivers' needs, and systematically responding to those needs during the disease process, nurses will be able to educate patients on management of their disease, treatment plans, signs and symptoms, while safeguarding patients' autonomy,[10-12] and in this way, take their advocacy role.

Neuro-oncology nursing, an example of patient advocacy

Neurology nurses play a key role in supporting patients and their caregivers: they have a frequent and intensive contact; and being closer to the patient and their caregivers, the neurology nurse may become a confidential adviser and counsellor. Participating in a multidisciplinary team, neurology nurses hear about treatment (im)possibilities, and have a complete overall picture. The nurse is able to simplify doctors' treatment plans, answer questions, meet needs, and get family members involved in the plan of care.[13] Besides supporting patients, families, and communities to achieve better health outcomes, the neurology nurse as part of a multidisciplinary team is in a position to advocate for partnerships between patients and healthcare professionals, to share information, and promote healthcare of good quality. The neurology nurse will be able to speak for the patient to the members of the multidisciplinary team, and sometimes on behalf of the patient even towards the caregiver and other relatives. In this way, the neurology nurse is in a unique position to act as an advocate. In Case study 9.1, several aspects of advocacy are addressed.

Case study 9.1 Advocacy during an incurable disease process—from diagnosis until death

A 42-year-old female presented with episodes of flashes in her right visual field of both eyes, accompanied with speech disturbances, confusion, headache, and nausea. Brain imaging showed a lesion in the left temporal lobe, mainly in the hippocampus and splenium of the corpus callosum. She was prescribed levetiracetam, and underwent a biopsy that showed a glioblastoma multiforme (without methylation of the MGMT-promotor). The patient started with chemo radiation followed by six adjuvant cycles of temozolomide.

At the end of the chemo radiation, the patient—accompanied by her two sisters—consulted the neuro-oncology nurse, and they addressed complaints of fatigue and because of that, difficulties in managing the household. The nurse contacted the GP to organize home care, and help for guidance for the two youngest children (11 and 9 years old). Four weeks later, the patient and her husband (originally from Morocco, away from home frequently, and not able to participate in the care for neither the children nor the household) came to the neuro-oncology nurse for the initiation of adjuvant treatment. They communicated that they decided not to start home care, because they believed that this would have disturbed their privacy. The eldest daughter—who recently gave birth to a boy—came to live with her parents, to support her mother. Besides, the sisters of the patient also helped the patient with her household, because of the apraxia and fatigue.

Before the start of the fourth adjuvant cycle, the patient was admitted to hospital because of a secondary generalized seizure. Postictally, she suffered from confusion, inertia, and speech disturbances. MRI—also made to evaluate the first three cycles—showed an increase of the tumour growing to the right temporal lobe and a satellite lesion in the left semiovale centre. At that time, the patient suffered from fatigue, inertia, worsened appetite, and memory problems. The neuro-oncology nurse advised for psychosocial support in the home situation by an oncology nurse besides, the patient gave her consent for a referral to the psychology outpatient clinic.

The patient was proposed new tumour treatment, which she agreed on, which existed of procarbazine, lomustine, and vincristine (PCV) chemotherapy. After the first cycle of PCV, the patient visited the emergency room together with her husband after a seizure. She had a speech arrest, was confused, suffered from hemianopia, and lab results showed a pancytopenia due to the PCV. A CT brain scan showed an increase in the lesions as compared to the latest MRI but no acute problems (e.g. herniation, hydrocephalus, haemorrhage). We wanted to admit the patient, but her husband wanted to take her home. PCV was put on hold, the anti-epileptic drugs were increased, and the patient went home.

After a month, the neuro-oncology nurse was contacted by the patient's sister, who stated that the patient was worsening: more severe headaches, more memory problems, more fatigue, and the patient was bedridden. Home care was still deterred, and the specialized oncology nurse had made several attempts to speak with both the patient as well as her husband, but appointments were subsequently cancelled by him. The neuro-oncology nurse contacted the GP, who visited the patient and prescribed pain medication.

With the consent of the patient, her sister contacted the neuro-oncology nurse again, reporting a rapidly deteriorating patient, and all appointments in the hospital were cancelled. The GP then became responsible for her care and prescribed dexamethasone and pain medication; the family was aware of the fact that the end of life was approaching. The patient spent most of her time alone, not being taken care of, not able to go to the toilet or eat or drink by herself. Because the patient's sisters were having problems with the lack of care from the husband, they withdrew their help and support to pressure him to allow home care to come. They asked the neuro-oncology nurse to intervene and arrange for hospice care, but shortly thereafter they withdrew this request because they were afraid of the husband and his anger about their involvement.

The incapacity of the patient to judge and to comprehend this situation, as well as the fact that she was at home and at a certain point was denied care by her sisters and home care nurses, placed the neuro-oncology nurse in a difficult position. It was difficult to intervene working at the outpatient clinic and being the contact person for care in the hospital. Besides that, the husband—who was her legal representative—never asked the nurse for help. Because of her knowledge of the severe situation, the nurse discussed the case with the neurologist. He suggested contacting the GP to arrange admission to the hospital ward. During admission, we would try to guide the patient and her family to transfer to a hospice. A social worker as well as an imam would try to speak with the couple. The spouse approved of this, and asked for his wife to have an MRI to be able to start chemotherapy again. During admittance, the patient became more clear and adequate after tapering pain medication, the responsible physician noted neglect at home, and a husband who refused delivered care. MRI showed progressive disease and leptomeningeal dissemination.

Patient, spouse, sisters, and the involved healthcare professionals came to an agreement that the patent could return home on the condition that care is accepted, and that they will contact the neuro-oncology nurse when the situation is deteriorating again, in which the GP plays an important role during the end-of-life phase.

Reproduced from Eur Assoc Neurooncol Mag, 4(2), Zwinkels H, Ethical Decision-Making in Glioma Patients, Copyright (2014), with permission from European Association of Neuro-Oncology.

Strategies for advocacy in neurology nursing

Competences and skills

Through active listening and relationship building to address the needs of the patient, the nurse will be able to advocate for the patient with his consent.[14] The nurse will need skills of informing and advising so that promotion and protection of patients' rights to be involved in decision-making and informed consent, can be pursued. Knowledge of the specific clinical field the nurse is dedicated to, and knowledge of the law and possession of ethical skills will help ensure nursing advocacy. Besides, acting on behalf of patients requires communicating and collaborating skills.[9] When nurses understand the scope of their practice, and are aware of the value nurses bring to patients and healthcare delivery, they will be able to articulate subjects that are important and need to stay the way they are, or that need to be improved.

Safe guarding patients' autonomy

Patients have a primary responsibility for their own health, and neurology nurses have the responsibility to respect and promote patients' health. When health becomes impaired, a patient needs to be able to make his own decision based on information about the diagnosed disease, so that he is able to give consent to treatment decisions. The patient in Case study 9.1 was supported by her husband and her sisters, they were the patients' advocate in finding information and resources during her disease trajectory. Nurses need to know in which kind of situations patients need an advocate; what patients' best interests are in a particular situation; and what kind of actions need to be taken to preserve, represent, and safeguard their situation, to be able to guide patients and their caregivers during the disease trajectory. The neurology nurse in Case study 9.1 advocated for the patient through communication with the treating physician, caregivers, the general practitioner (GP) and a home care nurse, in order to realize the best care for the patient. The neurology nurse's safeguarding of patients' autonomy involves helping patients to reason and deliberate their decisions, and in meeting the needs of the patient, giving the opportunity to express personal values, wishes, and treatment preferences (advanced directives), and to try to protect these even in the event of losing capacity to communicate.[15] The patient in Case study 9.1 needed to be admitted to realize respect for her autonomy. After analysing symptoms and needs, and subsequent communication between patient, caregivers, and healthcare professionals, an agreement was finally reached.

Acting on behalf of patients

When patients are not able or do not wish to represent themselves, nursing advocacy means taking actions that preserve and represent patients' values, benefits, and rights towards treatment and decision-making. This includes 'interceding', which means coming between parties, and intervening or mediating when necessary. Interceding can be between patients and healthcare providers, but also between patients and their family or significant others.[10] The patient in Case study 9.1 was not able to decide and act for herself, to use resources such as home care; she did not have enough insight and judgement to look at her situation and needed an advocate to have her needs addressed. Her sisters became her advocate, which resulted in their advocating for the patient via the nurse, by informing and supporting the patient and the caregivers, which enabled them to make decisions regarding healthcare.[16] When becoming a patient, an individual experiences a loss of control over his life, and an experienced loss of identity and initiative in patients with neurological disease is not uncommon. In this situation when facing concerns about health and possible separation from family, patients may be in need for an advocate, someone to speak for them, and in some cases, mediate on their behalf. The nurse in the centre of a multidisciplinary team would be able to advocate effectively for these patients, as a voice for the patient towards other healthcare professionals and their caregivers. When the nurse believes a better treatment option—or no treatment at all—for the patient exists, or when the patient disagrees with the treatment plan, the nurse will be able to advocate on behalf of the patient.

Provision and access of healthcare

The patient in Case study 9.1 was guided by the neuro-oncology nurse in accessing care in the hospital as well as in the home care situation. The nurse was responsible as a case manager for admittance in the end-of-life phase, to assure that all professionals and caregivers involved reached consensus on the necessary care to be delivered. When a multidisciplinary team for a specific patient group has a care navigator or case manager (e.g. a dedicated nurse responsible for continuation and coordination of care), this professional needs to know the clinical pathway of this specific patient group. Besides, the care navigator also needs to know the key players involved in this clinical pathway, and the organizational structure, to be able to execute nursing advocacy. Nursing advocacy is being able to effect changes not only on behalf of individuals, but also on behalf of patient groups or communities, so that inequalities and inconsistencies are identified and corrected in order to improve issues concerning health, health promotion, and education, for people who need medical treatment and support.[17]

Nurse care navigator and advocacy

Because of the complexity of patients' conditions and the multiple professionals and services involved in care, a good understanding of care coordination is necessary. Multidisciplinary healthcare has been the basis for several years within the healthcare system for diverse patient groups, such as oncology patients and patients with a chronic disease, such as neurology patients and rehabilitation care. The patient and his caregiver might need an advocate to help them navigate through the healthcare system. Nursing care navigators or coordinators are in a position to advocate and translate the voice of the patient towards the physician and the multidisciplinary team, and thereby improve outcomes for patients. Care coordination, which has been implemented in many countries in northern Europe, in Australia, the United Kingdom, and in the United States, consists of several core components. The nurse care navigator or case manager is a key contact for the patient, as well as for the healthcare professionals within the multidisciplinary team; is responsible for the coordination and continuation of care; assesses the needs of the patient, acting as an information and educational resource; provides patient-centred care and communicates through a multidisciplinary team.[18] Adjustment by the case manager towards a diagnosis by early and frequent education of patients in a supportive way, will help patients and their relatives foster adaptive coping.[19] The neuro-oncology nurse in Case study 9.1 deals with clinic scheduling, symptom management, medication (e.g. steroids, anti-epileptic drugs, chemotherapy), psychological support, and referral to other agencies as part of the process of patient care. Nursing care coordinators are rated highly by healthcare professionals providing care for brain tumour patients, as part of an important strategy for improving care.[20]

To advocate for the neurology patient

The neurology patient—who often has to deal with residual or permanent disability, due to their underlying disease—is in the centre of a multidisciplinary care team which includes physicians, nurses, physiotherapists, occupational therapists, speech therapists, social workers, and other healthcare professionals. Frequently the progress of the patient is evaluated by the team to review goals of care. Nurses—who are often at the patients' bedside—are increasingly involved in the treatment decision-making process, as well as patients, when compared to previous decades. Neurology patients often have complex supportive care needs, and to be able to understand and assess the needs of a neurological patient the nurse needs competences such as empathy, communication, collaboration, and adequate knowledge of neurology disease. It is even more important to be able to detect the needs of the patient, who is suffering from cognitive disturbances besides having a physical disability.

Being the voice of the patient—and their relatives—towards the multidisciplinary team and the responsible physician(s), is specifically for this patient group of the utmost importance. This is clearly understood in many nursing research papers about the adjustment and supportive care needs of patients and their relatives; for instance, in patients with primary brain tumours.[19,21,22] The basis of daily practice in the care for the neurology patient is a combination of individual and social efforts and actions, to ensure access to resources and opportunities, or assist increased reach towards them, that improves good health.

Difficulties and conflicts

The advocating nurse has to be self-confident, has to feel responsibility, and have the willingness to advocate, but also has to be aware of the fact that advocating for patients can create conflicts with, and implicate vulnerability towards the other healthcare professionals involved with a patient's care. The nature of relationships with other members of the healthcare team plays a significant role in the extent to which nurses will be able to advocate on behalf of patients.[14] Advanced nurse practitioners and clinical nurse specialists are cooperating intensively with physicians and take responsibility based on high competency levels and shared concerns in patient care. Thus, effective advocacy not only depends on attributes and skills of the nurse, but also on perceived receptiveness of the environment. Health policy, organizations, institutional cultures, multidisciplinary teams, and colleagues need to be supportive of the developing role of the nurse, and have consensus on the meaning of the nursing advocacy role.[23-25] Besides, within the nurse–patient relationship, which should be interactive and interconnected, the nurse needs to be aware of the fact that she has to empower the patient to make his or her own decision, and not persuade the patient or make decisions for him.[8]

Recommendations

Nursing advocacy implicates neurology nurses at positions in which they are able to navigate a patient and their caregivers through the disease process, with consent of physicians, and other healthcare professionals involved in the care for the patient. Nurses will aim at providing patient-centred care, by educating and informing the patient; by providing access to appropriate services; by coordinating care; and supporting and continuing multidisciplinary care. They aim at establishing an empathic nurse–patient relationship based on trust in which they assess a patient's symptoms and needs, and resolve issues to avoid unnecessary complications. Nurses try to identify patient-level barriers to care, and reduce delay in the provision of care.

References

1. **Curtin, L.** (1979) The nurse as advocate: a philosophical foundation for nursing. *ANS Adv Nurs Sci*, **1**(3), 1–10.
2. **Gadow, S.** (1980) Existential advocacy: philosophical foundation of nursing. In: Spicker, S., Gadow, S. (eds) *Nursing: Images and Ideals.* New York: Springer Publications, pp. 79–101.
3. **Kohnke, M. F.** (1980) The nurse as advocate. *Am J Nurs*, **80**(11), 2038–40.
4. **Mallik, M.** (1998) Advocacy in nursing: perceptions and attitudes of the nursing elite in the United Kingdom. *J Adv Nurs*, **28**(5), 1001–11.
5. **Mallik, M., Rafferty, A. M.** (2000) Diffusion of the concept of patient advocacy. *J Nurs Scholarsh*, **32**(4), 399–404.
6. **Mallik, M.** (1997) Advocacy in nursing–perceptions of practising nurses. *J Clin Nurs*, **6**(4), 303–13.
7. **Hewitt, J.** (2002) A critical review of the arguments debating the role of the nurse advocate. *J Adv Nurs*, **37**(5), 439–45.
8. **Water, T., Ford, K., Spence, D., Rasmussen, S.** (2016) Patient advocacy by nurses—past, present and future. *Contemp Nurs*, **52**(6), 696–70.
9. **Bu, X., Jezewski, M. A.** (2007) Developing a mid-range theory of patient advocacy through concept analysis. *J Adv Nurs*, **57**(1), 101–10.
10. **Baldwin, M. A.** (2003) Patient advocacy: a concept analysis. *Nurs Stand*, **17**(21), 33–9.
11. **Vaartio, H., Leino-Kilpi, H., Salanterä, S., Suominen, T.** (2006) Nursing advocacy: how is it defined by patients and nurses, what does it involve and how is it experienced? *Scand J Caring Sci*, **20**(3), 282–92.
12. **Vaartio-Rajalin, H., Leino-Kilpi, H.** (2011) Nurses as patient advocates in oncology care: activities based on literature. *Clin J Oncol Nurs*, **15**(5), 526–32.
13. **Tariman, J. D., Mehmeti, E., Spawn, N.**, et al. (2016) Oncology nursing and shared decision making for cancer treatment. *Clin J Oncol Nurs*, **20**(5), 560–3.

14. **MacDonald, H.** (2007) Relational ethics and advocacy in nursing: literature review. *J Adv Nurs*, **57**(2), 119–26.
15. **Shannon, S. E.** (2016) The nurse as the patient's advocate: a contrarian view. *Hastings Cent Rep*, **46** Suppl 1, S43–7.
16. **Chafey, K., Rhea, M., Shannon, A. M., Spencer, S.** (1998) Characterizations of advocacy by practising nurses. *J Prof Nurs*, **14**(1), 43–52.
17. **Fowler, M. D.** (1989) Social advocacy. *Heart and Lung*, **18**(1), 97–9.
18. **Bailey, A., Trad, W., Kastelan, M., Lamont, S.** (2015) Australian experience of neuro-oncology care coordination: a conversation. *Clin J Oncol Nurs*, **19**(5), 610–4.
19. **Cavers, D., Hacking, B., Erridge, S. C., Morris, P. G., Kendall, M., Murray, S. A.** (2013) Adjustment and support needs of glioma patients and their relatives: serial interviews. *Psychooncology*, **22**(6), 1299–305.
20. **Langbecker, D., Janda, M., Yates, P.** (2013) Health professionals' perspectives on information provision for patients with brain tumours and their families. *Eur J Cancer Care (Engl)*, **22**(2), 179–87.
21. **Janda, M., Steginga, S., Dunn, J., Langbecker, D., Walker, D., Eakin, E.** (2008) Unmet supportive care needs and interest in services among patients with a brain tumour and their carers. *Patient Educ Couns*, **71**(2), 251–8.
22. **Trad, W., Koh, E. S., Daher, M., et al.** (2015) Screening for psychological distress in adult primary brain tumor patients and caregivers: considerations for cancer care coordination. *Front Oncol*, **5**, 203.
23. **Seal, M.** (2007) Patient advocacy and advance care planning in the acute hospital setting. *Aust J Adv Nurs*, **24**(4), 29–36.
24. **Kalaitzidis, E., Jewell, P.** (2015) The concept of advocacy in nursing: a critical analysis. *Health Care Manag (Frederick)*, **34**(4), 308–15.
25. **ter Maten-Speksnijder, A., Grypdonck, M., Pool, A., Meurs, P., van Staa, A. L.** (2014) A literature review of the Dutch debate on the nurse practitioner role: efficiency vs. professional development. *Int Nurs Rev*, **61**(1), 44–54.

Chapter 10

Patient and caregiver advocacy

Helen Bulbeck

'The fight is so much harder than the diagnosis.'
Caregiver, United Kingdom

This chapter explores the role of advocacy, in both the patient and caregiver community, as it lives with brain cancer. When faced with a life-changing diagnosis, patients and caregivers will face many constraints which prevent them from accessing healthcare or from achieving the optimum quality of life. These constraints may be institutional, social, political, economic, and/or cultural; when one or more come into play, an advocate is needed to facilitate change, so that resilience, self-care, and empowerment become the norm. The goal of advocacy is to promote the development of capability so that the impact and effects of illness can be minimized, patients and caregivers can respond appropriately and become co-pilots in their care. Advocacy, in Chapter 1, has been defined as being political, educational, research-based, fundraising, support, and community outreach. All of these come into play when living with a brain tumour. Through an analysis of why advocacy is needed, what it looks like, and how it happens, this chapter will explore the impact advocacy can have for the brain tumour community, specifically for patients, caregivers, and for nurses and the challenges that advocacy brings.

Why is advocacy needed?

Brain cancer is an unrecognized clinical problem and is one of the most lethal human diseases; only 27% of people diagnosed with a glioblastoma will be alive at the end of the second year following diagnosis.[1] At five years this drops to 9.8%. Brain cancer is also the most prevalent form of solid tumour in children and the most common cause of cancer death in them.[2] It is different to other cancers; not only do patients and their caregivers have to come to terms with the diagnosis of brain cancer, but they do so in the knowledge that this diagnosis will certainly mean progressive neurological and cognitive deficit. Mukand[3] identified the following neurological complications in brain tumour inpatients:

- Cognitive deficits 80%
- Weakness 78%

- Visual-perceptual deficit 53%
- Sensory loss 38%
- Bowel/bladder 37%
- Cranial nerve palsy 29%
- Dysarthria 27%
- Dysphagia 26%
- Aphasia 24%
- Ataxia 20%
- Diplopia 10%

Some 75% of inpatients will have three or more of these neurological complications; 39% will have five or more.

In contrast to other cancers, patients and caregivers have a raw deal. Survival rates are appallingly low, and hundreds of lives year on year are lost and irrevocably changed by this devastating disease. Lehman et al.[4] acknowledge that in 80% of central nervous system tumours there is a need for rehabilitation. Any diagnosis of cancer is devastating, creating social, emotional, financial, and psychological problems. Patients are concerned about vitality, their identity and role, limitations, mental health, emotional well-being—all of these are important decision factors for patients. Caregivers feel unskilled, uninformed, and isolated. Even if individuals spend as much as 6 hours a year in a clinic or health professional's office with the patient, that leaves them 8,760 hours when they are on their own to manage the situation.

The following considerations resonate:

- Varying survivorship
- Variable trajectory, even for benign brain tumour diagnoses
- High frequency of disabling complications
- High severity of disabling complications
- Knowledge of increasing cognitive dysfunction
- Life context—where there is resilience or a lack of ability to cope

There is little support available through the usual clinical channels—only 47% of UK neuro-oncology multidisciplinary teams have access to neuropsychiatry services.[5]

Catt et al.[6] have identified that:

- Supportive care pathways for patients and their families differ between hospitals;
- Guidelines either omit important aspects of care and follow-up or are based on assumptions with little empirical support;
- As treatments of patients is often palliative, more efforts are needed to ensure good continuity of care;
- Current follow-up is failing to meet the psychological needs of patients and their caregivers;
- There is a need for developing innovative and integrated interventions that effectively support caregivers, such as proactive counselling or problem-solving services.

These points are echoed in the findings of a crowdsourcing project undertaken by *brainstrust* and createhealth.io.[7] Brain tumour patients and caregivers highlighted four main themes that would improve the quality of care for brain tumour patients post-surgery:

- A desire to know what to expect;
- Better mentorship, home care, and personal support;
- The importance of understanding and accessing long-term care;
- Increased uniformity in standard of hospital care from place to place.

What does advocacy look like for the brain cancer community?

This is complex—for a variety of reasons. Patient autonomy is a fundamental ethical principle, which should embrace the individual's right to choose goals and decide actions, based on the individual's context, attitude to risk, and values. However, healthcare systems have tended to empower large bureaucratic organizations and medical professionals rather than ordinary people. The big commissioning decisions are made by large organizations like the National Health Service (NHS) and clinical commissioning groups. Typically, how care is organized and managed is decided by providers such as large NHS trusts and general practitioner (GP) practices. Finally, the model of care is generally a medical one, whereby doctors hold most of the knowledge and power and patients are too often seen as passive and uninformed consumers.

Empowerment models

Empowerment models such as choice and entitlements have generally been seen as ways of better responding to a person's needs, rather than considering their capabilities. This is common across public services in developed countries, where services have been established with a 'deficit' mindset: hospitals exist to provide patients with medical treatment at times of acute need and doctors exist to diagnose illnesses and provide medications. This approach tends to infantilize and disempower people, creating dependency cultures, in which people's best hope for improving their lot is to wait for a paid professional to step in.

The presence of an adversary, in this instance, brain cancer, calls for advocacy. A good advocate will enable capability in the patient and mobilize people's 'relational power'; they will ensure that the patient is able to participate in their healthcare decisions and be agile and adaptive in the decisions that are made. Such approaches are still generally countercultural in our system, but some moves in the direction of shared decision-making share the same starting point. In particular, care planning under this model must start by discussing a person's needs and aspirations and then look at what resources are available to help meet them, taking into account their own skills and capabilities, as well as resources from the community before then looking at what can be provided by the state.

Patients and their caregivers live with their condition 24/7 hours and only spend a fraction of their time visiting clinical experts; the rest of the time they have to manage their condition themselves. So having the knowledge, skills, and confidence to manage one's own health is strongly related to a positive range of health-related outcomes.[8,9] Qualitative studies[10-13] show that some patients and the majority of caregivers want to be fully involved in understanding their illness, exploring their options for treatment, and for living with the illness and sourcing information, knowledge, help, and advice.

But this will mean different things to different people at different points on what is a very complex journey, covering prediagnosis, screening, diagnosis, therapeutics, follow-up, survivorship, progression, palliative care, end of life, and post-bereavement (Fig. 10.1). Following diagnosis and treatment for a brain tumour, patients will have differing trajectories, which may be predicted ranging from recovery, stable situation, or progression. Research shows that neuro-rehabilitation and neuro-psychosocial support improves outcomes for patients diagnosed with a brain tumour.[14] For improved survivorship, close collaboration is required between clinicians involved with neuro-rehabilitation, supportive care, quality of life, psychological, and palliative care to plan transition points in healthcare. This requires coordination of different specialties and expertise from symptom management to end-of-life care. Evidence shows that patients and caregivers who are coached through advocacy are better able to manage the complexity of their journey, have more resilience and a better quality of life. They are significantly more likely to attend screenings, regular check-ups, and significantly more likely to engage in healthy behaviours like eating a healthy diet[15-16] or taking regular exercise.[17-23] Conversely, less engaged patients are significantly less likely to have prepared questions for a visit to the doctor, to know about treatment guidelines for their condition, or to be persistent in asking if they do not understand what their doctor has told them.[17] They are also two to three times more likely to have unmet medical needs and to delay medical care compared with more highly engaged patients, regardless of income, education, and access to care.[19]

This illustration is based on the distillation of approximately 65 hours of research with diabetes and cancer patients from the United Kingdom and Germany to create a high-level patient journey which maps the patient's information-seeking behaviour. See more about Blue Latitude Health at www.bluelatitude.com.[24]

In addition, patients and caregivers with high confidence levels will become advocates for others. These patients and caregivers are highly knowledgeable on most aspects of their condition and the treatment options available. They tend to become advocates, and often influence other patients via support groups or even creating charities. They:

- are the expert on themselves
- are more than their condition
- understand what is happening and what is going to happen
- have a voice and are heard
- have control over their personal space
- know their values and what is important to them
- understand difference, respecting that not everyone has the same attitude to risk or the same values.

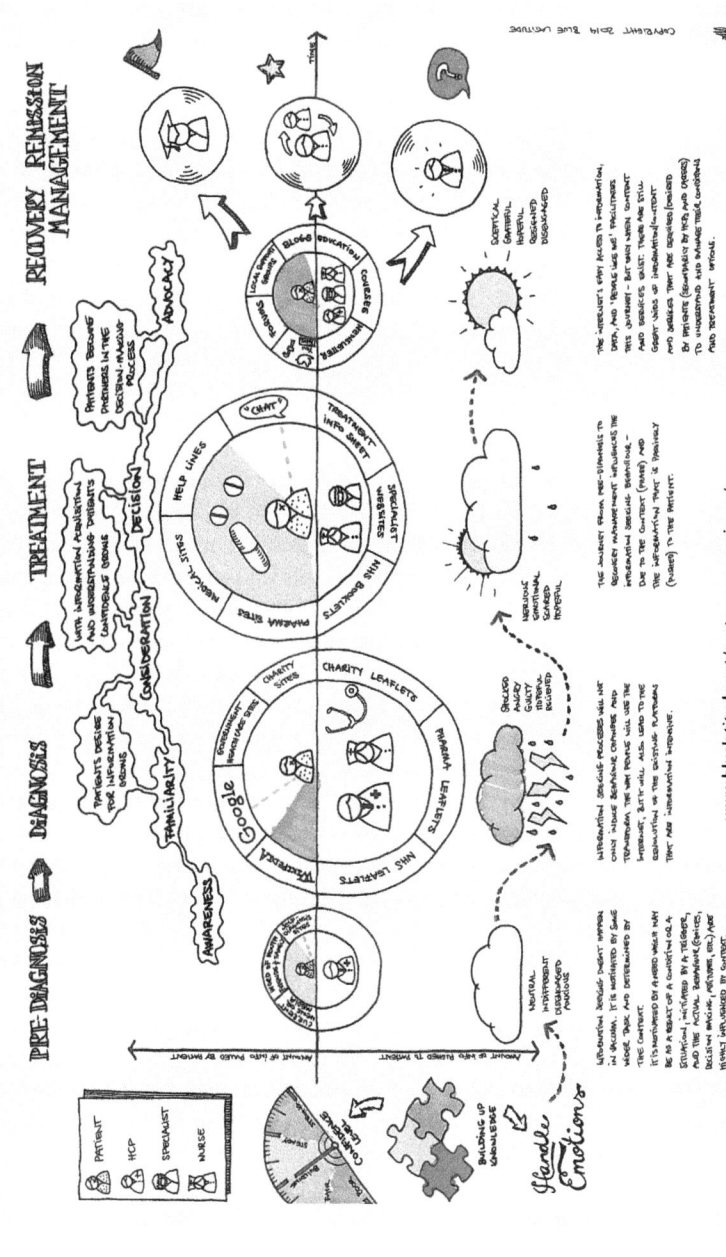

Fig. 10.1 The patient information journey.
© Blue Latitude Health 2014. This illustration is based on the distillation of approximately 65 hours of research with diabetes and cancer patients from the United Kingdom and Germany to create a high-level patient journey which maps the patient's information seeking behaviour. See more about BLH at https://bluelatitude.com

However, the advocate is likely to be a very small percentage (>5%).[25] The other two categories are the self-concerned (patients who tend to focus their knowledge on their own well-being) and the unengaged (patients who find it difficult to engage with their healthcare practitioners (HCPs) and their treatment): 50% of the patient population.

Therefore advocacy (having an advocate, or team of advocates) enables patients and their caregivers to play a more collaborative role[26-29]; patients and caregivers have more capacity to take control of their situation to secure the best possible outcomes; by being empowered through a variety of advocacy models they achieve greater autonomy, a better quality of life, and more satisfaction. Having greater control over our health and care is a good thing: autonomy, or the ability to exercise control over the forces that affect our lives, is an essential part of a good life. In healthcare, self-directed support is only now starting to break through into mainstream services, but there are strong grounds for extending it. Healthcare services, through advocacy, should support people to lead independent lives, rather than forcing them to fit their lives around the services on offer.

Patient activation

Strongly related to a broad range of better health-related outcomes is patient activation (having the knowledge, skills, and confidence to manage one's own health). Studies show that shared decision-making processes are more likely to result in people adhering with treatments and actions. Patients who are engaged in their health and healthcare—through health literacy, shared clinical decision-making, and self-management—are more likely to say that their healthcare is of high quality, and are less likely to report experience of medical errors.[30] We know that when people play a more collaborative role in managing their health and care, they can have better clinical outcomes.[27,31] We know too that patients who have the opportunity and who have support to make decisions about their care and treatment in partnership with health professionals are more satisfied with their care.[32] We also know that patients are more likely to choose treatments based on their values and preferences rather than those of their clinician.[33] They also tend to choose less invasive and costly treatments.[31] Most significantly, they are more likely to become advocates for themselves, and some become advocates for others.

There is also a health economic argument for advocacy: giving people the support and information they need to avoid getting ill, or when they have a chronic condition to self-manage it effectively. If people are not equipped and supported to self-manage, they are effectively left on their own and can end up with complications, health crises, preventable trips to the GP or A&E, avoidable suffering, and even premature death. Around 20% of emergency admissions to hospital are thought to be potentially preventable, and many of these involve chronic conditions.[34] The most robust evaluations of empowerment programmes focused on advocacy and redesigned consultations have been estimated to reduce acute care costs by 7%. Nesta estimates that this, which they describe as a conservative estimate, would save the NHS £4.4 billion a year across England.[35]

So, there is a straightforward moral case for empowering people in health and care through advocacy—but there is an instrumental case as well. Empowerment produces better health outcomes, more satisfied patients and caregivers, and much-needed financial savings.

How can advocacy be applied?

The attributes of a good advocate have been defined in Chapter 1 and it is acknowledged that advocacy can be taken up by many different persons and groups and different times on the patient journey. However, daily interactions with patient and caregiver experiences reveal that self-management practices, while being provided routinely in some places (by nurses, physiotherapists, GPs, health visitors, social workers, caregivers, healthcare assistants and others, in healthcare centres, people's own homes, day centres, or hospitals), tend to be on an ad hoc basis, reactive and unplanned. Patients and caregivers do not know what support is available to them, where to seek help, or what questions they should be asking.

Becoming empowered

A shift to becoming empowered begins at the point of diagnosis, with a collaborative and interactive relationship between patients and healthcare professionals, which empowers patients to take on responsibility for their condition with the appropriate clinical support. There remain major challenges to this change, for example, from moving from the position of seeing the healthcare professional just as an expert giving advice, to an advocate, an enabler who supports the person they are caring for to achieve their goals; and the challenge of patients seeing themselves as passive recipients of care, to becoming activated and taking responsibility for their own contribution to improving their health and well-being outcomes, and being empowered to do so.

Therefore, it is likely that the patient living with a brain tumour will identify different people within their team to meet varying and very different needs, which the brain cancer community has identified as being the following[13]:

- Clear signposting of care in the community
- The right information at the right time
- Public understanding
- Clear expectations
- A more equal relationship with my doctor
- More honest discussions sooner
- To know how to get what I want out of a discussion
- To not be alone
- To feel in control
- To know how to deal with death and dying

Communication

Communication is central to all of these. Without it, people cannot relate to those around them, make their needs and concerns known, or make sense of what is happening to them. It is concerned with informing and enhancing knowledge among the general public and people living with brain cancer, empowering them to express their needs and take action. In the context of brain cancer, advocacy can influence:

- policy changes and political and financial commitment;
- communication between caregivers and patients as well as communities;
- social mobilization to engage society in raising awareness about the challenges that come with living with a brain tumour.

Community support

Advocacy can secure the support of key constituencies in relevant local, national, and international policy discussions and prompt greater accountability from key players. Equally, encouraging providers to be more receptive to the expressed needs of the brain cancer community will make services more responsive to community needs. Social mobilization encourages communities to raise their knowledge of and demand for good-quality care and healthcare in general, assisting in the delivery of resources and services and strengthen community participation.

Advocacy roles are not mutually exclusive and could include:

- Navigator
- Information provider
- Mediator
- Anticipatory guide
- Spokesperson
- Referral resource
- Public relations[36]

Navigation

Navigation advocacy through patient clinic visits supports decision-making, improves understanding, and has been proven to be associated with better knowledge and understanding of diagnosis and treatment, improved ability to cope, and reduced distress. Qualitative studies[10-12] show that some patients and the majority of caregivers want to be fully involved in:

- understanding their illness;
- exploring their options for treatment and for living with the illness;
- sourcing information, knowledge, help, and advice.

Patients who were coached by a navigator advocate, by preparing through coaching for consultations, found that a discussion of personalized key issues, broader than the prime focus of the consultation, resulted. Patients felt more informed and utilized navigation materials to aid memory, information gathering, and understanding. Clinical feedback revealed that navigation led to more effective consultations and facilitated communication within consultations by giving insight into information gaps. Telephone follow-up was effective for information and support and psycho-education increased feelings of mastery.[37-38]

Information

Information provision advocacy provides knowledge, which builds power, but only if the knowledge is relevant and meets the needs of the patient and the caregiver. The information needs to encompass health information so that informed decisions can be made, respecting the patient's rights (e.g. for access to their health records), and signposting to relevant support.

As an example:

> 'I now realize that stuff like memory loss, not being able to articulate what's in your head and bone-aching tiredness that comes on without warning are not just my symptoms. Knowledge is coping, for me.'
>
> Patient

But this role is more than just an information provider; the advocate has to be objective, honest, and to not regard themselves as a 'fixer'. They should maintain a critical distance, understand that it is not within their gift to tell people what to do, otherwise they may gate-keep information and be selective in what they feel the patient and caregiver needs.

Types of advocacy

Mediation advocacy

Mediation advocacy argues the patient's and caregiver's positions, needs, and interests in a non-adversarial way. The advocate must know the context and the people involved, and be sensitive to where the power bases lie. They should know where barriers exist and work within the systems to enable the best outcomes. This role might find them mediating between the clinical team, the patient, the caregiver, and the family.

The role of the anticipatory guide is to encourage proactivity, rather than reaction. They build resilience so that the patient and caregiver are more comfortable living with uncertainty, by anticipating future challenges and needs before they arise. For example, looking at the disease trajectory, encouraging the elicitation of values, and planning for end-of-life care with the patient and their caregiver enables the family to manage this phase, so that the patient is where they want to be and the appropriate support is in place.

Spokesperson advocacy

The spokesperson advocate is a clear communicator who speaks on behalf of someone who is unable, or who does not want, to speak for themselves. They become their voice. They must be able to state the problem from a specific perspective in a succinct manner. This is not as straightforward as it appears, as there may be occasions when this problem is painful for a close person to hear. For example, there may be a caregiver who feels that their care is optimal, but in fact is not what the patient wants or needs at all.

Referral resource advocacy

The advocate who is a referral resource, also a sign poster, provides information that outlies the disease itself. Resources will include services in the community that will meet the patient's or caregiver's needs. Frequently now this advocacy role might be an online resource, such as the brain tumour hub (http://www.braintumourhub.org.uk). This is an authoritative, easy to navigate database of brain tumour support resources and UK-based brain tumour clinical trials. It is intuitive, easy to use, and developed with clinicians, patients, and carers, and provides advocacy on a range of community-based services for people living with a brain tumour.

Public relations advocacy

The public relations advocate works within the community building awareness of the disease, the challenges that this brings, support services, including advocacy and particular health-related topics, such as clinical research. One example of this advocacy might be presentations at support groups around a fatigue, or a workshop for caregivers.

Community advocacy

How these roles manifest themselves within the neuro-oncology community is varied and complex. Any individual may suddenly find themselves in the role of an advocate and not everyone will have the training for this role, nor is it always a role that they have applied for. This is true of the caregiver, who may well be the underpinning advocate for the patient. Becoming a caregiver for someone with brain cancer can happen abruptly or creep in slowly unnoticed, until one day you realize you are caring more for someone else than you are for yourself. This new role as a caregiver can become as frightening as the initial diagnosis of brain cancer.

So, the role of the community is as important for the advocate (whether the advocate is a healthcare professional, a caregiver, a friend, a work colleague, a relative) as it is for the patient. Being a less common cancer, patients and caregivers are unlikely to know someone in their local community or friendship group who also has a brain tumour. Therefore, advocacy from fellow brain tumour patients and caregivers is crucial as it is founded in shared experiences. As many as 79% of patients are not given a care plan, and 32% come away from their consultation without fully understanding the diagnosis.[39] At this point, feeling lost and scared, they desperately need someone to talk to, and someone who—having been affected by brain cancer—truly understands. The community advocate is necessary to enable them to find others in the same boat. Advocates working within communities:

- Enable patients to stand up for themselves and therefore secure better outcomes;
- Solve real problems collaboratively;
- Create the vision for patients and caregivers to help them understand how their care should be;
- Provide the community with a voice.

An example of the community in action is through the *brainstrust* meet up site:

https://www.meetup.com/brainstrust.[40]

'We have thoroughly enjoyed out time with everyone at the meet ups, a great idea to pull people together.'

Patient and caregiver

Creating a cohesive, vibrant, and useful healthcare advocacy community for brain tumour patients and their caregivers so that it transcends virtual and real-world boundaries (Fig. 10.2) results in an advocacy community where experts (HCPs, AHPs, patients, and caregivers) engage and take part in the discourse, and virtual world interactions can be taken offline into the real world.

Research has proven that a supportive network improves health outcomes for people with a wide range of conditions[41] including brain cancer.[14,42-47] Indeed, the availability of online health communities is especially appreciated by individuals with impaired mobility, busy schedules, or caregiver responsibilities that may prohibit them from receiving adequate face-to-face medical and emotional support.[48] In addition, research[49-50] focused on advocacy programmes proves that support from others who have been through a similar experience can help reduce the negative impacts of this disease. Using advocacy helps patients and caregivers to:

♦ Be an enabler for others;
♦ Be secure with uncertainty;
♦ Be open with not knowing and taking risks;
♦ Ensure that their inner dialogue is constructive;
♦ Be non-defensive by having nothing to prove and no agenda.

Continuous re-evaluation of the patient and caregiver advocacy needs and information is required as these change over time with disease progression.[51] Approximately half of distressed cancer patients do not access psychosocial services, with some blankly refusing as they see it as a sign of personal weakness.[52] Standards of care (including existential support) may be enhanced by moving towards a proactive approach, extending care goals beyond medical needs,[53] which may best be served by having one dedicated advocate and central point of contact for continuity of communication with a health professional.

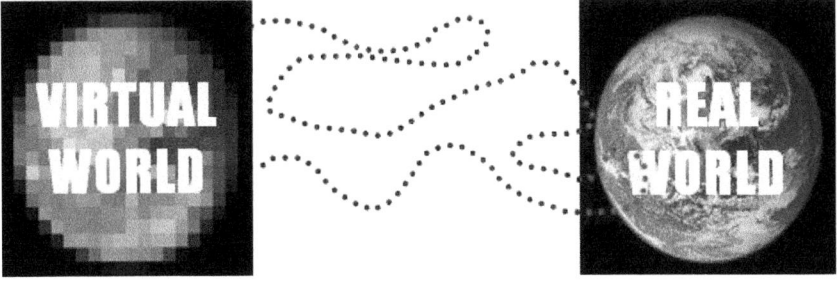

Fig. 10.2 Virtual world interactions can be taken offline into the real world.

Conclusion

Advocacy for patients and caregivers living with a brain tumour is fundamental to optimizing quality of life. Brain cancer is uniquely different from other cancers because it intersects three disease areas (cancer, rare disease, neurological disease) and significantly affects physical and cognitive abilities. Advocacy can take a variety of forms and will need to be agile as the disease progresses. This is unsurprising; when illness strikes, several structural and emotional skews will follow. Belief systems are challenged, roles are upended, and identities shift. The onset of a brain tumour diagnosis forcefully challenges the emotional and physical boundaries that we have spent a lifetime building. The tumour is an uninvited guest that we must somehow incorporate into our lives, while at the same time living with the undercurrent of threatened loss.

There is much too in this chapter which is relevant for advocacy in other neurological diseases. Having an isolating neurological diagnosis, and all that this entails, is not mutually exclusive to brain cancer. Being empowered through advocacy to:

- process and find ways of remembering information
- understand rights and choices
- make and communicate decisions
- access services
- access support groups to address social isolation
- live independently
- interact with health and social care professionals
- challenge assessments and care packages
- develop skills to be a voice

can help both patients and their caregivers to live with these challenges. A good advocate, no matter what the illness, will enable a deeper understanding of the condition, reduce isolation, and improve quality of life.

References

1. **Stupp, R., Hegi, M. E., Mason, W. P.**, et al. (2009) Effects of radiotherapy with concomitant and adjuvant temozolomide versus radiotherapy alone on survival in glioblastoma in a randomised phase III study: 5-year analysis of the EORTC-NCIC trial. *Lancet Oncol*, **10**(5), 459–66.
2. **Watts, C.** (2010) Brain cancer: an unrecognised clinical problem. *Oncology News*, **5**(2), 38–40.
3. **Mukand, J. A., Blackinton, D. D., Crincoli, M. G., Lee, J. J., Santos, B. B.** (2001) Incidence of neurologic deficits and rehabilitation of patients with brain tumours. *Am J Phys Med Rehabil*, **80**(5), 346–50.
4. **Lehmann, J., DeLisa, J. A., Warren, C. G., deLateur, B. J., Bryant, P. L., Nicholson, C. G.** (1978) Cancer rehabilitation: assessment of need, development, and evaluation of a model of care. *Arch Phys Med Rehabil*, **59**(9), 410–19.
5. **Rooney, A.** (2011) Challenges and opportunities in psychological neuro-oncology. *Oncology News*, **6**(4), 133–5.

6. **Catt, S., Chalmers, A., Critchley, G., Fallowfield, L.** (2012) Supportive follow up in patients treated with radical intent for high grade glioma. *CNS Oncology*, **1**(1), 39–48.
7. **Fellgate, T., Bulbeck, H., Hill, M., Jones, W.** (2014) Patient crowdsourcing: ideas that will improve the quality of life for people living with a brain tumour. In: *Quality of Life: What the Brain Cancer Community Needs*. October 2014. Available at: hhtps://www.brainstrust.org.uk
8. **Malak, A., Diramali, A., Yücesoy, K.** (2010) Effects of counseling on some care outcomes among patients with a brain tumour: pain, seizure, constipation, infection, dispatch conditions. *Nobel Medicus*, **6**(2), 25–31.
9. **Greene, J., Hibbard, J.** (2012) Why does patient activation matter? An examination of the relationships between patient activation and health-related outcomes. *J Gen Int Med*, **27**(5), 520–6.
10. **Cavers, D., Hacking, B., Erridge, S., Kendall, M., Morris, P. G., Murray, S. A.** (2012) Social, psychological and existential well-being in patients with glioma and their caregivers: a qualitative study. *CMAJ*, **184**(7), E373–82.
11. **Shepherd, S. C., Cavers, D., Wallace, L. M., Hacking, B., Scott, S. E., Bowyer, D. J.** (2012) 'Navigation' to support decision making for patients with a high-grade brain tumour. A qualitative evaluation. Proceedings of the British Neuro-oncology Society Conference; 27-29 June 2012; Manchester, UK.
12. **Brains Trust**. Available at: https://www.brainstrust.org.uk
13. **Brains Trust**. Campaigning to make quality of life a priority. Available at: https://brainstrust.org.uk/brain-tumour-support/our-campaigns/quality-of-life/.
14. **Bartolo, M., Zucchella, C., Pace, A., et al.** (2012) Early rehabilitation after surgery improves functional outcome in inpatients with brain tumours. *J Neurooncol*, **107**(3), 537–544.
15. **Hibbard, J. H., Mahoney, E. R., Stockard, J., Tusler, M.** (2005) Development and testing of a short form of the patient activation measure. *Health Serv Res*, **40**(6 Pt 1), 1918–30.
16. **Hibbard, J. H., Stockard, J., Mahoney, E. R., Tusler, M.** (2004) Development of the Patient Activation Measure (PAM): conceptualizing and measuring activation in patients and consumers. *Health Serv Res*, **39**(4 Pt 1), 1005–26.
17. **Fowles, J. B., Terry, P., Xi, M., Hibbard, J., Bloom, C. T., Harvey, L.** (2009) Measuring self-management of patients' and employees' health: further validation of the Patient Activation Measure (PAM) based on its relation to employee characteristics. *Patient Educ Counsel*, **77**(1), 116–22.
18. **Becker, E. R., Roblin, D. W.** (2008) Translating primary care practice climate into patient activation: the role of patient trust in physician. *Med Care*, **46**(8), 795–805.
19. **Hibbard, J. H., Cunningham, P. J.** (2008) How engaged are consumers in their health and health care, and why does it matter? *Res Brief*, **8**, 1–9.
20. **Hibbard, J. H., Tusler, M.** (2007) Assessing activation stage and employing a 'next steps' approach to supporting patient self-management. *J Ambul Care Manage*, **30**(1), 2–8.
21. **Hibbard, J. H., Mahoney, E. R., Stock, R., Tusler, M.** (2007) Do increases in patient activation result in improved self-management behaviors? *Health Serv Res*, **42**(4), 1443–63.
22. **Mosen, D. M., Schmittdiel, J., Hibbard, J., Sobel, D., Remmers, C., Bellows, J.** (2007) Is patient activation associated with outcomes of care for adults with chronic conditions? *J Ambul Care Manage*, **30**(1), 21–9.
23. **Blue Latitude Health**. The patient information journey. Available at: https://bluelatitude.com/our-ideas/the-patient-information-journey/

24. **Blue Latitude Health**. Available at: https://bluelatitude.com
25. **Del Gardo, E.** (2015) How do you solve a problem like non-adherence? (Part II). Blue Latitude. Available at: https://bluelatitude.com/our-ideas/how-do-you-solve-a-problem-like-non-adherence-part-ii/
26. **Van't Hooft, I., Norberg, A. L.** (2010) SMART cognitive training combined with a parental coaching programme for three children treated for medulloblastoma. *J Rehabil*, **26**(2), 105–13.
27. **De Silva, D.** (2011) *Helping People Help Themselves*. London: The Health Foundation.
28. **Boele, F., Hoeben, W., Hilverda, K., et al.** (2013) Enhancing quality of life and mastery of informal caregivers of high grade glioma patients: a randomised controlled trial. *J Neurooncol*, **111**(3), 303–11.
29. **Rosenberg, A., Dussel, V., Kang, T., et al.** (2013) Psychological distress in parents of children with advanced cancer. *JAMA Paediatrics*, **167**(6), 537–43.
30. **Edgman-Levitan, S., Brady, C.** (2013) Partnering with patients, families, and communities for health: a global imperative. *WISH Patient and Family Engagement Report 2013*. Available at: http://www.wish-qatar.org/app/media/387
31. **Hibbard, J., Gilbert, H.** (2014) *Supporting People to Manage Their Health: An Introduction to Patient Activation*. London: The King's Fund.
32. **De Silva, D.** (2012) *Helping People Share Decision Making*. London: The Health Foundation.
33. **O'Connor, A. M., Llewellyn-Thomas, A., Flood, A. B.** (2004) Modifying unwarranted variations in health care: shared decision making using patient decision aids. *Health Affairs*. Available at: http://content.healthaffairs.org/content/early/2004/10/07/hlthaff.var.63.long
34. **Blunt, I.** (2013) *Focus on Preventable Admissions: Trends in Emergency Admissions for Ambulatory Care Sensitive Conditions, 2001 to 2013*. London: Health Foundation and Nuffield Trust.
35. **Nesta** (2013) The Business Case for People Powered Health. Available at: https://www.nesta.org.uk/report/the-business-case-for-people-powered-health/
36. **Hummel, F.** (2006) Advocacy. In: Larsen, P., Lubkin, I. (eds). *Chronic Illness: Impact and Interventions*. London: Jones and Bartlett Publishers, pp. 375–402.
37. **Piil, K., Juhler, M., Jakobsen, J., Jarden, M.** (2016) Controlled rehabilitative and supportive care intervention trials in patients with high grade gliomas and their caregivers: a systematic review. *BMJ Support Palliat Care*, **6**(1), 27–34.
38. **Molina, I., Page, M., Patt, J., Chang, S.** (2014) Peer to peer support: a new way to support caregivers. *Neuro Oncol*, **16**(5), 211.
39. **Quality Health**. National Cancer Patient Experience surveys, 2010–2016. Chesterfield: Quality Health Limited. Available at: http://www.quality-health.co.uk/surveys/national-cancer-patient-experience-survey
40. **The Brainstrust Meetup Group** (2018) Available at: https://www.meetup.com/brainstrust
41. **Sarasohn-Kahn, J., THINK-Health** (2008) The wisdom of patients: healthcare meets online social media. California HealthCare Foundation. Available at: http://www.chcf.org/~/media/MEDIA%20LIBRARY%20Files/PDF/PDF%20H/PDF%20HealthCareSocialMedia.pdf
42. **Barakat, L. P., Hetzke, J. D., Foley, B., Carey, M. E., Gyato, K., Phillips, P.** (2003) Evaluation of a social skills training group intervention with children treated for brain tumors: a pilot study. *J Pediatr Psychol*, **28**(5), 299–307.

43. **Barrera, M**, **Chung, J. Y.**, **Fleming, C. F.** (2005) A group intervention for siblings of pediatric cancer patients. *J Psychosoc Oncol*, **22**(2), 21–39.
44. **Lindemalm, A.**, **Strang, P.**, **Lekander, M.** (2005) Support groups for cancer patients. Does it improve their physical and psychological well-being? A pilot study. *Support Care Cancer*, **13**(8), 652–7.
45. **Finocchiaro, C. Y.**, **Botturi, A.**, **Lamperti, E.**, et al. (2011) Privacy-solidarity conflict: the communication with the support group. *Neurological Sciences*, **32** Suppl 2, S225–7.
46. **Green, H.**, **Borwick, S.**, **Mihuta, M.** (2013) Cognitive rehabilitation interventions. *Asia-Pacific J Clin Oncol*, **9**(S3), 61–98.
47. **Gröntoft, M.**, **Westermark, M.**, **Hylin, S.**, **Stragliotto, G.** (2013) Psychosocial support by medical social worker is beneficial for patients with malign brain tumours. *Neuro Oncol*, **15**(Suppl 3), iii226–34.
48. **Im, E. O.**, **Chee, W.**, **Lim, H. J.**, **Liu, Y.**, **Guevara, E.**, **Kim, K. S.** (2007) Patients' attitudes toward internet cancer support groups. *Oncol Nurs Forum*, **34**(3), 705–12.
49. **Campbell, S. H.**, **Phaneuf, M. R.**, **Deane, K.** (2004) Cancer peer support programmes—do they work? *Patient Educ Couns*, **55**(1), 3–15.
50. **Hoey, L.**, **Ieropoli, S. C.**, **White, V. M.**, **Jefford, M.** (2008) Systematic review of peer-support programs for people with cancer. *Patient Educ Couns*, **70**(3), 315–37.
51. **Sterckx, W.**, **Coolbrandt, A.**, **Clement, P.**, et al. (2015) Living with a high-grade glioma: a qualitative study of patients' experiences and care needs. *Eur J Oncol Nurs*, **19**(4), 383–90.
52. **Golla, H.**, **Ale Ahmad, M.**, **Galushko, M.**, et al. (2014) Glioblastoma multiforme from diagnosis to death: a prospective, hospital-based, cohort, pilot feasibility study of patient reported symptoms and needs. *Support Care Cancer*, **22**(12), 3341–52.
53. **Janda, M.**, **Eakin, E. G.**, **Bailey, L.**, **Walker, D.**, **Troy, K.** (2006) Supportive care needs of people with brain tumours and their carers. *Support Care Cancer*, **14**(11), 1094–103.

Chapter 11

Patient involvement in European cancer societies: The example of ECCO—the European CanCer Organization

Françoise Van Hemelryck

Advocacy refers to activities which aim to influence decisions within political, economic, and social systems and institutions. Patient advocacy refers to the advocacy activities by the individual or by groups of patients to represent the interests of patients in decisions made by systems and institutions. Patient groups have come to the idea that patients are best placed to inform decision-makers about what is of value to patients in healthcare and to drive healthcare developments that is based on value to patients.

Patient advocacy has a long history in the field of oncology at a European level, with some patient advocacy groups already established in the early 1990s. Nowadays patient advocacy groups exist for most cancer types but differ very much in terms of their structure, governance, funding, or main focus of activity. Their work usually falls under the categories of direct support to patients, educational activities, and political activities aiming to influence health policies at a European and/or national level.

Increased emphasis is given to the patient perspective and the patient experience, to provide care that is of most value to patients but also an essential component of sustainable healthcare at a time when healthcare systems are facing sustainability issues (Box 11.1).

At a European level, patient advocacy groups are acting as advisors in most cancer care professional organizations. ECCO—the European CanCer organization created a Patient Advisory Committee (PAC) in 2008. Since 2012, the ECCO PAC Chair attends ECCO Board meetings and since 2016 has had a seat with voting rights.

Patient empowerment in cancer control

The literature provides numerous examples acknowledging the growing recognition of patient empowerment in cancer control as a key principle of patient-centred care.

The nature of cancer control is changing with an increasing emphasis on the patient experience during and after treatment. Informed patients expect a partnership model of decision-making and more responsibility to manage their own health and healthcare.[1]

> **Box 11.1 The scope of cancer in Europe and worldwide: Key facts**
>
> - Cancer is one of the leading causes of morbidity and mortality worldwide, with approximately 14 million new cases in 2012.
> - The number of new cases is expected to rise by about 70% over the next two decades.
> - Cancer is the second leading cause of death globally, and was responsible for 8.8 million deaths in 2015. Globally, nearly 1 in 6 deaths is due to cancer.
> - Approximately 70% of deaths from cancer occur in low- and middle-income countries.
> - Around one-third of deaths from cancer are due to the five leading behavioural and dietary risks: high body mass index, low fruit and vegetable intake, lack of physical activity, tobacco use, and alcohol use.
> - Tobacco use is the most important risk factor for cancer and is responsible for approximately 22% of cancer deaths.
> - Cancer-causing infections, such as hepatitis and human papilloma virus (HPV), are responsible for up to 25% of cancer cases in low- and middle-income countries.
> - Late-stage presentation and inaccessible diagnosis and treatment are common. In 2015, only 35% of low-income countries reported having pathology services generally available in the public sector. More than 90% of high-income countries reported treatment services are available compared to less than 30% of low-income countries.
> - The economic impact of cancer is significant and is increasing. The total annual economic cost of cancer in 2010 was estimated at approximately US$ 1.16 trillion.
> - Only 1 in 5 low- and middle-income countries have the necessary data to drive cancer policy.
>
> Reproduced from Media Centre: Fact Sheet: Cancer, Copyright (2018), with permission from World Health Organization. Available at http://www.who.int/mediacentre/factsheets/fs297/en/

Patient-centred care in cancer requires a multilevel approach in order to understand patients' concerns, needs, and expectations, all of which can change during the many stages and cycles of diagnosis and treatment.[2]

There are many aspects related to patients in the process of cancer care; the individual patient's view of his or her disease, as well as the treatment process; the interaction with the family, friends, and caregivers; the relationship with the surrounding society and culture; and finally, the communication barriers with the healthcare provider, especially with respect to unmatched health belief models and the understanding of treatment goals.[3]

Healthcare providers should adopt a partnership style with patients, and provide healthcare that is respectful of patients to support informed patient decision-making.[4]

The World Health Organization (WHO) uses the term 'responsiveness' in preference to 'patient-centred care'. Responsiveness describes how a healthcare system meets people's expectations regarding respect for people and their wishes.

Description of ECCO

Every cancer patient deserves the best: this is the philosophy of ECCO, the European CanCer Organisation. Through its 25 member societies, representing over 170,000 professionals, ECCO is the only multidisciplinary organization that connects and responds to all stakeholders in oncology Europe-wide.

ECCO is a not-for-profit federation that exists to uphold the right of all European cancer patients to the best possible treatment and care, promoting interaction between all organizations involved in cancer at European level.

It does this by creating awareness of patients' needs and wishes, encouraging progressive thinking in cancer policy, training, and education and promoting European cancer research, prevention, diagnosis, treatment, and care through the organization of international multidisciplinary meetings.

ECCO is uniquely positioned to provide the voice of consensus of European oncology professionals and engage with policymakers to ensure that cancer stays at the top of the EU agenda.

Providing a rallying point for Europe's community of oncology professionals, ECCO engages in planned and sustained interaction with EU policymakers as well as third-party stakeholders to anticipate and proactively shape EU policies in cancer control.

The core purpose of ECCO policy objectives are to:

- promote policies to underpin multidisciplinary in cancer care
- provide multidisciplinary recommendations to shape policymaking in common areas of concern

ECCO has been a partner in the recently released European Guide on Quality Improvement in Comprehensive Cancer Control (CanCon).[5]

The Guide aims to help reduce not only the cancer burden throughout the EU but also the inequalities in cancer control and care that exist between member states. The Guide is meant for governments, parliamentarians, healthcare providers and funders, and cancer care professionals at every level.

ECCO could bring the expertise of its membership and its Patient Advisory Committee (PAC) to this very important project. Among its key recommendations, the PAC stressed the importance of patient-reported outcomes to measure the quality of care and making sure that the cancer care structures recommended in the CANCON guide can be applied across all European countries. The PAC also stressed the importance of continuity of care, the need to address symptom management and psychological care during the entire disease trajectory to achieve the best possible quality of life.

Primary care professionals (including supportive care) can play an important role in providing care in these areas throughout the cancer care pathway and therefore more attention should be given to models of cancer management, whereby primary care and secondary care are joined-up.

ECCO is committed to widely promote the recommendations of this joint effort and seeks to actively engage all the European multidisciplinary oncology professional societies in its goal to improve the life of cancer patients and their carers.

Patient advocates are contributors to the ECCO position statements and debates on topical issues such as innovation in oncology. They are calling for greater involvement of patients in defining and assessing the value of innovation. Adopting a culture of innovation requires a multidisciplinary team approach—with the patient at the centre, and as an integral part of the team on both the individual patient and organizational advocacy level. It must take a whole-system and whole-patient perspective on cancer care, match unmet patient needs and patient-relevant outcomes, and be guided by high-quality real-world data that accurately reflect the impact of any innovation in clinical practice.

Suggestions were provided on the European Oncology Nursing Society (EONS) research protocol on the systematic review of the evidence of effectiveness and value of cancer nursing as part of the Recognising European Cancer Nursing (RECaN) project supported by ECCO. The PAC pointed to several types of oncology nursing interventions as well as outcome measures that are important to patients across the patient trajectory, and which should be part of the research protocol. The ECCO PAC believes this is a very important area as specialist cancer nurses do not yet exist in all European countries, but patient outcomes are better when specialized nursing is in place.

To position patients' interests at the core of its multidisciplinary activities, ECCO established the ECCO Patient Advisory Committee (ECCO PAC) in 2008. Since then, the ECCO PAC has played an increasingly important role in helping ECCO realize its vision. As already mentioned earlier, since 2012 the ECCO PAC Chair has attended ECCO Board meetings, and has had voting rights on the ECCO Board since 2016.

The people who comprise the ECCO Patient Advisory Committee (ECCO PAC) are expert patient advocates from a range of site-specific cancer entities and various European countries. PAC members have unique expertise in the field of patient advocacy including in-depth knowledge of medicines development, support issues, information provision, and regulatory/reimbursement issues. In addition, the composition of the Patient Advisory Committee seeks to reflect the wide variety of patient groups existing in Europe.

Patient advocacy groups in oncology

Representatives of the following patient advocacy organizations are members of the ECCO Patient Advisory Committee (2016–2018):

International Brain Tumour Alliance

The International Brain Tumour Alliance (IBTA; https://www.theibta.org) is a unique global network for brain tumour patient and carer groups around the world. It works alongside, and represents, members of our community—including researchers, scientists, clinicians, nurses, and allied healthcare professionals—to engage in advocacy, to raise awareness, and to share information.

Myeloma Patients Europe

Myeloma Patients Europe (MPE; https://www.mpeurope.org) is an umbrella organization of myeloma patient groups and associations from across Europe. MPE was formed following the merger in 2011 of the European Myeloma Platform and Myeloma Euronet.

Although myeloma is the second most common form of blood cancer, it only represents 1% of cancers. Myeloma does not cause tumours like many other types of cancer. Instead it causes damage to DNA during development of the plasma cells in the bone marrow, causing them to divide uncontrollably.

International Kidney Cancer Coalition

The International Kidney Cancer Coalition (IKCC; https://www.ikcc.org) is an independent international network of patient organizations that focus exclusively, or include a specific focus, on kidney cancer. It is legally incorporated as a foundation in the Netherlands. The organization was born from a very strong desire among various national kidney cancer patient groups to network, cooperate, and share materials, knowledge, and experiences.

Leukaemia Patient Advocates Foundation

The Leukaemia Patient Advocates Foundation (https://www.cmladvocates.net/about-lepaf) is a patient-led non-profit foundation connecting leukaemia patient organizations on all continents to strengthen their advocacy work. Its mission is to improve the lives and survival of patients affected by leukaemia as well as their relatives by supporting leaders in providing help and support. It is a platform for discussions and best practice sharing to leukaemia patient groups worldwide. The foundation collaborates with all stakeholders involved in research, treatment, and care of leukaemia patients.

EuropaColon and Global Colon Cancer Alliance

EuropaColon (http://www.europacolon.com) aims to unite patients, caregivers, healthcare professionals, politicians, the media, and the public in the fight against digestive cancers. The organization works with 43 groups in 32 European countries and has been recognized as the voice of colorectal cancer patients in Europe

Childhood Cancer International

Childhood Cancer International (CCI; https://www.childhoodcancerinternational.org; formerly known as the International Confederation of Childhood Cancer Parent Organizations) was founded in 1994, as an umbrella organization of childhood cancer grassroots and national parent organizations. Today, CCI is the largest patient support organization for childhood cancer. It is a global, parent-driven non-profit that represents 181 parent organizations, childhood cancer survivor associations, childhood cancer support groups, and cancer societies, in 90 countries, across five continents.

Europa Uomo

Europa Uomo (https://www.europa-uomo.org) is the European advocacy movement for the fight against prostate cancer. Europa Uomo's objective is to increase awareness of prostate cancer in Europe. Europa Uomo is a European coalition of patients supporting groups for prostate diseases in general and prostate cancer in particular.

European Men's Health Forum

The European Men's Health Forum (EMHF; https://www.emhf.org) is the only European organization dedicated to the improvement of men's health in all its aspects. Its vision is a future in which all men in Europe have an equal opportunity to attain the highest possible level of health and well-being.

Its mission is to improve men's health across all countries in Europe by promoting collaboration between interested organizations and individuals on the development and application of health-related policies, research, education, and prevention programmes.

EMHF is committed to gender equality, fully supports activities to improve women's health, and opposes the re-allocation of funding from women's to men's health.

Europa Donna

Europa Donna (https://www.europadonna.org) is an independent non-profit organization whose members are affiliated groups from countries throughout Europe. The coalition works to raise awareness of breast cancer and to mobilize the support of European women in pressing for improved breast cancer education, appropriate screening, optimal treatment, and increased funding for research. Europa Donna represents the interests of European women regarding breast cancer to local and national authorities, as well as to institutions of the European Union.

Lymphoma Coalition Europe

The Lymphoma Coalition Europe (LCE; https://www.lymphomacoalition.org) is the first regional branch of the Lymphoma Coalition (LC) created in 2015 to work more closely with LC European members (35 patient organizations in 27 countries) and European partners, focusing on issues of regional interest.

Lymphoma is a cancer of a part of the immune system called the lymph system. There are many types of lymphoma. One type is Hodgkin's disease. The rest are called non-Hodgkin lymphomas.

European Cancer Patient Coalition

The aim of the European Cancer Patient Coalition (ECPC; http://www.ecpc.org), under the motto 'Nothing About Us, Without Us!' is to represent the views of cancer patients in the European healthcare debate and to provide a forum for European cancer patient organizations to exchange information and share best practices.

ECPC works for a Europe of equality, where all European cancer patients have timely and affordable access to the best treatment and care available, throughout their life. ECPC believes that cancer patients are the most important partners in the fight against cancer and against all the cancer-related issues affecting our society. Policymakers, researchers, doctors, and industry should recognize cancer patients as co-creators of their own health.

Melanoma Patient Network Europe

The Melanoma Patient Network Europe (MPNE; https://www.melanomapatientnetworkeu.org) works to systematically and pragmatically address the problems European melanoma patients are facing in an independent, constructive, results-orientated, and collaborative manner. It aims to improve access to prevention, early detection, and effective treatment in melanoma across Europe.

Lung Cancer Europe

Lung Cancer Europe (LuCE; https://www.lungcancereurope.eu) is the voice of lung cancer patients, their families, and survivors at a European level. LuCE provides a European platform for already existing lung cancer patient advocacy groups and supports the establishment of national lung cancer patient groups in different European countries where such groups do not yet exist

MDS Alliance

Myelodysplastic syndromes (MDS) are a group of cancers in which immature blood cells in the bone marrow do not mature and become healthy blood cells. Early on there are typically no symptoms. Later symptoms may include feeling tired, shortness of breath, easy bleeding, or frequent infections. Some types may develop into acute myeloid leukaemia.

MDS Alliance (https://www.mds-alliance.org) is a global health initiative that aims to ensure MDS patients, regardless of their age, have access to the best multiprofessional care. This initiative aims to provide patients and their caregivers and the healthcare team with the training tools and the information about MDS, including current treatment options.

Sarcoma Patient EuroNet

Sarcoma Patients EuroNet Association (SPAEN; https://www.sarcoma-patients.eu), the international network of sarcoma, GIST, and desmoid patient advocacy groups, was founded in April 2009 with the aim of extending information services, patient support and advocacy to patient organizations for the benefit of sarcoma patients across the whole of Europe and internationally. Acting in partnership with clinical experts, scientific researchers, industry and other stakeholders, SPAEN is working to upgrade the treatment and care of sarcoma patients through improving information and support, and by increasing the visibility of sarcoma with policymakers and the public

A sarcoma is a rare kind of cancer. Sarcomas are different from the much more common carcinomas because they happen in a different kind of tissue. Sarcomas grow in connective tissue cells that connect or support other kinds of tissue in your body. These tumours are most common in the bones, muscles, tendons, cartilage, nerves, fat, and the blood vessels of your arms and legs, but they can happen anywhere.

Although there are more than 50 types of sarcoma, they can be grouped into two main kinds: soft tissue sarcoma and bone sarcoma, or osteosarcoma.

Patient perspective in ECCO multidisciplinary educational activities

The ECCO PAC members are partners to shape policy, define essential requirements in quality cancer care, and determine how the ECCO and ECCO member organizations evolve.

The patient voice in ECCO seeks to help healthcare professionals to better understand the 'desires' of patients rather than their perceived 'needs'.

Over the past couple of years, PAC members have provided the patient perspective in its annual workshop on methods in clinical cancer research. PAC members have directly communicated what matters to patients in clinical trials to the workshop's audience of junior clinical professionals managing cancer patients and involved in actual clinical trial design.

Since 2009, the biennial European Cancer Congresses (ECCs) have included a scientific programme track entirely developed by experts from the ECCO Patient Advisory Committee. This provides a high-level and widely publicized platform at the ECCs to proactively address issues and challenges faced by cancer patients, and leads to specific recommendations.

Patient care was at the centre of the European Cancer Congress 2013. A two-day track was devoted to patient advocacy with the overall theme of 'Collaboration' among all stakeholders involved in cancer care, including patient advocates as instrumental partners in the improvement of cancer outcomes. In the following list are the key themes and thoughts that emerged from the presentations and discussions within the track:

- The culture of research in Europe needs to change to stimulate data sharing and coordination;
- The patient advocacy community needs to demonstrate the value of patient involvement;
- Adherence to treatment is strongly influenced by the doctor–patient relationship;
- More and better-designed studies are needed to arrive at specific recommendations for life after treatment (e.g. in terms of diet), ideally providing tailored advice to different patient groups;
- Other key aspects affecting a cancer patient's return to normal life are physical activity, the unlocking of creative potential, and cancer support centres treating the person and not only the cancer;

- Palliation equals alleviation of symptoms, both physical and psychological, and should be addressed earlier on in cancer care;
- Molecular stratification can be successfully integrated into the healthcare system as shown by the French molecular testing initiative;
- Healthcare professionals need to engage more closely with patients in discussing treatment options, including possible personalized treatment;
- Healthcare services should tackle the huge differences in cancer survival between men and women across Europe;
- Networks of specialized centres, accreditation schemes, and transparent quality criteria may provide robust guidance to patients and reduce the risk of inequality of access to best quality cancer care;
- For young cancer survivors, the survivorship passport should be a standard of care. The survivorship passport provides every European childhood cancer survivor a document, paper and electronic based, containing cancer history and therapy information. Furthermore, based on the medical history of each individual as summarized in the passport, follow-up recommendations are included.

At the European Cancer Congress 2015, the following key messages and recommendations were made during the patient advocacy track:

- Good communication is a central component of clinical care.
- Genetic testing may reveal inherited mutations, and is giving rise to new ethical considerations.
- Patients should demand reliable biobanking.
- Biosimilar medicines can increase access to effective biologics.
- Children have rehabilitation needs specific to their age after cancer treatment.
- There is a need for official European protocols for best practice by employers.
- Multidisciplinary teams are the cornerstone of good care. One of the main challenges now is how to include patients and GPs in multidisciplinary teams.
- Clinical trials are a significant burden to patients. Patients in clinical trials may have a wholly negative experience. The process could be improved and patients' input from the early stages of trial conception, including in internal ratings based (IRB) discussions and grant panels, will help. Ultimately, randomized trials protect patients against beliefs that have taken hold in the medical community.

Conclusions

Care that is more patient-centred brings with it not only considerations of patient preferences and convenience, but also the whole-person approach that patients seek. Bringing the patient perspective is very much about bringing the human dimension into care, as care is given to human beings and not to organs.

Patient advocacy groups have an essential advisory role in oncology professional organizations to advocate for patient-centred approaches in science, education, and healthcare policies with the ultimate goal to provide patients with the care that is of most value to them, reflects their preferences, which does not necessarily coincide with the perception of their needs by healthcare professionals.

However, patient advocacy groups face several challenges. Demands for their involvement are growing in all types of healthcare organizations (professional organizations, regulatory agencies, pharmaceutical and medical equipment companies, and others) while the number of expert patients/patient advocates is limited. Their work is usually not remunerated and therefore many patient advocacy groups face issues of sustainability. Funding from pharmaceutical companies must be handled carefully to keep credibility and independence from commercial interests.

Adequate, significant, and valuable input from patient advocates will also come with the development of technical/medical knowledge in the areas where opportunities exist for patient advocates involvement. However, educational opportunities for patient advocates to develop their expertise in the different areas of care are limited. The European Patients' Academy (EUPATI) is a rare and good example of patient education on medicine development.

References

1. **Rubin, G., Berendsen, A., Crawford, S. M., et al.** (2015) The expanding role of primary care in cancer control. *The Lancet Oncology Commission*, **16**, 1231–72.
2. **Ben-Arye, E., Samuels, N.** (2015) Patient centered care in lung cancer: exploring the next milestones. *Transl Lung Cancer Res*, **4**, 630–34.
3. **Weeks, J. C., Catalano, P. J., Cronin, A., et al.** (2012) Patients' expectations about effects of chemotherapy for advanced cancer. *N Engl J Med*, **367**, 1616–25.
4. **Bravo, P., Edwards, A., James Barr, P. J., Scholl, I., Elwyn, G., McAllister, M., and the Cochrane Healthcare Quality Research Group**. (2015) Conceptualising patient empowerment: a mixed methods study. *Health Serv Res*, **15**, 252.
5. **Albreht, T., Kiasuwa, R., Van den Bulcke, M.** (2017) *European Guide on Quality Improvement in Comprehensive Cancer Control*. Ljubljana: National Institute of Public Health.

Chapter 12

Advocacy for neurology in migrants

Mustapha El Alaoui Faris

Introduction

International migration is a reflection of the world, resulting from the dynamics generated by changes in political, economic, and cultural structures. It reflects the advent of an interdependent world, stimulating new cultural and economic exchanges, contributing to the social reconfiguration of host and departure societies and the reconfiguration of national, social, and family assets within and beyond states.[1] Respect for migrants' right to healthcare reflects the acceptance of migrant populations in host societies. Migrants are both a vital demographic contribution in countries with an ageing population and their contribution to the economies of host countries is undeniable, although they are often confined to difficult and low-paid jobs.

Migrants have more health problems than the populations of the host country. They are more vulnerable to communicable diseases, maternal and child health problems, and mental disorders, but also to some non-communicable diseases such as diabetes or obesity. However, they seem to have fewer cancers. The prevalence of neurological diseases remains largely unknown among migrants.

Advocacy for the health of migrants must go through the development of legal rights and the application of existing legal provisions in the field of migration. A comprehensive policy for the health of migrants must take into account the special health needs of women and children and those of recent and second-generation migrants. Legal protection of the health rights of the most vulnerable migrants (undocumented migrants and asylum seekers) should be a priority at national and international levels.

Migration and health

Humanity has always known the migration of populations from one region to another. Recent migration, especially after World War II, was guided by several rules. First, migrants who are often from poor rural areas migrate for economic reasons to a richer border country (e.g. Italians and Spanish migrated to France, Mexicans to the United States). Secondly, migrations were also guided by the former colonial relations and by the fact that migrants could speak the language of the host country (e.g. the West sub-Saharan African migrates to France, the Indo-Pakistanis to the United Kingdom). Since the beginning of the twenty-first century migration has changed; in fact, 'in the past we migrated to survive, today we migrate to realize ourselves' wrote Philippe Fagues, director of the European Union Migration Policy centre (quoted in [2]). Currently, it is the educated middle classes endowed with high human capital and skills who migrate. These middle classes are increasingly numerous worldwide. The other migrant group whose numbers are constantly increasing are the students who go to study in a Western country and often do not return to their country of origin. Migration can have other causes such as political crises or civil wars in some parts of the world, as currently in the Middle East (Syria and Iraq), or the Sahel region in sub-Saharan Africa. In the near future, two particular situations will play an essential role in the migration of people around the world. First, climate change could create enormous refugee flows; and the ageing of the populations in the Western countries which, because of their low fertility and for obvious economic reasons, will need the immigrants from low- and middle-income countries (LMICs).[2]

The health of migrants is a global phenomenon that affects several million in the world. In this chapter we will mainly discuss the health conditions of migrants in Europe, especially those from the Middle East and Africa.

Health information systems in most European countries are generally not designed to identify people according to their migration status and the data collected in medical records rarely includes such information. The main exception in many European countries is mortality registers, which often include migration indicators. National death registers allowing correlations by migrant status for cardiovascular disease and diabetes exist in the majority of these countries. On the other hand, registries identifying the use of healthcare at national or regional level by migrants are only available in a few European countries. Thus, available data on the health of migrants in Europe are currently insufficient, making it difficult to identify the health problems of migrants and to develop prevention and care policies adapted to the immigrant population.

Difficulties in collecting information on the health of migrants include conceptual and methodological challenges, such as different definitions or understandings of who constitutes a migrant. Political sensitivities also exist, particularly around the collection of ethnic data that may be useful for understanding health problems. The data on health migrants may differ from one country to another. In France, for example, in accordance with the principle of the indivisibility of the Republic, routine data collection systems such as the national census refer only to nationality and country of birth and do not specify ethnic or religion of migrants. In Germany, no ethnic data are officially collected, partly because of the fear that such data may give rise to memories of the categorizations used within the framework of National Socialism and could be misused to incite racism and discrimination. In the Netherlands, data on the place of birth of migrant parents and grandparents are collected.

Most migrant health studies focus on differences with non-migrant populations in host countries. Migrants are often (at least initially) healthier than non-migrant populations in their host country (the so-called health effect of migrants) in particular because the act of migration usually requires good health. However, migrants face particular health problems, although some only become apparent after a long period. Where migrant health data are available, as in several Western European countries, they often point to contradictory directions due to the diversity of migrants in terms of age, sex, country of origin and destination, socioeconomic status, and type of migration.

In fact, many health gaps between migrants and non-migrants may disappear after controlling for socioeconomic status. However, the determinants of health have focused on socioeconomic factors, but largely ignored the role of migration which, due to the associated social exclusion processes, can be also a social determinant of health.

There are remarkable differences in health between migrants and non-migrants. Migrants appear to be more vulnerable to diabetes, communicable diseases, maternal and child health problems, occupational health risks, injuries, and poor mental health. These differences may have several explanations; for example, more frequent health risk factors, and higher prevalence of certain diseases in the country of origin (e.g. communicable diseases), difficulties in early childhood (e.g. poverty and malnutrition), poor living conditions in the host country, precarious and dangerous work, and psychological constraints related to the migration process.

Migrants face many barriers to accessing health services. In order to overcome these barriers, governments of host countries will need to decide on the appropriate balance between targeting patients (demand) and providers (supply). On the demand side, migrants may benefit from better information on health services and entitlements, as well as from education programmes to improve health literacy.[3] On the supply side, migrants often require extra interventions to ensure access. This typically involves improving the cultural competence of providers.

Neurology in migrants

Prior to the implementation of measures such as the disability-adjusted life year (DALY), the global burden of disease was primarily quantified in terms of mortality. With the advent of the DALY, the importance of neurological and psychiatric disorders became evident, accounting for approximately 28% of the global burden of disease.[4] The burden of neurological and psychiatric diseases in LMICs is very high.[5] The burden of neurological and psychiatric disorders in migrants coming from LMICs is probably as high as that in the countries of origin. But the weight of each disease would be different depending on the country of origin.[6] Many of the differences are explained by the wide variation in demography, culture, epidemiology, poverty, and genetics of different countries.[7] Adult migrants from LMICs who may have experienced early deprivation in their infancy and childhood are particularly vulnerable to subsequent neurological disorders and may still have a higher susceptibility to neurological and psychiatric illness that are reflective of the socioeconomic environment.[7,8] However, there is little statistical data available for the incidence and prevalence of different neurological diseases among migrant populations.[9]

Infectious diseases in migrants

Migrants have more infectious diseases than people from the host countries.[10] Tuberculosis has seen a re-emergence in Europe and is concentrated among migrants. It can cause neurological complications such as meningitis or intracerebral tuberculomas. Migrants arriving from North Africa and sub-Saharan Africa carry higher rates of hepatitis C and B which can be complicated by peripheral neuropathies. The prevalence of human immunodeficiency virus (HIV) is very high in sub-Saharan Africa migrants to Europe but the prevalence is very low in North African migrants. Sub-Saharan Africa migrants may have resistant profiles to HIV drugs,[11] and develop AIDS with cognitive disorders more frequently probably because of low economic status of sub-Saharan Africa migrants.[12,13] The diagnosis of these disorders requires cognitive tests adapted to the language and culture of the migrants.[14]

Epilepsy in migrants

Epilepsy affects quality-of-life in patients and their caregivers and can result in high societal costs through loss of work productivity and high medical care expenditures.[15] Cultural and religious beliefs in many developing countries, from which the majority of migrants originate, could make epilepsy underdiagnosed and often untreated. Incidence of epilepsy is higher because of the prevalence of brain birth injury and the frequency of neurocysticercosis in this population.[16]

The stigma against epileptic patients in some migrant communities must be taken into account in the care of epileptic patients.[17] Since the diagnosis of seizures for complex partial epilepsy is essentially based on patient questioning, if the patient does not speak the language of the host country and the neurologist does not understand the language of the patient, the diagnosis of epileptic seizure becomes hazardous and the epilepsy will be underdiagnosed.[18] An approximate and unclear medical history can take temporal seizures for psychiatric manifestations and direct the patient to the psychiatrist instead of the neurologist. Because myoclonus which is rarely spontaneously reported by patients will cause juvenile myoclonic epilepsy to be confused with generalized epilepsy, treatment with carbamazepine will increase the number of seizures and aggravate the condition of the patient.[19]

Multiple sclerosis in migrants

Some studies of multiple sclerosis (MS) have shown that migration from high-risk area to low-risk area at the beginning of life leads the reduction of MS risk. Evidence that migration in the opposite direction—from low-risk area to high-risk area—increases the risk of MS seems less obvious.[20] Several studies have shown that MS is much more severe in North African migrants than in the native French population.[21] These patients often present motor deficit or ataxia at the beginning of the disease and rapidly reach a progressive phase with permanent handicap. We also noted this finding in Moroccan patients with MS. The severity of MS in North Africans may require the use of second-line immunomodulatory treatments early in the course of their disease.

Behçet's disease in migrants

The prevalence of Behçet's disease is high in the native population of northern Africa and the Middle East but is rare in Europe. The neurological complications of Behçet's disease are little known by European neurologists, so the disease cannot be diagnosed in a migrant, especially since biological markers are not available and the diagnosis is based essentially on clinical features such as oral and genital aphthae.[22] European neurologists must be aware of the neurological disorders of Behçet's disease, which are suggestive of mesencephalo-diencephalic lesions well-identified by cerebral MRI.[23,24] The delay in the treatment of neurological complications can lead to severe motor and cognitive disorders.[25]

Neurogenetic diseases in migrants

Consanguinity and health in migrants

Consanguinity is widely practised in many parts of the world including North Africa, the Middle East, and South Asia. In fact, it has been estimated that couples related as second cousin or closer and their children account for 10% of the global population.[26,27]

The frequency of consanguinity in some migrant populations can be responsible for the high prevalence of some hereditary diseases with autosomal recessive transmission, usually rare in European countries. Woodcock et al.[28] found that children of Pakistani origin living in Yorkshire (United Kingdom) had three times more neuromuscular disorders than indigenous English children. Given the high prevalence of inbreeding in the North African population, some ataxias rare in European population are more frequent in North African migrants.[29] Consanguinity can also increase some psychiatric disorders, such as bipolar disorder in Egypt.[30]

Parkinsonism due to the *LRRK2* gene

The frequency of specific gene in a given population must be known in order to correctly diagnose and treat particular genetic diseases. For example, in the North African population, Parkinson's disease due to the mutation of the *LRRK2* gene is present in more than 30% of the patients. These patients are often young and have severe levodopa-induced dyskinesias, which should be treated by dopaminergic agonists and delay as far as possible the use of L-dopa.[31] The possibility of making a diagnosis at an asymptomatic stage and being able to follow the evolution of the disease by cerebral imaging will be a great contribution to the understanding of the pathophysiology of Parkinson's disease. Parkinson's disease due to the mutation of the *LRRK2* gene is a good example of the scientific contribution of a disease common in a given migrant population but otherwise rare.[32]

Stroke in migrants

Stroke is a real public health problem in migrants who are often from LMICs. Epidemiological studies show that due to the ongoing epidemiological transition, the stroke incidence in these countries is constantly increasing and constitutes a real global health problem. Given the high frequency of vascular risk factors in migrants such as hypertension, diabetes, obesity and smoking, and rapid acculturation and lifestyle change, migrants can have severe stroke at younger age with high mortality and persistent neurological disability.[33] Specific attention must be paid to the prevention of vascular risk factors, health education, and better lifestyle for migrants of first and second generations.

Migrants from sub-Saharan Africa or Asia may have specific causes of stroke that are very rare in Western countries, such as rheumatic heart disease that can cause severe stroke of permanent neurological disability in young adults.[34] The frequency of sickle cell anaemia in the sub-Saharan countries such as Nigeria should be known by neurologists and paediatricians in the host countries. These children require regular monitoring by transcranial echosonography to diagnose and monitor possible intracerebral vessel stenosis. This stenosis must be treated by repeated blood transfusions according to specific protocols in order to avoid the occurrence of stroke.[35] Migrants with cardiovascular disease or stroke may not have adequate treatment as reported in Bengalis patients with acute myocardial infarction[36] or in Mexican migrants in the United States with acute stroke who seem to be less likely to benefit from a treatment with thrombolysis.[37]

Cognitive disorders in ageing migrants

Another aspect of migrant neurology is the ageing of migrant population, with an increasing number having now reached the point where they are likely to have cognitive disorders. The elderly migrants sharing the same risk factors as older people in their home countries[38,39] have a higher likelihood of vascular dementia in addition to Alzheimer's disease.[40] However, cognitive disorders in elderly migrants are often underdiagnosed.[41] These people are usually of non-Western origin and are not fluent in the language of the host country. In such cases, the diagnosis of cognitive disorders requires specific neuropsychological tests adapted for every given population.[42] The care of migrants with cognitive disorders must take into account the cultural and religious beliefs of these patients. Moreover, it should not be forgotten that these patients may be subject to stigma.[43]

Advocacy for health in migrants

- Ask all European countries with a large population of migrants in their populations to adopt specific policies on the health of migrants.[44] Although there have been several attempts to put the health of migrants on the European political agenda, in particular during the Portuguese and Spanish presidencies of the Council of the European Union,[45] this has not led to any significant changes in the European countries' national regulations regarding the health of migrants. Thus, of 25 European countries, only 11 have adopted specific policies for the health of migrants at the national level.[44]
- Strengthen the legislative basis for protection of the rights of the most vulnerable migrants (undocumented migrants and asylum seekers) at the national level and to ensure their implementation.
- One of the major obstacles to the access of migrants to health services in Europe is the inadequacy of legislation on the health rights of migrants and the lack of political will to apply the existing one.[44]
- Ensure that international and European organizations, such as the International Organization for Migration, World Health Organization, and the Council of the European Union, play a crucial role in the commitment to the health of migrants.[46,47]

- Support non-governmental organizations and health professionals in Europe who defend the right to care for undocumented migrants and asylum seekers despite a difficult political context, and the passivity or even hostility of certain European governments.[48]
- Provide migrants with information about health and the health system of their host country in their own language.[49]
- Target language barriers in service delivery by the use of easily accessible and free professional interpreting services and train health workers in using them.
- Improve the health literacy of migrants through targeted health promotion interventions that take account of the different ways in which people perceive and experience health problems.
- Collect data on migration health status (e.g. country of birth, self-reported ethnic origin, nationality) accounting for the fact that migrants do not form a homogeneous population, but exhibit major variations according to religion, culture, language, ethnic origin, country of origin, and destination. The data on social determinants of health in migrants must also be considered.
- Collect data on neurological and psychiatric disorders in migrants by conducting epidemiological surveys on the incidence and prevalence of epilepsy, stroke, cognitive disorders in older people, neurological complications of infectious diseases and neurogenetic diseases.
- Appropriate genetic counselling should be provided to families who have had a child with neurogenetic disease, particularly in the case of parental consanguinity. Genetic counselling must take into account the language and culture of the parents, so that they understand the mechanism of the disease and prevent other children being affected.
- The rights of migrant women should be legally protected and they should have access to legal services and remedies, for instance, in reporting violence and workplace complaints. Legal services should be gender sensitive, and linguistically and culturally accessible and appropriate.
- Inclusion of all migrant children in existing paediatric programmes, to promote general immunization and to recognize potential risks for violence against children or harmful practices (including female genital mutation) and facilitate access to social services.
- A specific programme should prioritize the improvement of mental and neurological healthcare for migrants and ethnic minorities.

Recommendations

- All host countries should develop specific national policies aimed at improving migrant health. A transnational migrant health policy at the European Union scale will be a guarantee for health rights for migrants.
- Europe should tackle the considerable health inequalities between migrant and non-migrant people in different European countries by targeting specific obstacles

in accessing health services such as lack of information, cultural and linguistic barriers, and socioeconomic deprivation.
- Develop a strategy to combat discrimination in access to health services according to the culture or ethnicity of the migrants by allowing an intercultural opening up of the health system to identify the health needs of migrants.
- Collect data regarding different causes of mortality and morbidity in migrants according to age, genre, and socioeconomic level, and comparing these data with those of the host country and those of the country of origin.
- Migrant health policies can be targeted either for migrants in general but also on specific migrant groups, such as asylum seekers or undocumented immigrants.
- Policy should consider country of birth and to distinguish between different migrants and their descendants. Special policies should target the specific health need of second- and third-generation migrants. Particular attention should be paid to newly arrived migrants who can have specific health needs.
- Migrant women's human rights should be protected, and migrants provided with access to services and resources such as health, legal, and financial services. Governments should ratify international treaties and conventions promoting rights and protections for migrant women, as well as promote non-discrimination and women's access to labour markets.
- Generalize immunization to all immigrant children and integrate them into national child protection programmes.
- Prevention and treatment of neurological and psychiatric diseases should be a priority.
- The increasing importance of older migrants and the resulting need to develop culturally appropriate long-term care is another area that must be a priority.

Conclusion

The international community and the European Union should develop legal policies to guarantee the migrant's right to access the health system of host countries. This policy should target the obstacles to improvement of migrant health, such as lack of information, cultural and linguistic barriers, and socioeconomic disadvantages. Special attention should be given to women, children, recent and second-generation migrants; each of these groups may have specific health needs. Prevention of neurological and psychiatric disorders should be a priority.

References

1. **Mazzella, S.** (2016) *Sociologie des Migrations (Sociology of Migration)*. Paris: Editions des Presses Universitaires de France.
2. **Le Bras, H.** (2017) *L'âge des Migrations (Age of Migration)*. Paris: Editions Autrement, Paris.
3. **Netto, G., Bhopal, R., Lederle, N., Khatoon, J., Jackson, A.** (2010) How can health promotion interventions be adapted for minority ethnic communities? Five principles for guiding the development of behavioural interventions. *Health Prom Int*, **25**, 248–57.

4. **Whiteford, H. A., Alize, J., Ferrari, A. J., Degenhardt, L., Feigin, V., Vos, T.** (2013) Global burden of disease attributable to mental and substance use disorders: findings from the Global Burden of Disease Study 2010. *Lancet*, **382**, 1575–86.
5. **Gretchen, G. L., Meyer, A. N., Ogunniyi, A.** (2015) Nervous system disorders across the life course in resource-limited settings. *Nature*, **527**, S167–71.
6. **Ravindranath, V., Dang, H. M., Goya, R. G., et al.** (2015) Regional research priorities in brain and nervous system disorders. *Nature*, **527**, S198–S206.
7. **Bergen, D. C., Silberberg, D.** (2002) Nervous system disorders: a global epidemic. *Arch Neurol*, **59**, 1194–6.
8. **Davidson, L. L., Grigorenko, L. E., Boivin, M. J., Rapa, E., Stein, A.** (2015) A focus on adolescence to reduce neurological, mental health and substance-use disability. *Nature*, **527**, S161–6.
9. **Rinaldi, F., Nembrini, S., Concoreggi, C., Magon, M., Padovani, A.** (2016) Neurological diseases and health care utilization among first-generation immigrants. *J Neurol*, **263**(4), 714–21.
10. **Khyatti, M., Trimbitas, R. D., Zouheir, Y., Benani, A., El Messaoudi, M. D., Hemminki, K.** (2014) Infectious diseases in North Africa and North African immigrants to Europe European. *Eur J Public Health*, **24** Suppl 1, 47–56.
11. **The Antiretroviral Therapy Cohort Collaboration (ART-CC)** (2013) Higher rates of AIDS during the first year of antiretroviral therapy among migrants: the importance of tuberculosis. *AIDS*, **27**, 1321–9.
12. **Heaton, R. K., Clifford, D. B., FranklinJr., D. R., et al.** (2010) HIV-associated neurocognitive disorders persist in the era of potent antiretroviral therapy: CHARTER Study. *Neurology*, **75**(23), 2087–96.
13. **Birbeck, G. L., Kvalsund, M. P., Byers, P. A., et al.** (2011) Neuropsychiatric and socioeconomic status impact of antiretroviral adherence and mortality in rural Zambia. *Am J Trop Med Hyg*, **85**, 782–9.
14. **van Wijk, C.** (2013) Screening for HIV-associated, neurocognitive disorders (HANDs) in South Africa: a caution against uncritical use of comparative data from other developing countries. *S Afr J HIV Med*, **14**(1), 17–19.
15. **Asato, M. R., Caplan, R., Hermann, B. P.** (2014) Epilepsy and comorbidities—what are we waiting for? *Epilepsy Behav*, **31**, 127–8.
16. **Burneo, J. G., Cavazos, J. E.** (2015) Neurocysticercosis and epilepsy. *Epilepsy Currents*, **14** (1 Suppl), 23–8.
17. **Fiest, K. M., Birbeck, G. L., Jacoby, A., Jette, N.** (2014) Stigma in epilepsy. *Curr Neurol Neurosci Rep*, **14**(5), 444.
18. **Elafros, M. A., Mulenga, J., Mbewe, E., et al.** (2013) Peer support groups as an intervention to decrease epilepsy-associated stigma. *Epilepsy Behav*, **27**, 188–92.
19. **Genton, P., Gelisse, P., Thomas, P., Dravet, C.** (2000) Do carbamazepine and phenytoin aggravate juvenile myoclonic epilepsy? *Neurology*, **55**, 1106–1109.
20. **Alter, M., Kahana, E., Loewenson, R.** (1978) Migration and risk of multiple sclerosis. *Neurology*, **28**(11), 1089–93.
21. **Debouverie, M., Lebrun, C., Jeannin, S., Pittion-Vouyovitch, S., Roederer, T., Vespignani, H.** (2007) More severe disability of North Africans vs Europeans with multiple sclerosis in France. *Neurology*, **68**, 29–33.
22. **International Study Group for Behçet's Disease** (1990) Criteria for diagnosis of Behçet's disease. *Lancet*, **335**, 1078–80.

23. **Sefiani, D.** (2008) Neurological manifestations of Behçet's disease: study of 161 cases. Graduate Diploma in Neurology 2008. Rabat, Morocco: School of Medicine, Mohamed-V University.
24. **Aïdi, S., Benabdeljlil, M., El Alaoui Faris, M.** (2016) Neurological manifestations of Behçet disease. In: Chopra, J. S., Sawhney, I. M. S. (eds). *Neurology in Tropics*, 2nd edition. New Delhi, India: Elsevier, pp. 788–97.
25. **El Alaoui Faris, M., Rahmani, M., Boutbib, F., Aïdi, S., Benabdeljlil, M.** (2009) Neuro-Behçet's dementia: neuropsychological study of 12 cases. *J Neurol Sci*, **285**(S1), S155–339.
26. **Bittles, A. H., Black, M. L.** (2010) Evolution in health and medicine Sackler colloquium: consanguinity, human evolution, and complex diseases. *Proc Natl Acad Sci USA*, **107**(Suppl 1), 1779–86.
27. **Anwar, W. A., Khyatti, M., Hemminki, K.** (2014) Consanguinity and genetic diseases in North Africa and immigrants to Europe. *Eur J Public Health*, **24** Suppl 1, 57–63.
28. **Woodcock, I. R., Fraser, L., Norman, P., Pysden, K., Manning, S., Childs, A. M.** (2016) The prevalence of neuromuscular disease in the paediatric population in Yorkshire: variation by ethnicity and deprivation status. *Dev Med Child Neurol*, **58**(8), 877–83.
29. **El Euch-Fayache, G., Bouhlal, Y., Amouri, R., Feki, M., Hentati, F.** (2014) Molecular, clinical and peripheral neuropathy study of Tunisian patients with ataxia with vitamin E deficiency. *Brain*, **137**(Pt 2), 402–10.
30. **Mansour, H., Klei, L., Wood, J., et al.** (2009) Consanguinity associated with increased risk for bipolar I disorder in Egypt. *Am J Med Genet B Neuropsychiatr Genet*, **150B**(6), 879–85.
31. **Healy, D. G., Falchi, M., O'Sullivan, S. S., et al.** (2008) Genotype, and worldwide genetic penetrance of LRRK2-associated Parkinson's disease: a case-control study. *Lancet Neurol*, **7**(7), 583–90.
32. **Wile, D. J., Agarwal, P. A., Schulzer, M., et al.** (2017) Serotonin and dopamine transporter PET changes in the premotor phase of LRRK2 parkinsonism: cross-sectional studies. *Lancet Neurol*, **16**(5), 351–9.
33. **Ntsekhe, M., Damasceno, A.** (2013) Recent advances in the epidemiology, outcome, and prevention of myocardial infarction and stroke in sub-Saharan Africa. *Heart*, **99**, 1230–5.
34. **Wang, D., Liua, M., Lin, S., et al.** (2013) Stroke and rheumatic heart disease: a systematic review of observational studies. *Clin Neurol Neurosurg*, **115**, 1575–82.
35. **Galadanci, N. A., Abdullahi, S. U., Tabari, M. A., et al.** (2015) Primary stroke prevention in Nigerian children with sickle cell disease (SPIN): challenges of conducting a feasibility trial. *Pediat Blood Cancer*, **62**, 395–401.
36. **Barakat, K., Wells, Z., Ramdhany, S., Mills, P. G., Timmis, A. D.** (2003) Bangladeshi patients present with non-classic features of acute myocardial infarction and are treated less aggressively in east London, UK. *Heart*, **89**, 276–9.
37. **Hassan, A. E., Kassel, D. H., Adil, M. A., Tekle, W. G., Qureshi, A. I.** (2016) Are there disparities in thrombolytic treatment and mortality in acute ischemic stroke in the Hispanic population living in border states versus nonborder states? *J Vasc Interv Neurol*, **9**(2), 1–4.
38. **Bergen, D. C.** (2008) Effects of poverty on cognitive function: a hidden neurologic epidemic. *Neurology*, **71**, 447–51.
39. **Whalley, L. J., Dick, F. D., McNeill, G. A.** (2006) Life-course approach to the aetiology of late-onset dementias. *Lancet Neurol*, **5**(1), 87–96.

40. **Kalaria, R. N., Maestre, G. E., Arizaga, R., et al.** (2008) Alzheimer's disease and vascular dementia in developing countries: prevalence, management, and risk factors. *Lancet Neurol*, **7**(9), 812–26.
41. **Nielsen, T. R., Vogel, A., Phung, T. K. T., Gade, A., Waldemar, G.** (2011) Over- and under-diagnosis of dementia in ethnic minorities: a nationwide register-based study. *Int J Geriatr Psychiatry*, **26**, 1128–35.
42. **Goudsmit, M., Uysal-Bozkir, O., Parlecliet, J. L., et al.** (2016) The cross-cultural dementia screening (CCD): a new neuropsychological screening instrument for dementia in elderly immigrants. *J Clin Exp Neuropsychol*, **39**(2), 163–72.
43. **Liu, D., Hinton, L., Tran, C., Hinton, D., Barker, J. D.** (2008) Re-examining the relationships among dementia, stigma, and aging in immigrant Chinese and Vietnamese family caregivers. *J Cross Cult Gerontol*, **23**(3), 283–99.
44. **Pace, P.** (2011) The right to health of migrants in Europe. In: Rechel, B., Mladovsky, P., Devillé, W., et al. (eds). *Migration and Health in the European Union*. Maidenhead: Open University Press, pp. 55–66.
45. **Peiro, M.-J., Benedict, R.** (2010) Migrant health policy: the Portuguese and Spanish EU presidencies. *Eurohealth*, **16**, 1–4.
46. **Gushulak, B.** (2010) Monitoring migrants' health. In: **WHO** (ed.). *Health of Migrants— The Way Forward*. Report of a global consultation, Madrid, Spain, 3–5 March 2010. Geneva: World Health Organization, pp. 28–42.
47. **World Health Assembly** (2008) *Health of Migrants, Resolution 61.17*. Geneva: World Health Organization.
48. **Björngren-Cuadra, C.** (2010) *Policies on Health Care for Undocumented Migrants in EU27*. Country report Spain. Malmö: Malmö University.
49. **Ingleby, D.** (2011) Good practice in health service provision for migrants. In: Rechel, B., Mladovsky, P., Devillé, W., et al. (eds). *Migration and Health in the European Union*. Maidenhead: Open University Press, pp. 227–42.

Chapter 13

Advocacy for neurology: Local, regional, and national

Apoorva Pauranik

Introduction

The need for neurologists to get seriously involved in advocacy for their own profession and their patients cannot be overemphasized. Sadly, they fail on many accounts—their conviction, motivation, and imagination. There are myriad ways of doing advocacy. Some action plans may appear simple and trivial while others may be highly ambitious and challenging.[1]

There are stark contrasts between countries when it comes to the state of neurology services and education. The well-known reasons are historical, developmental, economical, ecological, and cultural. A wise reader sifting through this book's various sections will instantly realize that the limitations and roadblocks are more insurmountable in developing countries. It will also be apparent that neurology advocates and national neurology associations in developing countries have resorted to ingenious ways of advocacy. Accordingly, the priorities and models of advocacy will also differ. It is not an ideal world and will never be, but advocates for neurology will always be harbingers of hope.

Education and Awareness

Education is the single most effective tool for empowerment of patients, families, and healthcare providers. Increasing rates of literacy and the spread of media and the Internet have fuelled an insatiable hunger in the minds of people for more information about health. The right to health, good quality medical care, and relevant information are being recognized as fundamental. People are expected to take greater control of their lives. Enlightened social activism in the field of health is an encouraging phenomenon.

Public Neurology Education

The main aim of public neurology education (PNE) is the dissemination of neurological disease related knowledge to the widest possible number of people in the maximum possible detail and formats (see Box 13.1).

> **Box 13.1 Some examples of public neurology education (PNE)**
>
> - Polio vaccination drive in areas where it had been difficult to eliminate.
> - Iodized salt where hypothyroidism and mental retardation are endemic.
> - Awareness about warning symptoms of stroke and need for emergency treatment.
> - Persuading bikers to use crash helmets.
> - Messages about epilepsy—that it is common, treatable, non-contagious, not necessarily hereditary, not insanity, and not incompatible with employment, marriage, and parenthood.
> - Messages about dementia—that it is common, should be recognized early, need for compassionate care.
> - Learning disabilities, mental retardation, autism—that these conditions are common, need special care, and can be improved.
> - Neurological disabilities—that these are common, can be ameliorated to varying extent, physical and occupation therapy help, rehabilitation can be organized.

PNE has to be prioritized with respect to community burden, social and economic impact, myths and stigma, gaps in diagnosis and treatment, and potential for prevention. Its core messages should be crisp, brief, and salient.

Individual neurologists have been imparting PNE by radio, television, newspapers, magazines, and lectures. However neurology associations at regional and national levels may be in a better position to develop good-quality PNE material. Advertising consultants may be hired and government agencies can be approached for mass awareness and public education. In many countries, there are laws mandating a certain small percentage of airtime on radio and television channels to be set aside for disseminating public service announcements or messages of public interest.

Sadly this social responsibility is often overlooked by broadcasters.[2] It would be a triumph if individual neurologists or their associations are able to muster their advocacy skills in leveraging this provision.[3]

Neurology education for targeted groups

Apart from the general public there are many special interest groups that are potential targets for neurology education. The content and emphasis will vary with each group.

Neurology education for patients and their caregivers

In contrast to PNE, Patient Education (PE) can relate to common as well as rare disorders. It is not addressed through mass media, nor distributed randomly in a wide manner, but channelled selectively to persons suffering from specific ailments and facing specific disease-related issues.

An individual neurologist at the local level contributes by keeping a variety of handouts and brochures at his/her clinic or office related to common neurological diseases (Fig. 13.1). Many core messages can be displayed on LED screens in the waiting room of his/her clinic.

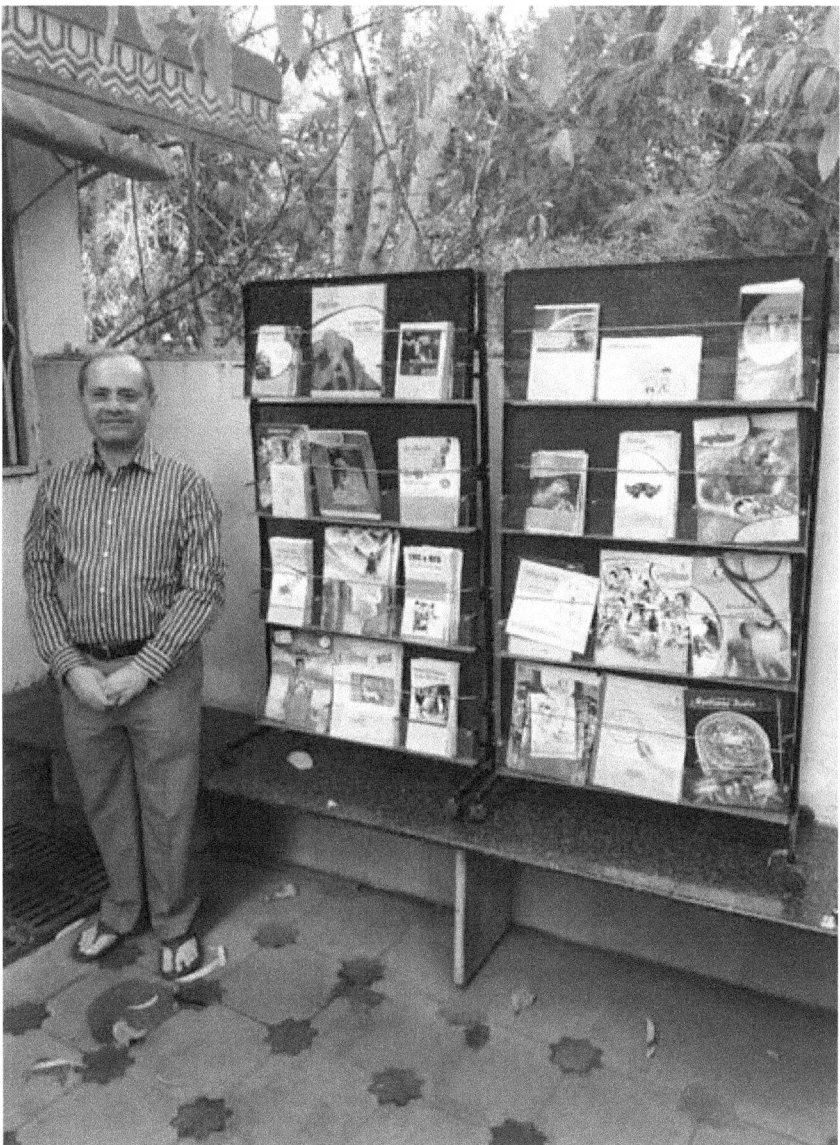

Fig. 13.1 The author with a display of brochures on neurology education.

> **Box 13.2 The main attributes of good PNE and PE literature**
>
> 1. Quality—authenticity, up-to-date, readability, engaging style.
> 2. Quantity—abundant and flowing.
> 3. Size—ranging from a few punch lines on a poster, a small paragraph on a flyer, a couple of pages in a brochure, a booklet to a full-length book.
> 4. Complexity and detail—from basic facts to simple scientific understanding to elaborate detail. Never underestimate the intelligence and interest of recipients.
> 5. Local languages—indigenous writers rooted in the culture and idiom of languages are needed.
> 6. Layout—good-quality paper, print, colours, graphics, formatting.
> 7. Electronic format—digital text, audio and video (online and offline).
> 8. Distribution—the literature must reach far and wide, up to remote areas, and in a sustained manner.

A wide variety of PE literature should also be displayed prominently in the outpatient waiting lounge, reception and registration counters, and consulting rooms of doctors and counsellors. Full-length books are also useful and should be available, perhaps for a small price (Box 13.2).

Neurology education for undergraduate and postgraduate medical students

It will be an important achievement of advocacy for neurology if a large number of students/doctors in training at undergraduate (UG) postgraduate (PG) levels develop interest in the subject and choose it as career option.[4] Even a slightly enhanced interest in and knowledge about neurology will always be welcome. The neurology component of medical education at the basic level should be high standard, evidence based, updated, and provided by trained and committed neurology faculty. Sadly, in many medical schools this responsibility is borne by internists or non-neurologists.

The National Neurology Association should oversee the development of a well-structured syllabus (theory and practical) for UG and PG students. Its drafts and recommendations should be regularly sent to medical education authorities at state and national levels.[5] Neurologists interested in teaching may offer their services as visiting lecturers to medical schools, where trained neurology faculties are not available.

The awareness and popularity of neurosciences among UG/PG medical students at local, regional, and national levels can be enhanced by an annual neurology quiz with attractive prizes (Figs. 13.2 and 13.3).

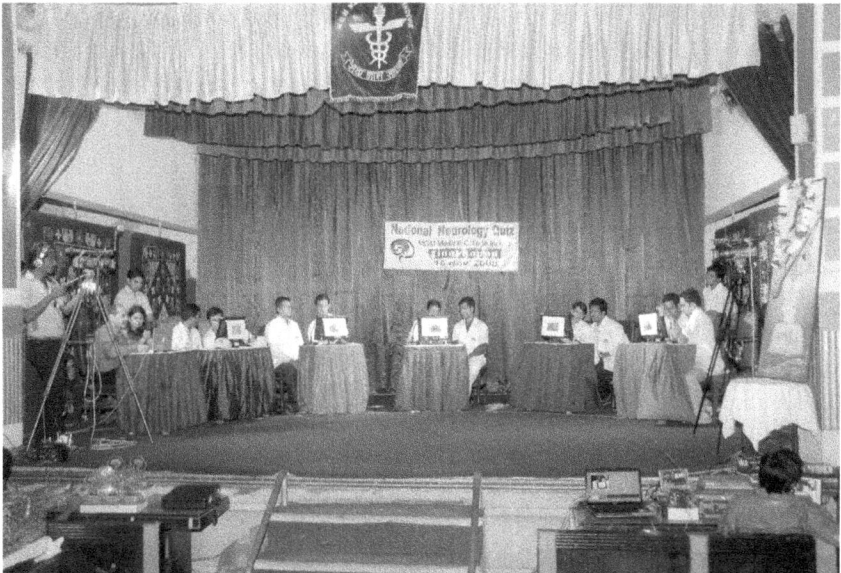

Fig. 13.2 The National Neurology Quiz for UG/PG medical students, at Indore, India.

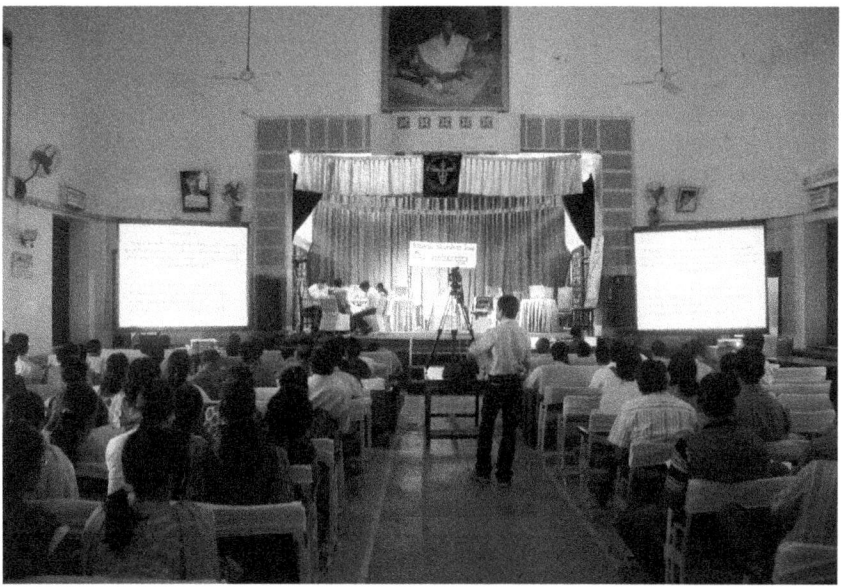

Fig. 13.3 The National Neurology Quiz for UG/PG medical students, at Indore, India.

Neurology education for internists and primary care physicians

The National Neurology Association must conduct a well-structured, focused, practical, and utilitarian update in neurology for internists and other non-neurologists.[6] A system must be put in place for CME-accreditation and certification for trainees as well as trainers. Outreach training can also be implemented through web-based self-assessment courses and mailings.

Neurology awareness for the media

Neurologists need to learn the skills of engaging with media. Clinicians and researchers should be able to talk and write about their work in an interesting and lucid manner. We need to shed our inertia, shyness, timidity, and lack of confidence when it comes to using media for advocacy.

Media is crucially important for awareness and type of information about any given neurological condition. For example, aphasia occurs as a long-term disability in about one-fourth to one-third of survivors of stroke. But few people know that it exists, let alone what it entails to have aphasia.[7]

A study investigated the quantity of aphasia-related news in the written media and compared it to Parkinson's disease (PD), multiple sclerosis, and muscular dystrophy. Aphasia was mentioned only once for every 27 PD-related articles. The amount of grants for research by foundations was skewed in similar proportions.[8]

The quality of information in media is also relevant. Often it lacks detail regarding the condition's complex nature, its effects on the person and their family, recovery, and rehabilitation. Media tends to focus on dramatic aspects.[9]

Neurologists should be vigilant about the ways and manner in which the media portrays myths and negative images about neurological diseases. We need to point out the fallacies and educate them in a decentralized manner through individual neurologists, and in a centralized manner through our National Neurology Association.

Sadly, unscrupulous practitioners, more so from so-called alternative systems of medicine, use media for ulterior motives. As a negative example, I want to mention the story of a self-proclaimed practitioner of Ayurveda in India, who portrayed himself as a saviour of patients with epilepsy through an expensive advertisement campaign. The National Neurology Association should take a united action against such quacks on multiple fronts. The same applies to charlatans who sell dreams in the name of stem cell therapy for many neurological disorders.[10]

Neurology institutes at local level and the National Neurology Association at national level must set up press offices, whereby trained writers will be able to influence which science and neurology stories will be picked by the media.

School children and teachers

Any advocacy effort will have a longer lasting multiplier effect if it is addressed to younger generations. Our issues must be chosen carefully, so that our input is not perceived as an extra burden.

Epilepsy, memory, and learning are subjects of interest for students and teachers. Popular lectures with interactive games hosted by neurologists visiting the schools help in countering many myths.

'Brain Bee' is a neuroscience competition for secondary school students. It begins with local city-based competitions that feed into regional, national, and world competitions. Neurologists should dedicate their time and expertise in organizing this in more places.[11]

This author has curated an exhibition on neuroscience for school kids, comprising of colourful posters, models, games, animations, videos, and brain-cutting demonstrations. Volunteer students are trained to act as interpreters at various stalls and kiosks. The National Neurology Association may multiply this activity all over the country.

Neurology advocacy with government institutions

In most of the developing and many developed countries, the state or public sector plays a dominant role in medical care and medical education. Advocacy for neurology will have to target the responsible authorities of government institutions.

White Papers (WP) on the importance of neurology

A White Paper (WP) is an authoritative report or guide that informs readers concisely about a complex issue and presents the issuing body's philosophy on the matter. It is meant to help readers understand an issue, solve a problem, or make a decision.

The national neurology associations should develop a WP or an official document, stating their vision and demands with a background of facts and justifications (Box 13.3).

The WP should be published in local languages and be adapted to regional needs. The full version will be supplemented by shorter formats like brochures, pamphlets, or flyers, and soft copy versions on flash drives and websites. The WP will be addressed to and presented before many people and institutions like ministers, secretaries,

Box 13.3 Suggested contents of a White Paper on neurology as an aid for advocacy

1. The definition of the field.
2. Community burden of neurological diseases.
3. Appallingly low ratio of neurologists in population and need for capacity enhancement.
4. Some scope of preventability of neurological diseases and a few action plans.
5. The huge unmet need for rehabilitation and paucity of paramedic professionals (physiotherapists, occupation therapists, clinical neuropsychologists, speech language therapists, and neuro-nurses.)
6. The need for public health education and PE programmes.
7. The value of nurturing of patient support groups (PSGs).

directors, media persons, politicians, members of parliament, opinion makers, social activists, and NGOs. The WP will serve as a handy document for all advocates, who will be encouraged to talk about core messages and demands before any of the abovementioned recipients, whenever and wherever they happen to meet them and submit copies of the document. The purpose of this exercise will be to marshal goodwill and make contact with every member of the national neurology associations at multiple fronts in a sustained and intense manner.

While drafting a WP, we will need authentic data and references from reliable sources like the World Health Organization, the World Federation of Neurology, the European Union, and the Global Burden of Disease study.[12]

Neurology services and more neurologists

Expanding the reach of neurology services to underserved regions of the world is one of the prime goals of advocacy for neurology. Neurology advocates need to engage public sector or government health departments at city, state, and national levels aided by the WP. The policymakers should be convinced about the community burden of neurological diseases and urged to make better provisions at more locations.[13]

Currently many parts of the world have only one neurologist for hundreds of thousands of populations.[14] The number of residency training programmes and neurologists being trained each year are highly inadequate. The neurology advocates and the national neurology associations will have to lobby hard with ministers, secretaries, and directors, trying to convince them about the need for establishment and the development of teaching departments at medical colleges.

Good neurology services in a comprehensive manner will become a virtuous cycle for advocacy. An increase in providers and facilities will in turn increase awareness, the feeling that needs are being met, and so on.

Health Fairs

Health fairs are sporadic or sometimes regular, events where patients get the opportunity for consultation, diagnosis, documentation, counselling, some simple investigations, medicines for a short period, some surgery, and referral to a higher centre. Even a piecemeal, non-recurring neurology service at a health fair serves a good purpose.

Health fairs are popular in many countries with poor infrastructure of medical services. They are organized by the government and social organizations. The locations should preferably be remote, rural, and underdeveloped. The people served are economically and socially less developed. Health fairs are a temporary, palliative, stop-gap remedy. Many neurologists in an individual capacity, and also as a member of a team, often provide free services in these camps. Potential patients are searched, screened, and brought to the venue by paramedic staff and volunteers. Prior publicity is necessary.

The present author was the recipient of an education grant from the International League Against Epilepsy (ILAE) in 1994 for conducting a massive public and PE campaign on epilepsy. Twenty-five health fairs for persons with epilepsy were organized at district places over a period of two years.

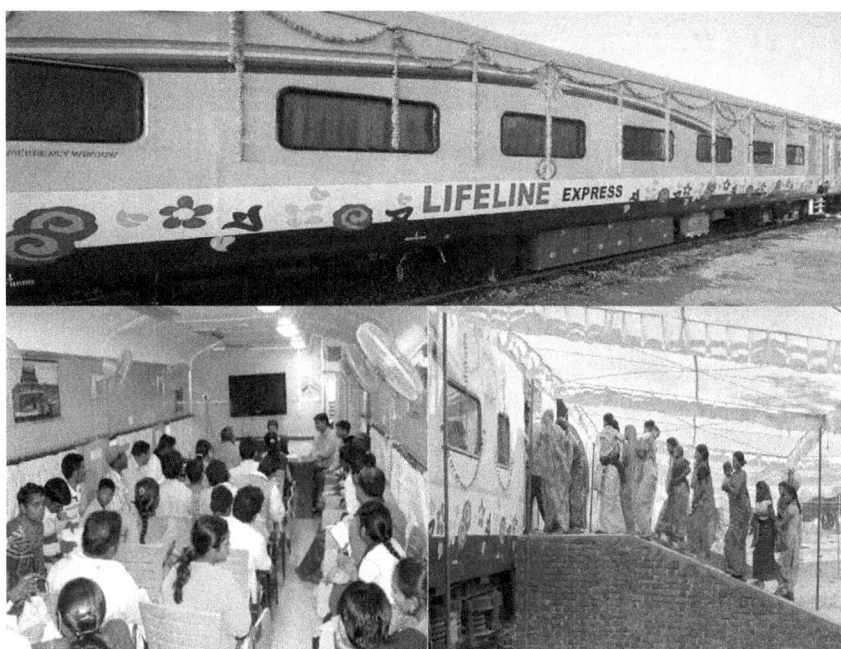

Fig. 13.4 Epilepsy camp on the Lifeline Express (Indian Railways).

The epilepsy clinic on Lifeline Express is an example of a private/public partnership, wherein neurologists and counsellors offer consultations at various stations on the Indian Railways network (Fig. 13.4).[15]

Working on legislations

Parliaments and congresses are empowered to enact laws, many of which may have bearing upon neurological practice and patient welfare. The national neurology associations can oppose or support bills depending on merit. The National Neurology Association should try to push for tabling and passage of acts (Box 13.4).[16]

One notable example is 'Neurology on the Hill' by the American Academy of Neurology. Imagine a scenario where a large number of neurologists, having been trained and motivated in advocacy, are constantly meeting representatives, briefing them about various issues, reminding and persuading them to take action by various means, such as tabling motions in the house and asking questions to governments.

The National Neurology Association should constitute a *Political Action Committee* with the tasks of: (1) writing the initial draft of the desired legislation; (2) searching and probing the legal advice; (3) seeking political support cutting across the party lines.

Engaging the judicial system

Judiciary can play a constructive role if approached in a right, timely, and professional manner. As an example, the Neurological Society of India lobbied hard in the 1980s

> **Box 13.4 A few examples of legislation as a means for advocacy in neurology**
>
> 1. Mandating the use of crash helmets for motorbike riders.
> 2. Launching a national epilepsy control programme.
> 3. Stroke Care Act—making provisions for emergency stroke care at district/county levels.
> 4. More scientific and updated definitions, and quantification of disability due to neurological diseases.
> 5. Mandating the establishment of district-level sheltered workshops for vocational rehabilitation.

with parliamentarians and judiciary for an amendment in law pertaining to the fallacious equivalence of epilepsy with lunacy or insanity and they were successful.

Public interest litigations (PIL) are sometimes resorted to in many countries like India. It has proved to be an effective tool, particularly when the executive arm of government often does not live up to its expectations. Better staffing of the neurology department at a medical college was achieved with the help of PIL in the State High Court.

Moves by governments to curb research on contentious issues like genetic modification, end-of-life care, animal experiments, and so on, on religious and non-scientific grounds have been opposed by the National Neurology Association through many means, including judiciary.[17] National Neurology Associations may sometimes have to give their opinion in controversial legal issues. The Terri Schiavo case was related to the question of consciousness and suffering, where in taking a stand on the scientific basis indirectly became an act of advocacy.[18]

Employment for persons with neurological disorders

The employment status of people with neurological disability is often suboptimal which is partly understandable. However, a tangible proportion of non-employment or underemployment is unwarranted. It occurs due to many myths, misconceptions, and biases. Employees with visible neurological disabilities are viewed less favourably.[19]

Neurology advocates in their individual, as well as collective, capacity should proactively lobby not only against negative discrimination of potential employees with neurological diseases, but also strongly in favour of affirmative action for the benefits of their patients.

'Code of good conduct for employers' has been created by some organizations working for persons with neurological diseases but needs to be popularized and implemented through persuasion.

Sheltered workshops are also useful in the rehabilitation of persons with neurological disabilities. We must strive for establishment of more such workshops in the public as well as private and charity sectors.[20]

Patient Support Groups

Man is a social animal. Common undercurrents behind social bonding are neighbourhoods, professions, religion, race, ethnicity, hobbies, political ideology, and so on. Joining and leading a community, based on a particular disease, has not captured the imagination of people barring a few exceptions. There is ignorance and apathy about the concept and role of patient support groups (PSGs), leading to lack of leadership among patients and caregivers.

The National Neurology Association must officially encourage and support the launch and growth of PSGs dedicated to common as well as rare neurological diseases in increasing number of cities, towns, and neighbourhoods. The websites of national neurology associations should have a section providing updated information about such groups and their members, along with the opportunity to join these online groups. The latter may then get converted into physical groups.

We must support and publicize these groups and hope that more spontaneous activities will follow (Box 13.5). The National Neurology Association may organize a yearly joint session of different PSGs so that members of each group may learn from the experience of others. The state and federal governments need to be persuaded to officially support PSGs by according them a legal status of Co-operative Societies.

Our advocacy efforts will have a greater impact in the minds of the people who matter, if we quote real life stories of patients. Our aim should be to set up a national coalition of several PSGs for as many neurological diseases in as many cities as possible. The activism arising from among patients will be the most powerful voice in favour of neurological sciences.[21]

Neurology as a branch of medicine has more varieties of rare ailments. Such patients and families fail to take advantage of social action due to their small numbers. We can gather larger groups of such families through our collective efforts and serve them

---

Box 13.5 Some examples of advocacy actions taken by Patient Support Groups

1. To foster a sense of kinship and solidarity with other patients suffering from similar disease.
2. To persuade local/state health authorities to ensure the regular uninterrupted supply of medicines (e.g. anti-epileptic drugs) in public hospitals.
3. To persuade local/state health authorities to make provision for the supply of expensive drugs for poor patients (e.g. intravenous immunoglobulin (IVIG), tpA).
4. To lobby for reduction in the cost of the drugs and devices by industry.
5. To lobby with national health authorities for policy matters, funding, and research.
6. To encourage more persons with neurological diseases to enrol in clinical research trials.

better. Lay societies dedicated to such orphan diseases* should come out in a bigger number. There is a voice in numerical strength. They will also be able to fight against the exorbitant increase in the cost of drugs.[22]

Role of non-government organizations, charities, and celebrities

Neurology advocates must explore funding from philanthropic foundations and industry. High levels of advocacy skills come into play when one or more neurologists seek grants from donors, explaining the merits of their project, and action plan. An Internet search easily provides lists of many organizations helping the cause of neurology.[23] For example, Rotary International (www.rotary.org) has been a major partner in the drive for eradication of one of the most common neurological diseases of the twentieth century: poliomyelitis.[24]

Conflict of interest and ethical issues may arise while seeking unrestricted grants for advocacy plans from pharma and device industry. The physician will have to take care of concerns like advertisements and endorsements. His or her own prescribing practices should not be influenced in lieu of such a support from industry. The product and their indications must be evidence based.

In a recent survey of patient advocacy organizations (PAO), a small but not insignificant number indicated that they received substantial support from industry and also that there may be pressure to conform their positions to the interests of corporate donors. However, most of the PAOs believed that their 'conflict of interest policies' were very good.[25]

Celebrities acting as brand ambassadors for one or more neurological conditions have been of great help for advocacy. Mohammad Ali did tremendous work for parkinsonism.[26] The ice bucket challenge was undertaken by thousands of common citizens and also by celebrities including President Barack Obama, raising awareness about amyotrophic lateral sclerosis.[27]

A celebrity may also support a cause if a family member has suffered with a condition, such as author J. K. Rowling aiding the Multiple Sclerosis Society in Scotland on behalf of her mother.

When famous actor Robin Williams died of Lewy body disease, his wife went public with his story, boosting the profile of the disease.

There are more examples of successful lobbying by NGOs and charities in North America, partly because many of them are headed and supported by eminent celebrities: Michael J. Fox and Muhammad Ali (parkinsonism); Julia Roberts (Rett syndrome); Christopher Reeves (traumatic spinal cord injury).[28]

---

* A disease that has not been adopted by the pharmaceutical industry because it provides little financial incentive for the private sector to make and market new medications to treat or prevent it. An orphan disease may be a rare disease (according to US criteria, a disease that affects fewer than 200,000 people) or a common disease that has been ignored (such as tuberculosis, cholera, typhoid, and malaria) because it is far more prevalent in developing countries than in the developed world.

Any neurologist may meet a celebrity at a local level and must not feel shy of requesting him/her to become ambassador for one or another neurological disease.

Advocacy within the National Neurology Association

The National Neurology Association should create a subsection for advocacy and must have an in-house programme to train members. A formal training and interaction with neurologists engaged in some sort of advocacy will boost the morale of members. Many skills must be learned and internalized. It helps if you receive a bit of training for engaging the media, giving interviews, submitting memorandums, using advertisements and propaganda, and addressing small or large groups.[29,30]

Joining hands with related organizations

The National Neurology Association should join other associations to strengthen the advocacy efforts, because many objectives are common (e.g. general practitioners, internists, psychiatrists, neurosurgeons, cardiologists (mainly for stroke), and epileptologists).

Mental health has recently been made a priority by the World Health Organization (WHO) and many governments. Neurology and neurosurgery are now part of the neurosciences along with psychiatry. If our cause is helped by the clubbing together of neurology with psychiatry or mental health (a sort of surrogate branding), we need not feel belittled.[31]

We want more budgets to be allocated for brain research, but changes in political landscape can have an unpredictable and detrimental effect on funding for healthcare and research.[32] Our coalitions of national associations must remain vigilant. It is necessary to lobby with parliament, congress, and executives in one loud voice rather than in many quiet ones.

Self-advocacy for neurologists

Though this book is mainly concerned with advocacy for patients, it would be prudent to mention that the skills of self-advocacy are relevant for neurologists also. Otherwise, we stand less chance of persuading more and better physicians to choose neurology as a career option.

Neurologists are sometimes justly concerned that their professional skills are not adequately recognized. There is an unfavourable bias towards procedures and investigation and a neglect of cognitive services and counselling.[33]

Protecting and expanding the turf of neurology practice is also important. Physician burnout is rather common and severe among neurologists compared to many other specialties. Advocacy to ward off and cope with burnout is one of the tasks for the national neurology associations.[34]

Concluding remarks

Table 13.1 summarizes a few examples of advocacy at different levels, under the framework of object (aim), agent (advocate), intermediary (medium), and beneficiary (recipient).

Table 13.1 Some examples of advocacy at various levels

OBJECT (AIM)	AGENT (ADVOCATE)	INTERMEDIARY (MEDIUM)	BENEFICIARY (RECIPIENT)
Advocacy mainly at local and regional level			
Health fair for one or many neurological diseases for clinical services and neurology education	Neurologist alone or his colleagues at local or regional level	Local NGOs, paramedical staff, district administration, city or village administration, volunteers	Patients suffering from neurological diseases, caregivers
Core messages for public awareness about common neurological ailments	Neurologist alone or, state/national association	Advertising professionals' government agencies, broadcasters	General public, whole population
To increase knowledge and awareness about neurosciences in high school boys and girls	Neurologist at city or state or national level	The school administration for exhibition and quizzes ('Brain Bee')	School kids and teachers
Advocacy mainly at regional and national level			
To enhance and safeguard opportunities for employment for persons suffering with neurological diseases	◆ Neurologist at city/state/national level ◆ Patient support groups or self-help groups at city/state/national level	◆ To draft, print, and distribute Code of Good Practice for employers ◆ To meet employers	Persons suffering from neurological ailments
Essential of neurology for primary care physicians	Neurologists in their individual capacity, or their associations at state or national level	Associations of primary care physicians through periodic courses	The basic doctors
Undergraduate and postgraduate neurology education	Neurologists or their associations at all three levels	Neurology quiz; neurology lectures	The medical students
Advocacy mainly at national level			
To oppose cuts in funding for research on non-scientific grounds (example—stem cells)	National Neurology Association	Members of senate, congress	The researchers and thereby the general public
To amend laws pertaining to epilepsy, (marriage, divorce, and its false equivalence with lunacy or insanity)	National Neurology Society (India)	Parliamentarians, judiciary (through writ petition)	Women and men suffering from epilepsy

Some neurologists do act as advocates, mostly in a personal capacity. It is considered by some as a deviation from primary professional duties and rather looked down upon as something non-academic, inferior, or secondary. It need not be so.[35]

Neurologists with inclinations and skills in leadership, lobbying, networking, and humanities will make better advocates. The importance of a little exposure to humanities (arts, literature, languages, social science, fine arts, philosophy) for medical students and practising physicians is being increasingly recognized, with the hope that it would make us better, more empathetic doctors.[36,37]

The writings of Dr Oliver Sacks and other authors served the cause of advocacy for persons suffering from neurological diseases in a unique manner.[38,39] More such popular clinical tales are needed. Not many patients, caregivers, and neurologists are good writers, yet we should persuade them to write their stories, which will increase the corpus of this type of literature and gradually good examples will emerge.

When advocacy and activism is targeted for a specific cause, it is a vertical approach. Various disease specific programmes (smallpox, malaria, tuberculosis, polio, HIV/AIDS, and now non-communicable diseases) are more likely to achieve success for their restricted goal. A horizontal approach is more general and holistic. Many NGOs work for overall improvement of health services. They plead for enhanced budget and reduced inequality of health. They say 'let all the boats rise equally with the tide'.[40]

It is argued that limited resources should be better spent on overall improvement. Disease-specific activism diminishes an already meagre budget. The more vociferous or powerful group garners larger than their fair share.

Where does advocacy for neurology fit into this debate? We believe that the community burden of neurological ailments is rather high and yet neglected.[41] There is valid reason to strive for neurology services and education. The twin approaches need not be mutually exclusive. Some degree of overlap or complementarity is inevitable, necessary, and useful. All advocacies for neurology will never belittle, ignore, or oppose the general horizontal efforts of advocacy—and the reverse is also expected.

Finally, a lingering doubt. Does advocacy work? Is it worth the time and resources? For those of us who have been active in this field, the intuitive and experience based answer is 'yes, it does'. But where is the evidence? There is paucity of research into efficacy of advocacy.[42] Studies are needed at regional and national levels seeking answers to well framed questions. As we have seen, advocacy is not homogenous. It has multiple facets at many spatial levels. Robust evidence will boost our morale and guide us to do better advocacy.

References

1. **Pauranik, A.** (2008) Advocacy in neurology. *Ann Indian Acad Neurol*, **11**, 60–5.
2. **O'Barr, W. M.** (2012) Public service advertising and propaganda. *Advertising & Society Review*, **13**(2), Project MUSE, muse.jhu.edu/article/484935.
3. **Stump, E., Kahan, M.** (2008) (The waiting room: our kind of women.) *Neurology Now*, **4**(2), 11.
4. **Solorzano, G. E., Jozefowich, R. E.** (2015) Neurophobia: a chronic disease of medical students. *Neurology*, **85**(2), 116–17.

5. **Charles, P. D., Scherokman, B., Jozefowicz, R. F.** (1999) How much neurology should a medical student learn? A position statement of the AAN Undergraduate Education Subcommittee. *Acad Med*, **74**(1), 23–6.
6. **Griggs, R. C., Dickinson, J. C.** (1992) Who teaches neurology to the non-neurologist? *Neurology*, **42**, 719–21.
7. **Engelter, S. T., Gostynski, M., Papa, S., et al.** (2006) Epidemiology of aphasia attributable to first ischemic stroke: incidence, severity, fluency, etiology, and thrombolysis. *Stroke*, **37**(6), 1379–84.
8. **Sherratt, S.** (2011) Written media coverage of aphasia. A review. *Aphasiology*, **25**, 1132–52.
9. **Collado-Vázquez, S., Cano de la Cuerda, R., Jiménez-Antona, C.** (2010) Deficiency, disability, neurology and cinema. *Revista de Neurologia*, **51**(12), 757–63.
10. **Shah, G.** (2016) Stem cell reality. *Neurology Now*, **12**(6), 50–3.
11. **International Brain Bee** (2016) **IBB press release, 5 July 2016**. Available at: https://www.TheBrainBee.org
12. **Chin, J. H., Vora, N.** (2014) The global burden of neurologic diseases. *Neurology*, **83**(4), 349–51.
13. **Janca, A., Aarli, J. A., Prilipko, L., Dua, T., Saxena, S., Saraceno, B.** (2006) WHO/WFN survey of neurological services: a worldwide perspective. *J Neurol Sci*, **247**(1), 29–34.
14. **Thakur, K., Tablane, E., Harper, M., et al.** (2016) The World Health Organization Atlas 2015: country resources for neurological disorders. *Neurology*, **86**(5) (16 Suppl), PL01–001.
15. **Prasad, C. A.** (2012) Train of hope, and a chance to train. *JAMA*, **307**(19), 2039–40.
16. **Editorial** (2017) Law: an underused tool to improve health and wellbeing for all. *Lancet*, **389**(10067), 331.
17. **Robertson, J. A.** (2010) Embryo stem cell research: ten years of controversy. *J Law, Med & Ethics*, **38**(2), 191–20.
18. **Bernat, J. L.** (2005) Neurology response to Terri Schiavo case. *Neurology Today*, **5**(8), P-4.
19. **Gouvier, W. D., Steiner, D. D., Jackson, W. T., et al.** (1991) Employment discrimination against handicapped job candidates: an analog study of the effects of neurological causation, visibility of handicap, and public contact. *Rehabil Psychol*, **36**(2), 121–9.
20. **Avitzur, O.** (2007) How to advocate for our disabled patients in the workforce. *Neurology Today*, **7**(15), 18–19.
21. **Kunkle, F.** (2016) Take action: for many patients and their families, advocacy is about helping themselves and others-and they say anyone can do it. *Neurology Now*, **12**(1), 24–6.
22. **Hartung, D. M., Bourdette, D. N., Sharia, A. M., et al.** (2015) The cost of multiple sclerosis drugs in the US and the pharmaceutical industry. Too big to fail? *Neurology*, **84**(21), 2185–92.
23. **National Institute of Neurological Disorders and Stroke (NIH). Support resources.** Available at: https://www.ninds.nih.gov/Disorders/Support-Resources
24. **Sever, J. L.** (2001) Rotary International: a partner in polio eradication. *Dev Biol (Basel)*, **105**, 105–8.
25. **Rose, S. L., Highland, J., Karafa, M. T., et al.** (2017) Patient advocacy organizations, industry funding, and conflicts of interest. *JAMA Intern Med*, **177**(3), 344–50.
26. **Avitzur, O.** (2016) Hero worship: Muhammad Ali was so much more than a boxing champion to the world and the Parkinson's disease community. *Neurology Now*, **12**, 4.
27. **Wicks, P.** (2014) The ALS ice bucket challenge—can a splash of water re-invigorate a field? *Amyotrophic Lateral Sclerosis and Frontotemporal Degeneration*, **15**, 479–80.

28. **[Leading edge]** (2003) Celebrities needed to promote brain research in Europe? *Lancet Neurol*, **2**(11), 647.
29. **Wasay, M., Hauth, E.** (2005) Advocacy training in leadership training improves the level of activity and impact of neurologist advocates. *J Neurol Sci*, **238**, S481.
30. **Wijeratne, T., DePold Hohler, A.** (2013) Residency training: advocacy training in neurology, lessons from the Palatucci advocacy leadership forum. *Neurology*, **80**(1), e1–e3.
31. **Agrawal, S. P.** (2006) Synergy among the neuro-specialties. *Neurol India*, **54**(1), 13–15.
32. **Katz, I. T., Wright, A. A.** (2017) Scientific drought, golden eggs, and global leadership—why Trump's NIH funding cuts would be a disaster. *N Engl J Med*, **376**, 1701–4.
33. **Donofrio, P. D., Barkley, G. L., Cohen, B. H., et al.** (2015) How neurologists are paid. Part 1: the Medicare payment system. *NeurolClinPract*, **5**, 397–404.
34. **Sigsbee, B., Bernat, J. L.** (2014) Physician burnout, a neurologic crisis. *Neurology*, **83**(24), 2302–6.
35. **Pauranik, A.** (2008) Entrepreneurs: teaching neurology to primary care physicians. *World Neurology*, **23**(4), 12.
36. **Shapiro, J., Rucker, L.** (2003) Can poetry make better doctors? Teaching the humanities and arts to medical students and residents at the University of California, Irvine, College of Medicine. *Acad Med*, **78**(10), 953–7.
37. **Michael, H. B.** (2005) Neurology and the humanities: reflections. *Neurology*, **65**(12), 176.
38. **Sacks, O.** (2009) *The Man Who Mistook His Wife for A Hat*. London: Picador.
39. **Pauranik, A.** (2016) Oliver Sacks: poet laureate of neurology. *Ann Indian Acad Neurol*, **19**, 165–6.
40. **Mill, A.** (2005) Mass campaign versus general health services: what have we learnt about vertical versus horizontal approaches. *Bull World Health Organ*, **83**(4), 315–16.
41. **Menken, M., Munsat, T. L., Toole, J. F.** (2000) The Global Burden of Disease study: implications for neurology. *Arch Neurol*, **57**(3), 418–20.
42. **Cornman, T., Michelle, I.** (2014) Advocacy training: blending classroom with experience. *Acad Med*, **89**(2), 196.

Chapter 14

Advocacy in the international arena

Raad Shakir

Introduction

If one looks at health provision across continents, we see the glaring discrepancy of financial commitment from the wealthy high-income economies to the poorest ones. If we compare the health expenditure per capita in a sub-Saharan African country to a Western European one, for example, with the Central African Republic to Norway, the difference is roughly 650-fold according to World Bank data from 2015. There are more than 50 countries in the world where the annual per capita expenditure on health, let alone neurology, is less than US$50 per annum. These countries are around the tropics concentrated in sub-Saharan Africa and Southeast Asia. Despite these huge discrepancies, all the countries and territories are members of the United Nations (UN) and the World Health Organization (WHO).

There are many ways of influencing governments to invest in neurological care. Direct contact is one, but this is difficult as non-governmental organizations (NGOs) like the World Federation of Neurology (WFN) must have a massive web of contacts which is not practical. Another way of doing this it to go to the regions with the most need. There are regional multinational organizations which are geographically dispersed to look after the needs of a group of nations with similar background economies, geography, and demographics; for example, the African Union (AU), Association of South East Asian Nations (ASEAN), the Arab League (AL), and others. It may be more advantageous to go through the regional associations for support for neurology; however, the health sections of these organizations tend not to be as well-developed when compared to the WHO and its regional offices. Be that as it may, such regional bodies may have more flexibility and target certain areas when the WHO may find it difficult to engage.

The WFN is primarily an organization which promotes neurological education and training. Advocacy and health promotion is an additional goal, which we are trying to achieve. It took many years of collaboration and thinking to decide that the WFN needs to be represented at the WHO at the highest possible level. This was a goal several WFN presidents have cultivated. The relationship is now well established and flourishing.

It was apparent from the beginning that accurate statistics are the cornerstone of every scientific collaboration, without which progress cannot be made. In 1990, the

WHO produced the International Classification of Diseases, Tenth revision (ICD-10). The ICD-10 has been used across the world to report back to the WHO the mortality, morbidity, and prevalence of diseases. It was clear to the neurology community that there were obvious flaws in the classification. Major neurological conditions were wrongly placed and therefore disease attributions were totally incorrect. It can be argued that this may not affect the outcome, but it really does!

Resource allocation for the provision of healthcare, training nurses, doctors, medicines supply, and other governmental expenditure depends on the WHO statistics which are so far misleading to say the least. As an example, see the European region of the WHO (Fig. 14.1). The projected disability-adjusted life years (DALYs) lost, 2008, 2015, and 2030 in countries of the European region, by major cause and income level. Stroke is mentioned when combined with cardiovascular diseases under the rubric or cardiovascular diseases. Moreover, the combination of 'neuropsychiatric disorders' mixes all neurodegenerative disease including the dementias and epilepsy with less common psychiatric conditions. There are numerous other examples which needed rectification. This muddies the concept of healthcare provision for mental health, neurology, and cardiology. In the twenty-first century, with hyper acute treatment readily available for myocardial infarction and ischaemic stroke, it is crucial to have the correct statistics to provide facilities to save lives.

The process of reviewing ICD-10 is a massive collaborative effort of specialists in various fields of neurology. The WHO and the WFN came together and established a neurosciences topic advisory group (TAG). The smaller group consisted of seven members who had to be drawn from all six WHO regions. I had the honour of chairing the TAG. Our first meeting was in June 2009 and we communicated regularly and met annually. The group drew on the expertise of nearly 50 specialists from all fields. Many neurology and neurosurgery specialty organizations were involved and their advice was given to the group and passed on to the WHO. The work involved financial support from the WFN to employ fellows to work on the project and consolidate information. There were ten such fellows from various parts of the world during the years.

The ICD-11 production is cumbersome to say the least. Each section needed to be looked at not only from the specialist point of view, but from the user's viewpoint as well. The main aim is to be able to use the classification in the field by non-medical users as well as those highly qualified medical scientists working in more advanced teaching and research institutions. It is important to emphasize that the TAG's main aim was inclusivity and simplicity. This meant that at times the specialists' views influence in advanced genetics had to be tempered with the reality of data gathering on morbidity and mortality in the field. It is also important to clarify to every neurologist or neurosurgeon involved in the work that they must think about the wider applicability of the classification, making sure that the primary goal is fulfilled.

For those not involved with coding and classification as some were when the process started, there was a sharp learning curve. The basic classification will enable an individual coder, whether medical or non-medical, to state that this person died of say an ischaemic stroke, or provide the code that the person was left disabled by such a diagnosis. This is the Mortality and Morbidity section of the ICD-11. This so-called Joint Linearization of Mortality and Morbidity (JLMMS) is the most commonly used part

ADVOCACY IN THE INTERNATIONAL ARENA | 155

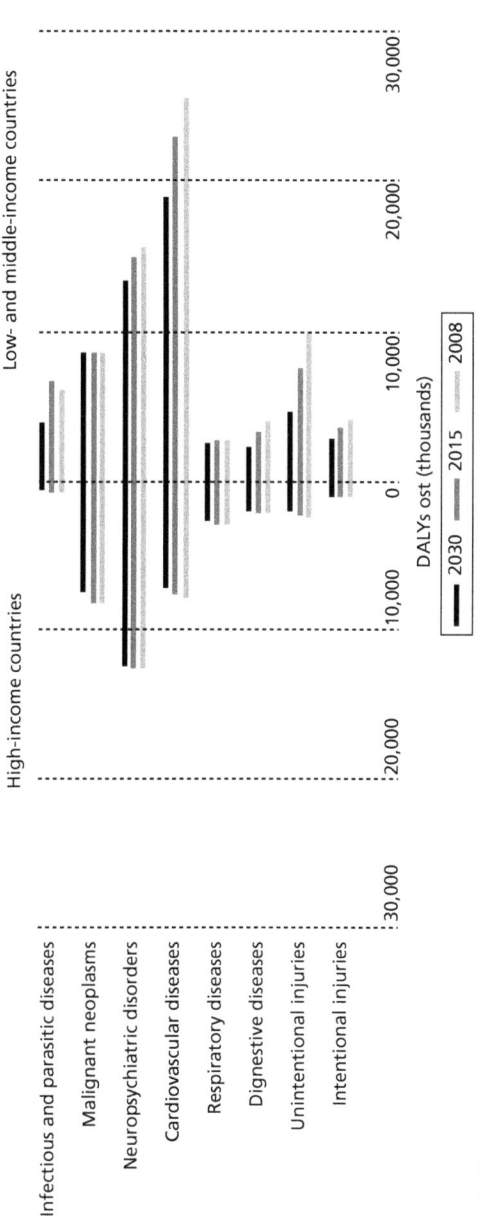

Fig. 14.1 The European health report: charting the way to well-being 2012.
Reproduced from The European health report 2012: Charting the way to well-being, Copyright (2013), with permission from World Health Organization. Available at: http://www.euro.who.int/__data/assets/pdf_file/0004/197113/EHR2012-Eng.pdf

of ICD-11. It is important to remember that all ministries of health who are members of the WHO report back annually to the appropriate WHO department for distribution and publication. Therefore, it is crucial to get the statistics correct. However, the second 'foundation layer' goes in more detail of conditions and this is for the knowledgeable coder who will report finer details of the JLMMS diagnosis. As an example, the JLMMS coder might report a basic 'cerebral ischaemic stroke' but this is not complete, as a more detailed coder will additionally report 'ischaemic cerebral stroke due to extracranial large vessel atherosclerosis'. There is a clear argument for both reports. The first captures the diagnosis and is crucial in the statistics of ischaemic stroke. Health economists will be delighted to map out the incidence of stroke and look for trends of mortality and morbidity. However, the more detailed reporting will in addition help us further understand the exact nature of diseases and in case of those with a genetic anomaly background will certainly help detailed epidemiology.

The neurosciences TAG consulted widely among specialists. Their advice shaped the classification. The ICD-11 beta review is now open to the public for comment. It is most important to state that the WHO Statistics and Informatics department makes the final decisions and our roles are advisory.

There are several changes in ICD-11 compared to ICD-10. The most glaring example is cerebrovascular disorders. These have been primarily placed under circulation disorders on the assumption that they affect blood vessels. This decision was made in 1955 when ICD-7 was published. The issue has muddied statistics as heart attacks were lumped with strokes. The first contact we made was with our cardiology colleagues who had the same issue. An agreement was reached and the advice given to the statisticians was that heart attacks and brain attacks need to be separated and placed in the appropriate chapters in ICD-11. The close collaboration, support, and assistance of the World Stroke Organization (WSO) has been and continues to be a massive help to the neuro TAG in shaping the WHO's decisions in the field of cerebrovascular diseases. It just shows that when two major NGOs (i.e. WFN and WSO) work closely together, obstacles tend to disappear. It took several years to effect the change and in 2017 the decision was made that cerebrovascular diseases are placed and counted as neurological diseases. This is a major achievement and will lead to appropriate allocation of resources for the second most common cause of death. One can now say that cerebrovascular diseases have come home after six decades.

Working with the WHO takes times and requires close collaboration and funding. In a way, neurology is 'fortunate' to be in a smaller WHO department with mental health and now with non-communicable diseases (NCDs). The WHO and UN have taken an excellent stance on NCDs and there is now a clear policy to combat NCDs both in their causation and management. Neurological disorders are the second commonest cause of death and the first cause of DALYs. This is now very clear in the Global Burden of Disease study.[1-3]

The WFN has closely collaborated with the WHO in joint production of the publication *Atlas: Country Resources for Neurological Disorders*, which was first published in 2004.[4] Data on manpower, resources, financing, availability of medicines, and social support were collected from all over the world. The second edition was published in

2017. Atlases on country resources were published for epilepsy (2005), multiple sclerosis (2008), and headache (2011).

The WHO and WFN collaboration is also exemplified in the publication of *Neurological Disorders: Public Health Challenges* in 2006.[5] This document, which is 232 pages long, emphasizes the public health issues of neurological diseases. There are chapters discussing major topics such as epilepsy, dementia, headaches, infections, nutritional disorders, Parkinson's disease, traumatic brain injury, and stroke. This information is provided to policymakers and raises awareness for neurological disorders.

The WHO is heavily involved with the issue of combating NCDs. It is most important that in addition to cancer, diabetes, chronic respiratory diseases, and cardiovascular diseases, all other neurodegenerative diseases are included in the process.[6] Although due to the ICD-10 classification of diseases cerebrovascular diseases include stroke, all other disabling conditions such as all dementias, Parkinson's disease, multiple sclerosis, epilepsy, muscular dystrophies, post-traumatic brain and spine disabilities, motor neuron disease (amyotrophic lateral sclerosis, ALS), congenital and developmental cognitive and physical disabilities, to name but a few, are not included.

Dementia affects 47.5 million individuals globally and the WHO recommended the World Health Assembly (WHA) to approve the plan on global action on the public health response to dementia. The plan was approved by the WHA on the 29 May 2017. The WFN is delighted with the plan and has added its own comment on the role of neurologists in the early diagnosis and treatment of the causes of dementia. It was pointed out in the statement that the causes of certain types of dementias are diverse and that early observation of clinical characteristics is essential to guide future treatment.

Neuroscience is moving full steam ahead in a better understanding of basic molecular pathology and progression. It naturally follows that once therapy is to be trailed, neurologists are the specialists in brain diseases who should be at the forefront of guiding appropriate diagnosis and management. The need for more neurologists is most important to provide the best care possible for all causes of dementia.

The role of non-governmental organizations is crucial in raising awareness through provision of correct statistics to healthcare providers, which anchors their decisions on how best to deal with all forms of diseases, which vary greatly in communities. Neurology continues to need public recognition and support, as it is the discipline dealing with conditions leading to the second cause of death and the first cause of disability across all ages.

References

1. **GBD 2015 Disease and Injury Incidence and Prevalence Collaborators** (2016) Global, regional, and national incidence, prevalence, and years lived with disability for 310 diseases and injuries, 1990–2015: a systematic analysis for the Global Burden of Disease Study 2015. Lancet, **388**, 1545–602.
2. **Murray, C. J. L., Lopez, A. D.** (1996) *The Global Burden of Disease: A comprehensive assessment of mortality and disability from diseases, injuries and risk factors in 1990 and*

projected to 2020. Geneva: The Harvard School of Public Health on behalf of the World Health Organization and The World Bank.

3. **Kassebaum, N. J.**, **Arora, M.**, **Barber, R. M.**, **et. al.** (2016) Global, regional and national disability-adjusted life years (DALYs) for 315 diseases and injuries and healthy life expectancy (HALE), 1990–2015: a systematic analysis for the Global Burden of Disease study 2015. *Lancet*, **388**, 1603–58.
4. **World Health Organization** (2004) *Atlas: Country Resources for Neurological Disorders*. Geneva: WHO.
5. **Aarli, J. A.**, **Dua, T.**, **Janaca, A.**, **Muscetta, A.** (2006) *Neurological Disorders: Public Health Challenges*. Geneva: WHO.
6. **Shakir, R.** (2016) Brain health: widening the scope of NCDs. *Lancet*, **387**, 518–9.

Chapter 15

Working with others, the lesson of the European Brain Council

Jes Olesen and Frédéric Destrebecq

Introduction

The European Union organizes the support for research in so-called 'framework programmes'. Currently the eighth framework programme—renamed 'Horizon 2020'—is at a halfway point. The first five framework programmes were dominated by cancer and cardiovascular diseases, and brain research (then called 'neuroscience') played a very minor role. During the 1990s, as vice-president and subsequently president of the European Federation of Neurological Societies (EFNS), one of the authors (JO) attended several meetings in Brussels. These were organized by basic neuroscientists with the aim of increasing the focus on neuroscience. All came to nothing and for a neurologist that was easy to understand. Politicians are like the general population when it comes to understanding the importance of science. While neuroscientists can see the beauty of new enzymes, new receptors, and new findings in genetics, it is difficult for politicians and other decision-makers to see the consequences of this kind of research for their voters. In other words, it is very difficult to conduct advocacy from molecule to man. JO decided that advocacy must be done from man to molecule. Furthermore, he observed that during these meetings, the interest in how to cut the pie was greater than the interest in increasing the size of the pie. There was a division and competition between basic science and clinical science, and between neurology, psychiatry, and neurosurgery. Furthermore, the most important element in the chain of advocacy was missing: the voice of the patients. But how could all these thoughts be put into action? JO decided to form a collaborating organization that for the specific purpose of advocacy united the following groups:

- Patient groups from within neurology and psychiatry, at the forefront of advocacy.[1]
- Societies representing neurologists, psychiatrists, neurosurgeons, and basic neuroscientists, underpinning the scientific evidence in this advocacy.
- The research-oriented pharmaceutical industry, which provided support to the involved groups involved.

What is in a name?

When it comes to advocacy, terminology proves to be of crucial importance. Experience demonstrates, for instance, that 'neuroscience' is not ideal insofar that it does not generate the necessary appeal.

It has a distinct flavour of basic science and few neurologists would say that their clinical research is in neuroscience. There have been attempts to talk about clinical neuroscience and basic neuroscience but in general it does not fly. It is even worse for psychiatrists and the wider mental health community who, in most cases, cannot identify their own research as neuroscience. It may be that English-speaking people understand the word neuroscience better, but non-English-speaking people definitely do not.

The World Health Organization uses the term 'nervous system', but this terminology bears a connotation of 'nervousness' and also is not understood by the general public.

The obvious term is of course 'brain research'. One obstacle to that name was that a significant part of neurological and basic science was focused on the spinal cord, the peripheral nerves, and muscles. Nevertheless, the words 'brain research' and 'brain diseases' were selected for the newly unified organization, which was then called the European Brain Council (EBC). In a footnote, it was stated that research on spinal cord, peripheral nerves, and muscles was included in the terms 'brain research'.

This terminology also has many advantages. The general public usually understands the importance of the brain and all the players in the field (with the above-mentioned exception) can identify themselves with brain diseases and brain research. The brain is the driving organ in the human body and it is what makes us human as compared to animals. All our other organs can be replaced by animal organs if problems of immunity can be solved, but not the brain. If it were possible to switch brains between two persons, who would then be the new person—the one with the body or the one with the brain? Thus, it was decided to create not only a new organization but also a new terminology, although this debate has been surfacing within the organization on a regular basis.[2]

Creation of the European Brain Council

Uniting all players with an interest in brain diseases and brain research seemed an almost impossible task but, because JO was President of the EFNS—now united within the European Academy of Neurology, EAN,[3] with the full support from its management committee—sufficient administrative support was covered by the EFNS. Unlike cardiovascular diseases which in most countries have one and only one heart association, neurological and psychiatric diseases were collaborating with a multitude of disease-specific patient organizations. Spearheaded by Mrs Mary Baker and with the administrative and moral support of the EFNS, the European Federation of Neurological Advocacy (EFNA[4]) was established as an umbrella organization of neurological patient organizations. In psychiatry, the Global Alliance of Mental Illness Advocacy Networks-Europe (GAMIAN-Europe[5]) proved to be an ideal and relevant partner to represent patients. It focused primarily on depression but also on other psychiatric diseases and, in this capacity, accepted participation.

The psychiatrists also had different organizations but were, in the beginning, represented by the European College of Neuro-Psychopharmacology (ECNP[6]) and later also by the Association of European Psychiatrists (AEP), which then became the European Psychiatric Association (EPA[7]). The neurosurgeons were represented by the European Association of Neurosurgical Societies (EANS[8]), and the basic neuroscientists by the Federation of European Neuroscience Societies (FENS[9]).[10] There was also an attempt to bring the pharmaceutical industry on board though their umbrella organization (European Federation of Pharmaceutical Industries and Associations—EFPIA) but it was not possible to gain its support as such. However, a group of pharmaceutical companies that were willing to participate and support the initiative individually was constituted to support the activities of the newly established organization.

With this level of support, the organization was formally established as a non-profit organization in Brussels on 22 March 2002 and got its permanent office there.

Advocacy for FP6

At the time of preparing for the EBC and before its incorporation, action was urgently needed to influence the draft proposal for FP6. In former framework programmes, little attention had been paid to brain research and a preliminary version of the programme proposal for FP6 showed no positive development. There was not a single word about brain research or brain diseases. Despite the fact that the EBC was not formally established or in function as yet, EBC representatives managed to get a meeting with the then EU commissioner responsible for research (1999–2004), Mr Philippe Busquin, and his director Mr Bruno Hansen. In preparation for this meeting, data on the burden of brain diseases had been developed, on the basis of the Global Burden of Disease study of the World Health Organization.[10] These data demonstrated an enormous impact of brain diseases on the European society. In further discussions with the Commission, it proved possible to have a mention of brain diseases in the written programme and eventually FP6 had substantially increased funding of brain research. Table 15.1 demonstrates that, in financial terms, support to brain research tripled between FP5 and FP6, from €115 m to €431 m, for that period of time.

Table 15.1 Level of investment (in €) spent under the successive European Union's framework programmes for research and development

	FP5 (pre-EBC)	Total in FP6	FP7 2007–2013 (figures updated 15/03/2017)
Brain	115 m	431 m	**4.2b**
Cancer	235 m	914 m	2.2b
Cardiovascular	54 m	232 m	737 m

Advocacy for FP7

After the urgent action for FP6, it was immediately time to prepare the negotiations for FP7. For that purpose, it was decided to generate more solid evidence to support our arguments for increased research funding, the most effective being the economic argument. World Health Organization (WHO) data on the burden of diseases at the time were measured in disability-adjusted life years—but what does that tell politicians and other decision-makers? To create a striking argument to politicians, figures had to be in real money terms, in Euros. JO therefore initiated a huge study entitled the 'Cost of disorders of the brain in Europe'. This study was a collaboration effort involving more than 100 experts, partly clinicians with expertise in epidemiology and partly health economists. Patients were of course also represented. A multidisciplinary task force was formed for each of the major brain diseases and the results were presented in two distinctive groups: as cost for each disease in Europe and as cost in each of the European countries.[11-13] The document was of course shared with the relevant stakeholders and institutions and it proved to have a huge impact on the European Commission's Directorate-General for Research and Innovation in advance of the final programming for FP7. It was now clear that brain diseases had substantially higher socioeconomic impact than either cardiovascular diseases or cancer. With the cost documented, we then worked on an analysis of the funding of brain research in Europe. This work was mostly done by health economists but was supported by the EBC and by a grant from the EU. It turned out that comparing research funding to the cost of the disorders, brain research was poorly funded throughout Europe and it was also possible to document that this was the case in each single country.[14] Funding for each disorder relative to its socioeconomic cost was calculated. Having documented the enormous cost of brain diseases and the low funding of brain research, we aimed to show to decision-makers what could be achieved if increased funding were available.

In another major collaborative effort, we developed the document entitled 'Consensus document on European brain research'.[15] We used a standard template to describe for each of the major disorders the background, past achievements in Europe, proposals for future research, and significance of increased research. The document was very well-received by the Commission and was actually successfully used to formulate some of the calls in FP7. Besides carrying on advocacy to European institutions in Brussels, it was also key for EBC to convince national governments, particularly as the great majority of the funding for brain research is organized or provided at a national level. We therefore also developed cost papers for each country in Europe to be used locally in advocacy for brain research.

Funding for brain research in FP5, FP6, and FP7

Advocacy for brain research is obviously not the only factor behind the enormous increase in European funding of brain research that took place in FP7, and it is impossible to determine exactly how big an influence EBC's advocacy has had. For those involved, it seems obvious that the effort of the EBC contributed greatly to the general wave of awareness leading to increased funding. In the following, we refer to data from the Commission so that figures are unbiased. Table 15.1 shows funding for brain research in the successive framework programmes. For comparison, data are provided for brain, cardiovascular system, and cancer. It is obvious from these figures that advocacy for brain research at the European level has been incredibly successful.

FP8-Horizon 2020

This framework programme started in 2014 and the EBC naturally worked for several years before its inception to maintain momentum and funding for brain research. The cost of the disorders of the brain document mentioned here[12] was extensively revised and updated. Several diseases could now be included because new data became available, as had several cost parameters for already included diseases. The new document resulted in the conclusion that the cost of brain disorders in Europe was a staggering burden, as it was almost 800 billion Euros per year. This was demonstrated to be more than heart diseases, cancer, and diabetes put together. Again, we were successful in completing this document in a draft version early enough for the data to be considered in preparation of the framework programme.[11,12] We also revised the document of consensus in brain research.[16]

Once adopted, it turned out that Horizon 2020 has a completely different structure as compared to the previous framework programmes, and at the time of writing it is still only halfway from its end term. It is therefore challenging to have a clear picture as regards the funding for brain research.

Preparing for FP9 and future actions

Reaching above the bar of 3 billion Euros for brain research under FP7 was of course seen as a major achievement for EBC and its constituency. However, this satisfaction was tempered by the fact that:

- Such massive investments were still not matching the actual needs arising from the burden of brain diseases.
- The translation and implementation of research outcomes still needed to be improved.

These are elements that EBC has emphasized when developing its new consensus document on 'The need to expand brain research in Europe'.[17]

With its new consensus document, EBC—while recognizing the efforts made—redefined European research priorities and restated clear expectations across and beyond brain disorders. On that basis, EBC called on the European Commission and EU Member States to tackle brain health in an integrated manner, increase support to basic and clinical research, optimize funding opportunities, and ensure concrete translation of basic research.

While this document was presented and disseminated in the EU Council and European Parliament[18] such advocacy again needed to be supported by solid arguments (i.e. brain disorders were involving more than a restricted community of patients, researchers, and clinicians, and had an impact on society as a whole). This is why, EBC decided to run a new study on the socioeconomic impact of brain disorders in Europe on the basis of its previous work. This is how the current EBC project on 'The value of treatment for brain disorders in Europe' (VOT) was born.[19]

Through the analysis of nine case studies (schizophrenia, dementia, idiopathic normal-pressure hydrocephalus, stroke, Parkinson's disease, epilepsy, headache, multiple sclerosis, and restless legs syndrome), this project aims to identify the treatment gap in each of the conditions examined. On that basis, the clinical intervention that is identified as necessary will undergo a socioeconomic impact evaluation in order to demonstrate its benefits. As its end outcome, the project came up with a white paper to provide the necessary policy recommendations to revisit the model of care for brain disorders in Europe.[19] The closing conference of the project was on 22 June 2017 in Brussels under the auspices of the Maltese Presidency of the EU.

The last element of EBC's current advocacy was the launch of a 'Call to Action' in November 2015. This call supports a longer-term campaign aiming at the adoption of national brain plans to be coordinated under the aegis of a European framework, as per the recommendations made by the European Commission in conclusion to the European Month of the Brain organized by DG Research in May 2013.[20]

A reflection process is being run in order to identify the key features for such national plans, taking as examples the recent success stories of cancer and diabetes. Ideal models for these plans should encompass: bringing together various stakeholders; streamlining existing resources; coordinating sectoral policies; improving patient care; addressing cross-cutting themes such as stigma, prevention, research, carers, economics, or education.

The European Brain Council pledged to make 2014 the Year of the Brain (YOTB) in Europe with the overall aim to increase awareness within society about nurturing, preservation, and protecting the brain through diet, exercise, and safety measures. Through enhanced understanding of brain disease, improved treatment, and promotion of brain health, the burden to society and the health economy could be substantially reduced.

This initiative quickly gained significant support from over 200 organizations representing patients, scientific communities, healthcare professionals, and industry in all areas of brain disorders.

Combined with support from several European Commissioners, the project also received significant and enthusiastic support from within the European Parliament and EU Member States.

The purpose of the YOTB was to change the way people think about their brains and the conditions which affect it.

This was achieved through coordinated efforts as well as by stimulating many other parties—governments, professional societies, patient groups, industry, pressure groups, trusts, individuals, and a multitude of other organizations—to be part of this ongoing campaign which was closed with a conference on depression in the workplace on 9 December 2015.[21]

Key players in supporting EBC's advocacy during the YOTB and more recently through the call to action consensus document or VOT project, undoubtedly were the National Brain Councils.

The National Brain Councils (NBCs) were created as mirror organizations to EBC, gathering national organizations or societies in order to represent patients, clinicians, and science at national level.

With time, NBCs have built up their role and some have become extremely active and influential and managed to set concrete examples for those countries lagging behind. This culminated with the admission of the Belgian, French, and Serbian Brain Councils as observer members of EBC on 1 January 2017, which were followed by the Dutch, Norwegian, and Spanish Brain Councils on 9 February 2017.

In order to support their efforts and contribute to building their respective capacity of influence, EBC established an annual meeting of what is now recognized as the 'Academy of NBCs', where delegates can share their experience and good practices but also meet with experts and guest speakers.

With this work completed at the national level, EBC managed to increase its impact, particularly as the balance of decision-making at EU level is shifting increasingly to the member states.

In 2017, EBC will be celebrating its fifteenth anniversary. On this occasion, policy events and awareness opportunities will be organized throughout the year.[22] In order to support this effort and the necessary communication around it, a new brand 'I Love My Brain' would be created. It emphasizes the importance of our brain as the key organ in our body that we need to nurture, preserve, and maintain. Under the label 'I Love My Brain', EBC aims to spread the word. It invites member organizations to take ownership of this vision and use it in all the activities that they will organize and that meet these objectives. First and foremost among these will be the concept of early detection and early intervention for brain disorders.

Conclusions

The example of the EBC demonstrates that concerted action is highly effective. Politicians and other decision-makers are turned off by divisions and lack of unity among the stakeholder community. However, unity stimulates and is a driving force when trying to convince decision-makers. Brain research proved to be a much better terminology than neuroscience when it comes to advocacy, and persistent and continued efforts over decades are incredibly important. Brain diseases have gained recognition as the most expensive and debilitating diseases and funding for brain research has finally reached a level which is getting closer to commensurate with their cost. Advocacy does pay off but it is only effective when supported by solid data and truthful argumentation. In this regard, sharing a vision with politicians that expands beyond the boundaries of one single disease, profession, or activity can prove to be extremely powerful. This is why EBC's work on demonstrating the societal impact of brain disorders is so invaluable and will be continued under different formats.

References

1. **Olesen, J.** (2007) Collaboration to promote neurological research—the European Brain Council experience. *Nat Clin Pract Neurol*, **3**(6), 298–9.
2. **Olesen, J., Freund, T. F.** (2006) European Brain Council: partnership to promote European and national brain research. *Trends Neurosci*, **29**(9), 493–5.
3. **European Academy of Neurology (EAN)**. Available at: https://www.ean.org/

4. **European Federation of Neurological Associations (EFNA)**. Available at: http://efna.net/
5. **GAMIAN-Europe**. Available at: http://www.gamian.eu/
6. **European College of Neuropsychopharmacology**. Available at: https://www.ecnp.eu/
7. **European Psychiatric Association.** Available at: http://www.europsy.net/
8. **European Congress of Psychiatry**. Available at: http://www.eans.org/pages/home/
9. **Federation of European Neuroscience Societies.** Available at: http://www.fens.org
10. **Olesen, J., Leonardi, M.** (2003) The burden of brain diseases in Europe. *Eur J Neurol*, **10**(5), 471–7.
11. **Olesen, J., Gustavsson, A., Svensson, M., Wittchen, H. U., Jonsson, B.** (2012) The economic cost of brain disorders in Europe. *Eur J Neurol*, **19**(1), 155–62.
12. **Gustavsson, A., Svensson, M., Jacobi, F., et al.** (2011) Cost of disorders of the brain in Europe 2010. *Eur Neuropsychopharmacol*, **21**(10), 718–79.
13. **Andlin-Sobocki, P., Jonsson, B., Wittchen, H. U., Olesen, J.** (2005) Cost of disorders of the brain in Europe. *Eur J Neurol*, **12** Suppl 1, 1–27.
14. **Sobocki, P., Lekander, I., Berwick, S., Olesen, J., Jonsson, B.** (2006) Resource allocation to brain research in Europe (RABRE). *Eur J Neurosci*, **24**(10), 2691–3.
15. **Olesen, J., Baker, M. G., Freund, T., et al.** (2006) Consensus document on European brain research. *J Neurol Neurosurg Psychiatry*, **77** Suppl 1, i1–49.
16. **Di, L. M., Baker, M., Corradetti, R., et al.** (2011) Consensus document on European brain research. *Eur J Neurosci*, **33**(5), 768–818.
17. **Morris, R. G., Oertel, W., Gaebel, W., et al.** (2016) Consensus statement on European brain research: the need to expand brain research in Europe–2015. *Eur J Neurosci*, **44**(3), 1919–26.
18. **European Brain Council (EBC)**. Report on outreach activities. Available at: http://www.braincouncil.eu/activities/news/meeting-of-the-ep-interest-group-on-mental-health-well-being-and-brain-disorders/
19. **European Brain Council (EBC)**. *The Value of Treatment for Brain Disorders in Europe: exploring the potential for a holistic care model for brain disorders to close the treatment gap in Europe: development of a workable care model and case studies analysis.* Available at: http://www.braincouncil.eu/wp-content/uploads/2016/01/EBCdiscussionpaperA4FINAL3.pdf [The policy white paper is available at: http://www.braincouncil.eu/wp-content/uploads/2017/06/EBC_white_policy_paper_DEF26072017_Low.pdf].
20. **European Brain Council (EBC)**. *Call to Action*. Available at: http://www.braincouncil.eu/wp-content/uploads/2015/11/EBC-Call-to-action2.pdf
21. **European Brain Council (EBC)**. *Year of the Brain*—closing conference. Available at: http://www.braincouncil.eu/activities/news/year-of-the-brain-how-to-reduce-the-burden-of-depression-in-the-workplace/
22. **European Brain Council (EBC)**. EBC planned events. Available at: http://www.braincouncil.eu/activities/events/

Chapter 16

SOS Children's Villages: Rediscovering advocacy to increase relevance and impact. A high-level case study

Richard Pichler

From a charity to a development organization

Start as a service provider with a big vision

SOS Children's Villages was founded in 1949 in post-World War II Austria out of the need for care for children who had lost parental care or could not stay with their parents. The founder Hermann Gmeiner was of the conviction that the traditional large orphanages were no adequate answer to the needs of children. He wanted to provide care for children in a family-oriented way. His original intention was to showcase his SOS Children's Village model and spread it in Austria. Hermann Gmeiner wanted to offer the model, show its practical feasibility, and invite others to copy while maintaining his organization, which continues to operate the model. Through this, he also wanted to reform the way that children without parental care are cared for in general. He was a tireless advocate for family-oriented care where children can have a reliable relationship with a person who cares for them, which was typically the SOS mother.

Soon the model was a publicly recognized success first in Austria, then in Europe, and from 1960 onwards also on the other continents. However, its public success also brought significant opposition from professional circles, academia, and authorities. The reason for this opposition can be found, on one hand in its success and public recognition, and on the other hand, in the lack of scientific proof for the model and the missing discourse with academia and the professional circles.

Very prominent opposition was, for example, found in the partly harsh criticism towards SOS Children's Villages in Germany through the AFET[1,2] ('Allgemeiner Fürsorgeerziehungstag', which was the leading conference of academia, authorities, and service providers in the area of child welfare), which concluded in its annual meeting in 1964 based on an earlier evaluation that 'the SOS Children's Villages are not in the position to fulfil essential professional, pedagogic and legal requirements of institutional care'.

No matter if some of the criticism in the early days was well founded or not, today there is no longer any doubt that the traditional orphanages did, in many instances, a lot of harm to children and influenced their development negatively. Small family-like settings, foster care, kinship care, and adoption are considered to be in the best interest of the child who is not able to grow up with biological parents.

The organization itself engaged only slowly in academic discourse in a few countries (particularly in Germany and Austria) in the 1970s and 1980s. On the international level it showed even more reluctance to do so, and rather continued with scaling up service provision. It was absent from the international discourse on topics of alternative childcare. In doing so, it continued to develop qualities and standards for its own work in what technically is referred to as 'alternative care' for children.

The consequences

The concept, the results, and the impact of the model remained little known in relevant international platforms and with key influencers, policy- and decision-makers. Even on the national level, in particular in countries where the work of the organization was mainly funded through sources abroad, there was little knowledge in national professional fora on the concept and its impact. The professional experience of the organization, which was there in abundance, was not asked for or leveraged, nor was it proactively offered. Silently, it was taken for granted that the alumni of the organization's care performed well, but little was asked about the reasons for it.

Major global developments started without involvement and little knowledge of the by then already largest child care organizations in the world (e.g. the global de-institutionalization process, development and implementation of the Millennium Development Goals, funding strategies of major grant-givers in the global North). These developments were even perceived internally to obstruct the successful further development of the organization. Combined with the significant external pressure put on the organization due to the HIV/AIDS pandemic, with millions of children being orphaned by AIDS, the organization had to rethink some strategies.

Why could the organization flourish despite quite a detachment from discourse?

Of course, it was most relevant to have a visionary and charismatic leader, well-developed teams and structures. However, without the necessary financial resources it would have been hardly possible. The organization was blessed with funding for the good cause of caring for children in need from the private donor market due to its innovative fundraising technique. The donors saw in the model a very worthwhile endeavour to support and since the organization also produced results, the funding continued.

For that reason, there was very little need to exchange with professional circles and authorities. One was very self-determined so long as there was no significant need to negotiate for resources with authorities.

Stocktaking around the year 2000

By then, the organization was a very successful service provider globally, recognized by a large donor base and by a small group of experts and authorities seeking out their own successful solutions in the field of child welfare. Governments were generally satisfied with the performance of SOS Children's Villages, which was taking a load from their shoulders in childcare. However, particularly outside the industrialized nations, there were no significant signs of larger scale reforms in their policies to improve the situation of children in alternative care. Internally the organization was content and convinced of doing good work, which was also proven by the alumni leaving its care. It was, however, detached from global, regional and, in most instances, national discourse, which has moved on substantially in the last decades and has firmly established exchange platforms, definitions, and its own language/terminology.

The programme portfolio of the organization was with few exceptions focused on service provision in direct care, and essential services in health and education. A minority group within the organization started to recognize the fact that the organization could and had to increase its impact if it wanted to remain relevant and contribute at a commensurate level to its size in global development. The following two directions were the result of the internal global thinking process:

a) Based on data collected by default upon admission of children into care the organization found that if it proactively reaches out to vulnerable families 8–10 years before children are referred for long-term care, it could support and strengthen family structures to overcome difficulties and avoid disintegration, violence, and abuse largely. This could, therefore, avoid the situation of these children needing its care to begin with.

b) The organization has practical experience in the care of children in over 100 countries. It should engage with policymakers and society, and push for improvement of the national policy and legal framework for children in alternative care, as well as strengthen public services and access to public support for vulnerable families.

After some internal discussions around 2005, family strengthening and advocacy was added next to direct care as an integral part of the programme portfolio of the strucure in all national organizations. It was significantly easier to add the family strengthening programmes to the portfolio, since they are a more practical aspect and have more direct visible impact. It was also easily understood in its cause–effect relationship: if one supports a family earlier, it is more likely that the family keeps caring for its child.

Including advocacy was much more difficult. There were quite some barriers since it was felt early on by large parts of the organization that it is a too political, too theoretical, and too difficult to measure engagement for an organization known for its track record in quality care and tangible results. Questions arose, like 'Will a dilution of the existing programmatic concept happen, will the donor accept that one uses funds for advocacy, will existing programmes get into difficulties if the organization engages in advocacy . . . ?'. Finally, it became part of the five-year strategy to make initial steps.

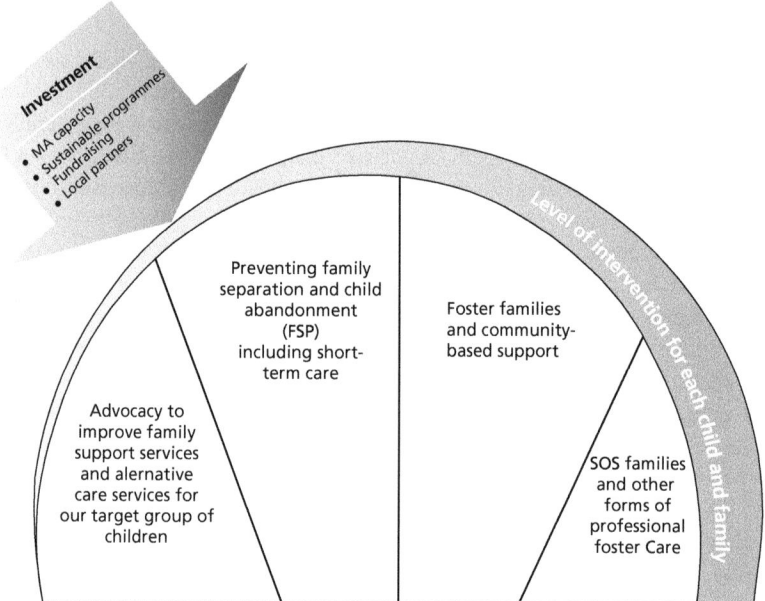

Fig. 16.1 The programme portfolio of SOS Children's Villages, 2016.
Reproduced from the programme portfolio of SOS Children's Villages, Copyright (2016), with permission from SOS Children's Villages International.

The focus of advocacy was placed on the rights of children, with a particular emphasis on children in danger of losing parental care or who had lost parental care. This is illustrated in Fig. 16.1.

Key challenges and achievements of advocacy as part of the programme portfolio of SOS Children's Villages during the last 25 years

Internal challenges

Initially there was very little know-how on doing successful advocacy. Although there were many people in the organization who, with the right training and mindset could have been very successful advocates, it was difficult to make use of this resource. The concept and the benefit needed to be made known to a broader internal public. Skills needed to be built, partly also through hiring new staff from outside. With these new staff members, who by tendency were younger, with high technical skills and of quite some critical thinking, one saw that the process of including these new colleagues in the existing workforce needed quite some attention. They brought discussions, which so far largely happened outside the organization, to the inner core of it. Common practices of the organization were put to question, and one had to rethink several arguments one had used thus far to explain the work the organization was doing. One also had to review a number of policies for non-compliance with commonly accepted international frameworks.

For example, one can take the claim of SOS Children's Villages in those days to offer 'a permanent home for children'. While the United Nations (UN) Convention on the Rights of the Child clearly refers to the biological family as the best place for children to grow up, what would SOS Children's Villages do if a family recovers again in a way that it can care for the child earlier placed into the care of the organization? Following this thought, the organization decided it should engage in, or support the building of the capacity of the families and when successfully achieved, reunite the children with the biological parents. In logical consequence, this had to lead to the reformulation of the claim to 'a long-term placement for children'. This, in turn, created a lot of debate in the organization, since it potentially threatened or destabilized the successful implementation of the care programmes building strongly on the child to rely on permanent relationships.

Without these and other discussions and necessary adaptations in the policy frame, it would have been futile to engage in advocacy, since external criticism would have easily weakened even the best arguments put forward by SOS Children's Villages with the simple reference to practices which even do not fulfil basic international practices.

Another example is the attitude towards independent research. The organization had, for many years, done internal research to assess its progress. Only in combination with external independent research can arguments be used as a powerful advocacy tool. The organization also had to learn to deal with this and at times unfavourable research results with a need to improve practices.

Tied in internal arguments and equipped with limited resources, it was also difficult to produce showcase results to underpin the value added by advocacy. It was finally those parts of the organization which became under significant threat from outside, who did the swing and saw the benefit of advocacy—namely the countries significantly touched by the deinstitutionalization process.

Advocacy had therefore first to help the organization in getting ready for successful advocacy. In the case of SOS Children's Villages this also meant that in earlier years, until a point of no return, the advocacy colleagues were at times not shown due appreciation by a broad internal public. In retrospect, however, the new colleagues contributed significantly to a refreshment of the organizational culture and a more self-reflected mindset throughout the years.

Successes on an international level

The deinstitutionalization process

In the late 1990s after the opening up of Eastern Europe, reports about disastrous conditions in huge government orphanages resulted in an accelerated deinstitutionalization process (DI-process) in childcare.[3] This process had started in the course of the early 1990s and focused on dissolving or converting orphanages with institutional features (large, closed-in, staff on 8-hour shifts, little to no personal relationship and bonding with children). Due to its previous absence from the discourse, SOS Children's Villages was not known in many professional circles for its concept and qualities. If it was known, it was only some superficial institutional features of the model that were at the forefront of people's minds. Therefore, SOS Children's Villages was commonly associated with 'institutions'. Having worked already for over a decade in several countries behind the former 'iron curtain', the organization was suddenly confronted with a threat and an opportunity. The threat was to be closed, and the opportunity was to contribute in the DI-process with its so far internally kept experience and quality standards. The organization decided to rapidly step up its advocacy efforts in these countries and contribute know-how in this process to help avoid a one-dimensional solution of pushing children into foster care and adoption only, while disregarding a key principle of the Convention on the Rights of the Child which is 'the best interest of the child'.

Based on the learning from Eastern Europe, the organization could pre-empt and much more constructively engage in the processes, which followed in the other continents thereafter. For example, it engaged from the outset (2000 onwards) in an alliance of like-minded organizations in Latin America to drive this process with advocacy means from the continental and national levels.

UN guidelines on alternative care for children

Around the year 2005 it became evident that the Convention on the Rights of the Child fell short in recognizing the special needs of children in alternative care.[4] This knowledge was built partly through the findings in the DI-process. Key stakeholders, including the UN Committee on the Rights of the Child/Geneva, among others, built up momentum to advocate for the development of a complementary reference document next to the convention with the goal of defining new common practice standards in national child rights policy. SOS Children's Villages took this opportunity and engaged in a leading role together with like-minded organizations and governments to draft the document 'UN guidelines on the alternative care for children'. This engagement offered four big strategic opportunities:

a) To contribute and make transparent the quality standards the organization has been developing over six decades. The minimum standards could be brought into the discussion and most of them also made it into the document.

b) To engage in a profound discussion with other organizations and governments participating in the formulation on the relevance of each standard. This significantly contributed to the strengthening of the profile of the organization in professional circles. It gave ample opportunity for the exchange of professional arguments, understanding the views of other organizations, and validating the organization's own strength.

c) To influence the direction of future policies relating to children in alternative care globally and nationally, based on the organization's long-standing practical experience in its work with the target group, which should be followed by authorities in the best interest of children in alternative care. It also relates to issues outside the direct work of the organization, to the framework conditions under which children are placed in alternative care; for example, the principles of necessity (is it necessary at all) and appropriateness (there is not one standard solution but a range of options which have to be looked at in the best interest of the child) of placement into alternative care was a key result, which have far-reaching impact on children of the target group.

d) To understand and learn about how on highest international level policy comes into place.

The document was finally welcomed by the UN General Assembly in September 2009. Today, these guidelines have been adopted by over 70 governments internationally as the policy reference for alternative care and every year more governments are coming on board. It is now the key reference document for the organization's advocacy work, as well as being next to the UN Convention on the Rights of the Child as the binding document on the programmatic engagement of SOS Children's Villages.

Advocacy in the development of the UN Sustainable Development Goals 2015–2030

Had the organization been surprised in 2000 by the release of the Millennium Development Goals through the UN, it applied the lessons learnt ten years later.[5] It decided early on that the next set of global goals needed to have the needs of most vulnerable children much better represented, ideally through an orchestrated push of several like-minded organizations and other stakeholders. Together with the other globally active child-focused non-governmental organizations (NGOs), SOS Children's Villages engaged in this development throughout a period of four years through targeted advocacy activities.

The goal was to position the issue of most vulnerable children who lost parental care, or are in danger of losing parental care prominently in the new set of goals in order to have in the implementation phase sufficient arguments to link to. This is particularly necessary for:

a) *Further advocacy activities*—for example, it was common agreement in the negotiations that one reason for neglect of the needs of most vulnerable children in a society is that children without parental care often are not part of the normal statistical household surveys. For that reason, they are not part of official statistics and do not appear as a vulnerable group in official data. One of the first actions after approval of the Sustainable Development Goals was to focus advocacy on including children without parental care in the official statistical data collection.

b) *Funding possibilities*—government spending but also philanthropic focus will align in subsequent years with the Sustainable Development Goals. Causes not supported by the goals will have great difficulties accessing these major funding sources.

Soon it became clear that other sectors (e.g. the business sector) were already quite progressed in well-prepared advocacy strategies. It needed a bigger effort and joined-up thinking among several organizations to balance this. Some 20 of the largest civil society organizations in the world—among them also the child-focused organizations—teamed up and put down a six-point joint programme for advocacy, which was presented early on to the UN. The child-focused organizations could utilize the six points well emphasized, and added their particular concerns. Each of the child-focused organizations pushed through its contact channels individually and some activities were done jointly. While in the early phase it was still an objective to have a stand-alone goal for children as a result of the process, it was soon discovered that this would have had less chance to be accepted with heavy competition from various other causes. One chose the strategy of jointly working on a mainstreaming of issues relevant for the healthy development of children, so that children's issues were the integral part in the various goals. This has proven to be a successful strategy.

When the Sustainable Development Goals 2015–2030 were approved by the UN General Assembly in 2015 it could be recognized that the joint efforts had paid off and the needs of most vulnerable children were strongly represented in these goals. With these results, SOS Children's Villages, as well as the other child-focused agencies, has a significantly better perspective from which to provide services and further advocate for realizing and improving the rights of children. This is illustrated in Fig. 16.2.

Lessons learnt for successful advocacy

- Understand the cause–effect cycle of societal issues—advocacy action—societal/policy change. Laws and subsequent implementation rules are the expression of government policy. Lawmakers are exposed to public opinion. Usually the law-making process is accompanied by an input process from various stakeholders. In addition, public opinion is influenced through opinion leaders. Stakeholders engage with advocacy methods to influence both—laws and public opinion. If one does not engage actively, one implicitly accepts that other stakeholders shape prevailing opinion.
- Create internal readiness—it needs advocacy for advocacy. As a service provider, the organization had to re-learn the value added of advocacy for its mission. This can be considered an organizational development process and needs collective will in an organization to make it happen.
- Advocacy is an essential strategy to increase the impact and create multipliers for a cause. If you are a service provider you always have limited reach with limited resources. If you want to scale up and increase your impact, you need to go beyond your own business environment and influence others to act in a certain way, which brings the desired results.
- Advocacy needs to be evidence based. To make arguments powerful, you need to back them up with strong research. Without independent research, one risks losing the advocacy battle early on.
- It needs dedicated resources. No matter if it is an ongoing engagement or a time-limited action, one needs to have explicit resources assigned for the time one wants to have impact.
- It is an attitude, which needs to be lived first and foremost by leading people of the organization. This is particularly relevant in a civil society organization where usually a significant part of the programme is to further develop policy frames, so

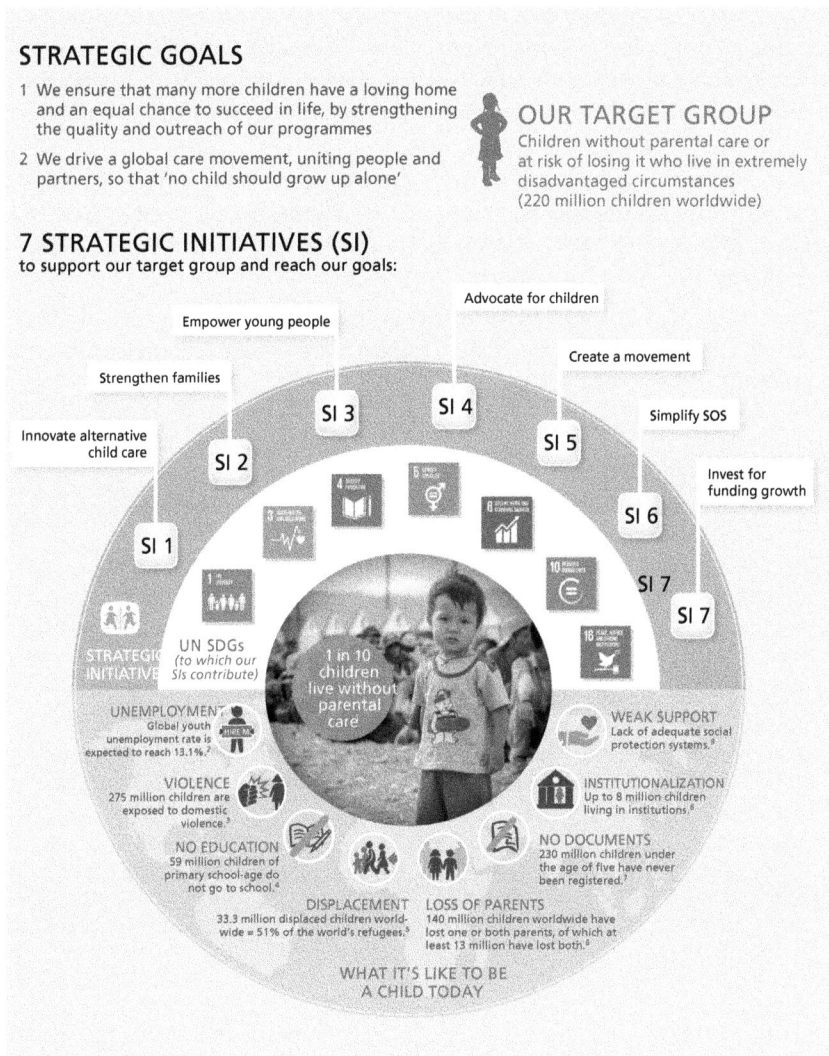

Fig. 16.2 Strategy 2030 of SOS Children's Villages, with reference to the Sustainable Development Goals.
Reproduced from Strategy 2030 of SOS Children's Villages, reference made to Sustainable Development Goals, Copyright (2016), with permission from SOS Children's Villages International. Available at https://www.sos-childrensvillages.org/getmedia/a396383a-c537-4a59-a0cc-b73151e4775f/SOS-Children-s-Villages-2030Strategy.pdf

that everybody in the organization stands for the cause. Therefore, everybody is also an agent of advocacy, even at a minimal level. This aspect is particularly relevant for leadership staff, since they are the official communication source of the organization.

- Depending on the resources available, you can create waves to ride on or you ride on existing waves with your advocacy goals. Sometimes advocacy is also an opportunistic undertaking. Certain windows of opportunity are opening and closing again. If one does not use them, one might have to invest significantly larger amounts than when using the windows of opportunity.
- Successful advocacy is also about successful alliance building. If there are others who are like-minded, why not trying to do it together even if in other areas one might be competing. You can usually use a bigger network and have more resources available.
- Define the goals and regularly check on progress. To avoid unfocused advocacy, define clear goals. It can be a long-term goal or a shorter-term target which is achieved after a limited period.

References

1. **European Parliament's Committee on Foreign Affairs (AFET)** (1972) Allgemeiner Fürsorgeerziehungstag. Evaluation.
2. **Flitner, A.**, **Bittner, G.**, **Vollert, M**. (1966) *Pädagog Probl Kinderdorfs Umrisse Einer Praxisbegleitenden Unters*. Sonderdruck.
3. **Bakhshyan, A.**, **Poghosyan, M**. (2011) *Deinstitutionalization Process*. Regional Conference on Inclusive Education for Children with Disabilities. Moscow: Russian Federation, 27–29 September 2011. Available at: https://www.unicef.org/ceecis/1.Bakhshyan.pptx
4. **CELTIS Centre for excellence for looked after children in Scotland** (2013) *Moving Forward: Implementing the 'Guidelines for the Alternative Care of Children'* (cited 2 June 2017). Available at: http://www.alternativecareguidelines.org/Home/tabid/2372/language/en-GB/Default.aspx
5. **United Nations (UN)** (2017) Sustainable Development Knowledge Platform (cited 2 June 2017). Available at: https://sustainabledevelopment.un.org/topics/sustainabledevelopmentgoals

Section 3

What tools can be used for advocacy?

Chapter 17

Project management techniques for advocates

Walter Struhal and Thomas Grisold

Introduction

'Your beliefs become your thoughts, your thoughts become your words, your words become your actions, your actions become your habits, your habits become your values, your values become your destiny.'

Mahatma Gandhi

This book presents a broad spectrum of advocacy efforts and techniques. This chapter deals with the basics and focuses on the operational side of advocacy. In many ways, planning and implementing advocacy projects is different to working in common clinical environments, and this chapter sets out to present tools and techniques that help with staying focused and getting advocacy projects done.

In doing so, we will first answer the question; *What is needed for doing advocacy?* This question is crucial because in many ways, doing advocacy requires a different mindset and different tools compared to working in a clinical environment. Physicians and nurses will find it hard to apply their best practices in a straightforward manner. Thus, being an advocate is not only about learning how to do new things, but also about *unlearning* established ways of seeing and doing things.[1]

What are the major challenges when working on advocacy projects?

First and foremost, advocacy projects are initiated because they do not exist for some particular issue so far. Thus, we often face a lack of structure and infrastructure, respectively. Whereas clinical environments have clear hierarchies and communication directions, advocates have to build up reliable structures themselves. For example, they need to find target groups and provide resources that can be used.

Furthermore, advocacy projects start with a higher-order purpose or general concern but they should have concrete goals and well-defined milestones. Advocates need to come up with realistic scenarios, expectations, and goals in order to know how to achieve them, when they are successful, if they should adjust them.

Third, common working environments specify what is needed and should be achieved (e.g. through directives or policies). Advocates, defining and pursuing projects on their own, lack external goals and requirements. They need a high level of intrinsic motivation and it is crucial that advocates are aware of what is driving them and how to continue when objections appear. For example, they can be confronted with procrastination and it is important to know how to deal with that.

We use these challenges to organize our chapter into three main parts.

In the first part, we explore how we can prepare the grounds for an advocacy project and create an appropriate infrastructure.

The second part will focus on how we can create goals and milestones.

Finally, in the third part, we will deal with the aspects of motivation and procrastination.

This chapter utilizes the extensive and valuable know-how provided by the Donald M. Palatucci Advocacy Leadership Forum of the American Academy of Neurology.[2] It also integrates findings from other fields.

Preparing the ground and creating an infrastructure

Taking a proactive mindset

Advocacy takes the right mindset. Advocacy is a proactive way of transforming ideas into actions and actions into meaningful reality.

To advocate for a goal, it takes a lot of initiative. In general, people rather react to any situation or act on their issues. Proactive behaviour is necessary to lead a project. When facing challenging situations, people may be tempted to think 'I can't . . .', or 'I could if only this or that was different . . .'. Proactive thinking means remaining focused and optimistic and not to worry about things that one has little control over. The focus is solely put on aspects that one can influence. Proactive people think in terms 'I do . . .', 'I prefer . . .'; they take control and feel fully responsible for what is happening.

Target audience

A project needs to be planned with a target audience in mind and project resources must be aimed at that audience. For example, in order to speak to the public, one needs media contacts (similarly, to influence politicians, one needs to have reliable contacts). The advocate has to ensure that the advocacy project is within the current scope of actions of the politician in mind; for some projects, one might need the support of national specialist organizations.

'Sound bite'

Many projects fail due to communication failures. Communication serves special needs—it transmits information and it persuades. However, communication is not only a synonym for talking. In many cases, it entails the opposite. Peers or team leaders, who feel the urge to keep talking, may lose the attention of the audience, and losing attention can cause lack of communication. Quite counterintuitively, talking can be the best way of losing attention. The paradoxical solution to this fact is that if one wants people to listen, he/she should follow a piece of simple advice: 'Think what you have to say, say it, stop talking.'

In analogy to Eastern philosophy, which emphasizes that taking an action includes the possibility of *not* taking an action,[3] we argue that people can be highly persuasive when they voice a well-thought-through opinion but do not talk otherwise.

A good training to learn how to communicate short and well-thought-through statements is to practice 'elevator pitches', which is a standard training to managers, sales people, policymakers, and others. An elevator pitch is a short summary of one's statement in 20 seconds to 2 minutes. The name comes from the idea that one might eventually run into an important person (e.g. a politician) during an elevator ride. The brief but persuasive summary should provide a simple outline of an advocacy plan and how it supports the target group. In this limited time, one should be able to promote the advocacy plan successfully. One might have only one chance to gain the attention of someone important.

Resources

Resources need to be considered from the very beginning of any advocacy project. Resources are usually one or more of the following:

- Human resources: one's working time and working time of others who contribute to the project.
- Financial resources: costs that may arise and funding that is needed.
- Information resources: information that is needed during the project (address lists, business controlling figures, epidemiological data of insurance companies, and so on).
- Peer resources (peers in the form of senior politicians, senior specialists, and others): peers are needed to support the project's goals.
- Media resources: media coverage that is necessary to carry out the project and respective kinds of media.
- Online resources: Does the advocacy project profit from online footage (e.g. website/subwebsite of a hospital, social media channels)?

If the advocacy project is not a stand-alone initiative but attached to a hospital/ an institution/a national specialist organization, commitment from this other side is mandatory. A series of regulations may influence the advocacy initiatives needed to be taken into account. Participating institutions and organizations must approve the plan prior to the project's inception.

Creating goals and milestones

Any project needs concrete goals and results to be achieved. Before developing goals, one has to have a vision or any other longer-term purpose that should be achieved. We begin this section with methods to come up with a project vision. Subsequently, we suggest how such a vision can be broken down into concrete and achievable goals.

Creating visions and long-term goals

One way to create visions is by learning from an envisioned future. Learning from an envisioned future is a technique that is used in various contexts, including coaching and innovation research.[4,5] The basic idea is that to a large extent, our cognitive processes depend on experiences depend that we have made in the past. We are 'driven by the past'[6] in the sense that we tend to repeat what has worked for us while we avoid what has caused unwanted experiences. While this makes sense for how we behave in our daily lives (e.g. when children avoid touching the hot stove because they remember that it causes pain), this cognitive disposition can hinder our ability to think big and come up with radically new ideas and solutions.[7] Thus, when creating a vision that is compelling and inspiring, we have to set our own experiences, best practices, and expectations aside.

Creating an advocacy plan for the future requires two people: one who performs a mental time travel visualization and another who serves as a facilitator. One of the two should create a vision. He/she is encouraged to undertake 'mental time travelling' where he/she envisions an ideal future point in time (e.g. in 20 years) where *anything* can be possible.[8] The other one serves as a facilitator. He/she has to ensure that one can think of whatever he/she wants; the facilitator should give the feeling that the even the 'craziest ideas' can be possible. He/she should help the mental time traveller to interact with this future state and ask questions, such as 'How does it feel to be there?', 'How does it look like?', 'What happens next?', and so on. The facilitator takes notes of what the mental time traveller reports. In the context of advocacy, the mental time traveller might envision that there is a future state where no one will suffer from a disease that could be avoided when potential victims are sufficiently educated.

In the next step, both facilitator and mental time traveller jointly work on ways that could lead to this future state. This is done via 'back-casting'.[9] The idea here is to start with the latest event, respectively, then look for the previous event which led to this event. Thereby, one learns from the future and realizes ideas in the present. This approach is similar to the '5 Why's' where engineers can find the root of a problem by asking the question 'Why?' 5 times in a row.[10] The goal of back-casting is to reach a present state, while having several steps at hand on how one should proceed.

Consider our example from before. While back-casting, the mental time traveller may report that before everyone was educated and free of a specific disease, a campaign was implemented that attracted everyone's awareness; before the campaign had attracted everyone's awareness, the campaign was launched on the right channels; before it was launched on the right channels, it was created in a way that the target group appreciated the idea and design of the campaign; to do so, it was first ensured that the designers had a good understanding of the target group and a sample of them was invited to judge the idea, and so on.

This technique is applicable to all kinds of scenarios and projects.

'Higher altitudes'—perspective list

Similar to a vision, a higher altitude goal reports on a long-term purpose. The time perspective is longer (e.g. 2–5 years) in order to achieve a given goal. An example could be a young neurologist aiming 'to build a hospital for those in need and get public funding for it'. 'Higher altitudes' are goals a person wants to achieve in the long run.

Another simple method to identify long-term goals and visions is to write a letter to yourself while pretending that this letter will be sent in around ten years ahead.

One should ask, 'What kind of person will receive this letter?', 'How do you imagine this person to be seen by others?', 'What did this person achieve during this time?'

These questions help putting one's ideas into context and identifying central values. They also help to define the higher vision of what someone wants to achieve.

Preprocessing and setting an advocacy goal

While the previous sections focused on how visions or some higher-order goals can be created we will now pursue the question of how we can break them down into concrete and achievable goals.

At first, large goals and visions might appear scary and risky. As a popular analogy, imagine that you have to eat an elephant; bearing in mind that the goal to eat the elephant can be important but at the same time, might quickly cause frustration and end in frustration. The problem is that the task appears too challenging and one does not know where to start. This is why one should think of eating the elephant by 'one bite at a time'. The following chapter will try to provide advocates with tools to eat the elephant by many—and effective—bites.

SMART

Any objective needs some preprocessing before one is able to start working on it. It is quite effective to first check objectives in whether they are SMART (Specific, Measurable, Attainable, Realistic, Timely).

Specific—it is important that any goal is specific. Formulating an object like 'I want amyotrophic lateral sclerosis (ALS) patients to have access to counselling' is unspecific. Instead, it should entail a specific objective: 'ALS patients (*who*), by the end of 2020 (*when*), will have a counselling group helping them to deal with their everyday problems (*what*) in Central Austria (*where*)'.

Measurable—any objective needs to be measurable with respect to quantity (in numbers) and quality (in comparison to similar structures). 'To become the best intensive care specialist of my country' might be an encouraging objective, but it is not measurable; it is not clear when and under what circumstances someone is the best intensive care specialist. A better way to put this is to 'to improve the intensive care at my unit' and 'obtain the certification of a national reference centre'.

Attainable—any objective must be within in the reach of one's own limits. If it exceeds the limits, one has to redefine the issue, divide one issue into several issues, and/or start with some attainable goal in the first place. For example, 'to provide access to palliative care for all ALS patients throughout the EU' is probably not an attainable target. However, 'to provide access to palliative care for all ALS patients throughout my country' might be. From there, one may be able to plan subsequent goals; a next objective could be 'to advocate the advantages of palliative care for ALS patients to all counties of my country', and so on.

Realistic—goals should be built on realistic expectations, and one should have the means to pursue them. It might be unrealistic that a basic science teacher does an advocacy plan in neuroimaging for brain tumours; a neurologist or neurosurgeon is the most suitable person for pursuing this aim.

Timely—goals should be attainable within a specific time frame. For this, it needs both a deadline and interim deadlines (milestones). Planning a deadline is tricky. One way to define a deadline is to go through the project outlines and infer how long this might take from one's own experience. However, studies show that only 20% of projects are finished within the predicted time frame[11]; the phenomenon that is referred to as a 'cone of uncertainty' has been observed at NASA and in many other contexts, and it can be crucial for planning advocacy projects. It is advisable to consider at least five scenarios, which could potentially delay the deadline; by adding the time that is needed to deal with longest delay can be helpful for defining a realistic deadline. Milestones are intermediate goals that are needed to achieve the overall goal. They are necessary to further pursue the final goal and to follow the plan of the project.

Here is an example of how a goal can be divided into milestones:

- 22 March: Convincing hospital administration to provide free rooms for ALS counselling within the outpatients' department.
- 1 May: Finding 2 neurologists, 2 nurses, and 1 psychologist and committing them to meet once a month with an ALS group.
- 1 July: Having a subwebsite on the administration's website promoting the meeting.
- 1 July: Making calls to all ALS services throughout the county promoting the ALS initiative and convincing them to recommend the website to their patients and their care givers to spread information on the service.
- 30 September: Having the first ALS counselling meeting.

Finally, writing down a short summary of the initial intentions will maintain focus on this goal.

To-do lists

Most people use to-do lists in one way or another. A to-do list helps us to not forget tasks, and, it keeps one's mind free of distress that something might be overlooked. However, if not done right, a to-do list can be a major source of frustration as it leaves items that have not been done on there for a long time (please also refer to https://gettingthingsdone.com and stephencovey.com).

How to write a to-do list and what it is for

First it is important to understand the difference between *projects* and *tasks*. Tasks are single items that are done in a single session. If something cannot be done in a single session, it is a project, and a project consists of several tasks. To avoid frustration, one should never put projects on a to-do list. Projects should be placed on a separate project list; the to-do list is for tasks only.

Projects list

The next thing to do is having a second look at the projects list. Within this second look, it is wise to check whether they are SMART (see earlier section, 'SMART'). If the project is large enough to have milestones, those need to be on a project list as well.

If there are projects on the list that are not SMART, there is a good chance that the project is just a perspective. This again should be deleted from the project list and placed on a personal perspective list.

Dealing with lists

By following the above considerations, one will end up with three kinds of lists: to-do lists, project lists, and higher altitudes lists. While the higher altitudes list will serve as a source of motivation or occasional adaptation, it is important to deal with the other two lists appropriately.

Working on the to-do list

The to-do list does not entail any projects but only tasks. Adding a heading 'inbox' finalizes the first collection of tasks. One should also add any new incoming task to the 'inbox'. As a rule of thumb, one should not add tasks that can be done within 2 minutes; such tasks should just be done immediately or regarded as non-important.

The next step is to select tasks from the 'inbox' that need to be done within a week. Those tasks are transferred into the 'week's list'. Many clinicians feel that their main daily work is *not* their to-do list as they might have to get their patients work done before they can follow up their to-do list. A good strategy can be to not have more than 10 items on a 'week's list'. If they are done by the middle of the week, one can still add 'inbox' items to the 'week's list'. However, one should not add too many tasks to 'week's list' as this can be a source of stress and frustration and chances are high that the lists will not be worked down.

Once a task is completed, it is important to take some seconds to define the next step and the next task on the 'inbox' list. At this moment, it takes the least time to think about what is needed next to pursue the project, and it may save time at a later point in time.

Reviewing lists

The 'week's list' requires daily review until all tasks are completed.

The 'inbox' and 'projects list' only require weekly review. This is also a good point to define the next action for a project on the project list, and add that to the 'inbox'. If resources are needed for getting a task done, such as an address list or some information from elsewhere, the task should be added to the 'inbox'. If a task was delegated to someone else, the task should be kept in the 'inbox', and eventually turned into a task which entails sending out a reminder to that person.

The platform does not matter

These simple tools should enable anyone to manage complex projects. It does not matter what platform one uses to keep these lists. The easier and faster, the better. It is important to have a platform or paper and pencil available at all times. One should develop a habit of writing down new tasks that float in and immediately adding them to the 'inbox'. If one prefers handwriting, it is better to keep those lists in a notebook than on a bunch of single papers. Marking undone tasks with a '–', and turning them into a '+' when completed is a simple trick that may add motivation.

Nowadays, many tasks float in as emails and one might prefer to organize them there. Simple tools will help with that. One can create a 'projects' subfolder, a 'weeks' subfolder and an 'inbox' subfolder in the mailbox. This can be done on almost any smartphone. Incoming tasks are simply moved into the inbox and further processed from there.

Keeping the wheel turning—motivation and procrastination

While goals and visions are important to initiate and keep track of a project, there can be challenges while working on it. This section will explore how we can get things done successfully.

Make doing tasks a habit

One challenge is to create a habit for working on tasks. As soon as doing tasks on a daily basis becomes a habit, it does not need much motivation to work on them. How does such a thing become a habit? The simple answer is: by working on it every day. One popular method to achieve this behaviour has been invented by Jerry Seinfeld, a famous comedian in the United States.[12] He suggests putting a large calendar at a prominent place in one's house or office. Subsequently, one uses a large red marker pen, and every day that is used to work on tasks should be crossed out with a large 'X'. After several days, one realizes that the series of X looks like a chain. From this day onwards the guiding principle should be: 'Don't break the chain'. Soon it may become a habit.

Procrastination

Procrastination deserves special attention as we often find ourselves in environments that can distract us. Typically, a neurologist works with a laptop and has a smartphone at hand. These two items are also a calendar, a telephone, a television set that plays one's favourite shows, a computer game, a postbox where letters (emails), short texts and image snippets (social media) pop up constantly, and so on. Interestingly, procrastination tends to appear during small or seemingly unimportant tasks; it can be defined as 'letting the low-priority tasks get in the way of high-priority tasks'.[13] Furthermore, procrastination has been linked to intrinsic and extrinsic motivation. *Extrinsic* motivation depends on external contingencies (such as monetary reward) and *intrinsic* motivation results from an internal drive. It has been found that intrinsic motivation correlates with lower degrees of procrastination (e.g. see[14]). In the context of advocacy, this means that one should always envision why he/she is doing something and what purpose he/she is trying to achieve; this can help to overcome perceive burdens that could potentially trigger periods of procrastination. It can also help in cases where greater challenges appear. In that regard, we find it inspiring to refer to neurologist and holocaust survivor Viktor Frankl, who claimed that one can master anything as long as he/she is aware of the purpose; that is, why he/she is doing it.

There are many ways to fight procrastination. In the following, we will present two techniques that employ conditioned reflexes to make task completion a habit.

Start your work

If one is about to start with a task, he/she should take a second to think about the next task. Then, he/she should enact a movement pattern, such as standing up, taking some steps around the chair and sitting down; then to immediately start with another task. Once you have commenced your task, you will work on it. Repeating the procedure (short focus with closed eyes and movement pattern) will condition you to focus on the next task.

Stay focused and take regular breaks

A simple method for mixing creativity with recreation is the 'pomodoro method'. The only tools that are needed are a simple kitchen clock and any piece of paper. Deciding on the task one wants to work on and setting the kitchen clock to 25 minutes is the first step. Subsequently, one works on the task until the kitchen clock rings. If any distractions occur during this period, one should note them down on the piece of paper; this is referred to as the 'junk journal'. One should immediately return to the task. Once the clock rings, there will be a 5-minute break. During that break, one can do whatever he/she likes, also things that have been written down in the junk journal. After the break, the clock should be set to 25 minutes and one returns to the task. After doing four 'pomodoros', there is a longer break of 15–30 minutes.

After applying the pomodoro technique for a while, one will find it much easier to focus. Rewinding the timer triggers attention to focus on the task. The ticking sound of the kitchen clock externalizes one's wish to complete the task. Focus will become a conditioned reflex coupled with the mechanical stimuli of the kitchen clock.

Motivation and fighting procrastination—lessons learnt by Churchill and Eisenhower

Winston Churchill was famous for both being focused and working through a tremendous pile of work. He had several important rules that can be interesting for working on advocacy projects.

1. He never focused on more than one subject and one or two side subjects. He did not allow any intrusions into his work and that way, he mastered procrastination.
2. He used two types of priorities. He tagged his memos by 'respond today' or by 'respond in three days'. That might be far from how one works in clinical environments but the important point is that he only used two types of priorities: important and not important. The simpler the rules to follow in project management, the more effective they are.
3. Churchill did not accept responses that were longer than one single typewriter page. Nowadays, we receive emails. Trying to keep them as short as possible (an email should not be longer than a few lines), and making a phone call for one specific action saves precious time for both the sender and the recipient.

Dwight Eisenhower invented a productivity method that is called the 'Eisenhower Box'. He assigned two types of priorities to any task: important/not important and urgent/not urgent.

Important tasks target one's goals. Urgent tasks call for immediate action.

Why can this box be helpful? It provides a simple means to focus on tasks that have direct impact on one's goals. Another interesting finding is that urgent tasks fulfil someone else's needs, while non-urgent tasks are set for oneself. Therefore, the proactive advocates will find the most important tasks in the 'important/not urgent' quarter. Those tasks need special attention. The 'important/urgent' quarter is important for teamwork but it may stress one's personal resources that are needed for the 'important/not urgent' quarter. Therefore, an important strategy to save resources is to spare items from this quarter. While 'not important/urgent' tasks do not help reaching one's goal, someone else depends on them. Therefore, those tasks should be delegated. The 'not important/not urgent' tasks are distracting. One should not work on them at all.

Every clinician, medical doctor, or member of any other medical discipline has to take many important decisions. Decision fatigue is a common problem for clinicians and other advocates. With respect to decision fatigue, Barack Obama once commented: 'I don't want to make decisions about what I'm eating or wearing. Because I have too many other decisions to make.' Decision fatigue can be prevented by focusing on decisions that really matter.

Note-taking techniques help to record meetings and stay focused. Any medium suffices as long as it does not cause distractions. Therefore, laptops might be a bad choice.

Bill Gates relied on taking notes. Despite being a computer-literate, a skilled person who could even hire an assistant to take notes, he takes the notes himself, and it is said that his notes are extremely detailed. He does so by splitting a page into quadrants where each quadrant conveys different kinds of information (e.g. references, questions, to-do items). A similar system is the Cornell note-taking method, which should help students to take notes.

While there may be a number of other techniques, any effort to learn how one can take efficient notes is important.

Discussion: Why projects fail

So far, we have presented techniques and methods that support advocates in carrying out projects successfully and efficiently. In that regard, it is important to consider common causes for project failures. While failures are inevitable to some extent and can even be a valuable source for learning and improving projects (see Chapter 18), common problems can be avoided when advocates focus on them exclusively.

General sources of failure

Failures can be assigned to one of the following categories:

- poor communication (e.g. being unable to make the goal of the projects clear and easily understandable to the project team)
- bad cooperation (e.g. team leaders are unsuccessful in holding committed people together and keeping them motivated)
- insufficient quality or communication (e.g. leaving different team members with different expectations, eventually decreasing team motivation and commitment)

Leadership failures

Insufficient leadership can also lead to failures (please also refer to [15]) under the following reasons:

- no clear roles provided to team members
- responsibilities are not well defined
- unrealistic team planning and commitment imagination
- poor risk awareness
- misinterpretation of risks as results (and eventually making team members responsible for it)
- choosing too complex a process to reach the goal, if similar results may be reached with less effort
- reacting to any problem as soon as they occur instead of situation analysis and 'triaging' problems
- poor resource planning
- lack of 'situation awareness' leading to insufficient consequences

Poor scheduling

Another reason for failures can be poor scheduling when

- not choosing a good compromise in high quality and time resources (tighter schedules often cause poorer quality; overestimated quality expectations may destroy any scheduling and end in project failure);
- there is poor risk management, or risk assessment AFTER scheduling.

Problems are part of any project and they should not provide reasons to cancel a project. It may be helpful to look at how emergency departments deal with patients: before treating any patient, they triage incoming emergencies while setting aside the urgency of the disease. It is important to collect sufficient context information and start tackling problems in a triage-like system. For the context of project management in advocacy, it can be helpful to redefine the operational steps that are necessary to reach the goal, and eventually adapt the project strategy.

If one cannot get the project on track again, one should immediately stop putting any resources into the project and clearly communicate the decision to the team. The project should not be regarded as failed but it can be resumed as soon as there are realistic chances for a successful implementation.

However, if success is unlikely, the project needs to be terminated. It has to be communicated that the project is not pursued anymore. In such cases, advocates should reflect on why a project failed since negative experiences can be valuable for any project that will follow.

Conclusion

'Continuous effort—not strength or intelligence—is the key to unlocking our potential.'
                                                                                                    Winston Churchill

We set out to focus on the operational side of advocacy. Stressing that advocates can face a number of challenges when working on their projects, we collected and presented various tools and strategies that might be helpful for planning and implementing ideas. We presented tools and project management techniques that are easy to implement.

One challenge can be that there is no or malfunctioning infrastructure. Thus, we suggested how advocates can define their target group, communicate effectively, and organize their resources.

Another challenge can lie in the fact that there are no concrete goals and milestones. We explored how advocates can create visions and higher altitude goals. Furthermore, we argued that effective goals follow distinct patterns and to-do lists can be effective means to keep track of any project.

We identified a third challenge with respect to motivation and procrastination. Being prepared for scenarios when procrastination kicks in can be essential for anyone who is doing advocacy.

While we placed emphasis on efforts that should be taken before or during a project, we did not consider the post-hoc analysis of advocacy projects. Advocates should carefully revisit their plans and notes after they have carried out a project. By understanding what actually changed and did not adhere to prior predictions, one can develop more realistic plans for subsequent projects.

The toolkit we have provided is applicable to various contexts. However, a toolkit should not become the project itself. Often, people tend to spend too much energy in defining tasks. For example, websites offer a number of recommendations of adding a range of tags to one's tasks (e.g. tagging by 'circumstances', adding 'due' dates, 'ID' lists, and so on). It is important to consider that the more work one has with defining tasks, the less time will be spent on actually achieving them.

References

1. **Grisold, T., Kaiser, A.** (2017) Leaving behind what we are not: applying a systems thinking perspective to present unlearning as an enabler for finding the best version of the self. *J Organ Transform Soc Change*, **14**(1), 39–55.
2. **American Academy of Neurology**. Palatucci Advocacy Leadership. Available at: https://www.aan.com/public-policy/palatucci-advocacy-leadership-forum/
3. **Brook, C. et al.** (2016) On stopping doing those things that are not getting us to where we want to be: Unlearning, wicked problems and critical action learning. *Hum Relat*, **69**(2), pp. 369–389. http://journals.sagepub.com/doi/abs/10.1177/0018726715586243
4. **Scharmer, C. O.** (2001) Self-transcending knowledge. Sensing and organizing around emerging opportunities. *J Knowl Manag*, **5**(2), 137–150.
5. **Kaiser, A., Kragulj, F., Grisold, T., Walser, R.** (2016) Learning from an envisioned future—an empirical account. *Electron J Knowl Manag*, **14**(1), 18–29.
6. **Seligman, M. E. P., Railton, P., Baumeister, R. F., Sripada, C.** (2013) Navigating into the future or driven by the past. *Perspect Psychol Sci*, **8**(2), 119–41.
7. **Grisold, T., Peschl, M. F.** (2017) Why a systems thinking perspective on cognition matters for innovation and knowledge creation. A framework towards leaving behind our projections from the past for creating new futures. *Syst Res Behav Sci*, **34**(3), 335–53.

8. **Markley, O. W**. (2008) Mental time travel: A practical business and personal research tool for looking ahead. *Futures*, **40**(1), 17–24.
9. **Dreborg, K. H**. (1996) Essence of backcasting. *Futures*, **28**(9), 813–28.
10. **Chiarini, A**. (2013) *Lean Organizations: From the Tools of the Toyota Production System to Lean Office*. Milano: Springer.
11. **Little, T**. (2006) Schedule estimation and uncertainty surrounding the cone of uncertainty. *IEEE Softw Los Alamitos*, **23**(3), 48–54.
12. **Trapani, G**. (2007) *Jerry Seinfeld's Productivity Secret*. LifeHacker. Available at: https://lifehacker.com/281626/jerry-seinfelds-productivity-secret
13. **Vij, J**., **Lomash, H**. (2014) Role of motivation in academic procrastination. *Int J Sci Eng Res*, **5**(8), 1065–70.
14. **Chu, A. H. C**., **Choi, J. N**. (2005) Rethinking procrastination: positive effects of 'active' procrastination behavior on attitudes and performance. *J Soc Psychol Phila*, **145**(3), 245–64.
15. **International Project Leadership Academy**. 101 Common Causes. Available at: http://calleam.com/WTPF/?page_id=2338

Chapter 18

International advocacy: Case studies and lessons learnt

Wolfgang Grisold, Anna Klicpera, and Thomas Grisold

Introduction

Advocacy activities aim at taking the voice of patients to inform, protect, and support them. This book shows that advocacy can take on various forms in different contexts (e.g. for specific diseases or regions) and on different levels (e.g. micro, meso, and macro). In this chapter, we emphasize yet another dimension that is important to consider: advocacy on an international level as compared to advocacy on a national level. We believe that this is crucial because as soon as we talk about international advocacy, there are more dimensions to be taken into account. Think of cross-cultural communication, for example, which does not only yield language barriers but also requires us to rethink how we talk to potential recipients. Another example may be different culture based negotiation styles that, when one is unaware of them, can be surprising and unsettling at times.

Naturally, we can differentiate between two kinds of outcomes: success and failure. Success stories motivate us to start with projects and push them through. At the same time, failures can equip us with important insights and make us aware of issues that we might overlook otherwise. While we may tempted to report on accounts which actually worked well and proved to be successful, we also want focus on the possibility of failure. We are confident that the question '*What has not worked for us in advocacy projects?*' will be equally enlightening to anyone who is planning activities on an international level. What is more, by allowing a *culture of failure* among physicians and advocates, we hope to raise awareness of the importance of being open as this allows us to avoid setting unrealistic goals and have discussions about possible threats. An example, which we find inspiring in that regard, is Princeton professor Johannes Haushofer's 'academic CV of failure' which sparked an open and stimulating discussion about the strengths and weaknesses of academia.[i,ii]

---

[i] https://www.theguardian.com/commentisfree/2016/may/02/cv-of-failures-rejections-success-not-guaranteed

[ii] https://www.nature.com/naturejobs/science/articles/10.1038/nj7322-467a

How can advocacy work on an international level? This is the question we will pursue from multiple perspectives. Essentially, the main goal of an international (and any other) advocacy activity is to draw attention to and take actions with respect to health-related issues. However, since there are countless possibilities to enter an international sphere, we will point to different kinds of activities.

This chapter is structured as follows. We will first present two different advocacy activities that we consider a success on an international level. Subsequently, we will present cases where we were involved and reflect on what has worked and what has not. Finally, by clustering insights from the first two sections, we present some lessons learnt that should be taken into account when practising international advocacy.

International advocacy in neurology

The following two cases illustrate two kinds of advocacy on an international level. First, we will present what we refer to as a 'classical' advocacy activity. Starting from the observation that some patient groups may be in need of advocacy, advocates plan political activities to reach their goals. Second, we will show a 'modern' and disruptive approach, which utilizes the outreach of social media.

The treatment of stroke

Stroke for a long time was a disease that went 'unclaimed' by several medical specialties, including neurology. The reasons being that stroke is a devastating disease, remedies were very few, and it concerned mainly elderly persons, which had few supporters. Often, as voiced by a neuropathologist, all one could ask and hope for in the case of stroke was to have 'a good nurse'. This was, and is reflected also in the old World Health Organization (WHO) ICD 10 classification, where due to the 'causality principle' stroke was mainly a vascular disease and which neglected its neurological aspects, care, and rehabilitation. But in recent years, several steps at different levels allowed important improvements. What led to this growing awareness and subsequent success in this case? In addition to some important medical advancements (such as thrombolysis and treatment of occlusion of large vessels), important activities took place (and still do) that we today label 'advocacy'.

First of all, *statistical analyses* have made it clear that 'non-communicable diseases' are the greatest burden in high-income countries and are becoming also an increasing burden in low- and middle-income countries countries.[1]

Second, by taking a historical perspective,[2] the concept of a *stroke unit* emerged in Europe in the 1990s. There are still controversies about the exact structure, purpose and procedure of a stroke unit but it was shown that stroke units improve patient treatment as compared to conventional units. The use of stroke units has been accepted as an improvement with the main argument of special care and attention.

Finally, *neuro-rehabilitation,* which not only focuses on motor and sensory deficits but also covers the wide range of neuropsychological and neurocognitive changes, has become more and more important. Its significance has been underestimated and the concept of neuro-rehabilitation in stroke patients is increasingly used.[3,4] Particularly patients which do not suffer from clearly recognizable deficits as motor and sensory symptoms, but subtler neuropsychological and neuropsychiatric disorders benefit from neuro-rehabilitation. Several centres were established. The concept of further rehabilitation was introduced to both patient/carer and neurologist and its acceptance continues to grow.

These efforts taken together led to increasing awareness within neurologists of the importance of caring for their patients beyond their medical duties. Such endeavours go on until today, promoting efforts towards better recognition, classification, treatment, rehabilitation, and prevention of stroke. Following the distinction made in Chapter 1, this campaign was implemented on a meso-level, as the focus here was on local developments in Austria. Nevertheless, it had a strong backing in the international development. It was a global success that stroke was moved from its classification as a vascular disease to a neurological disease in ICD 11. It also shows that many changes on several levels can be implemented,[5] which will help to make stroke treatment globally more efficient; this is further discussed in Chapter 14.

The ice bucket challenge

An example of a modern approach to advocacy can be seen in the 'ice bucket challenge'. This campaign created a global craze in 2014. By encouraging Facebook users (including influential celebrities) to pour cold water over their heads, the campaign was aimed at increasing awareness and acquisition of resources to fight amyotrophic lateral sclerosis (ALS), which is a rapidly progressive incurable neurological disease. Within a few days and weeks, this campaign attracted worldwide attention and found many imitators.[6-8] The campaign started on Facebook and its spread was described as a 'roller coaster' effect[9] and a 'viral infection',[10] and it is generally considered a success for scientific research funding.[11] International and national societies dealing with ALS were the beneficiaries and according to reports,[8] money devoted to research could be accrued. For the purpose of this chapter, the most striking point about this campaign was that it disrupted the conventional way of doing advocacy. There was no one pushing through the message that ALS research should be supported but rather, the community took over and made it their own concern. By that, people were made aware of this disease which might not have happened otherwise. This example illustrates that social media is a powerful instrument, also in the context of advocacy.[12]

At first glance, the two cases—stroke and ALS—differ in various respects. Yet, both share two aspects that we want to highlight.

First, both campaigns responded to the needs of the time. Stroke was a disease that could not be treated well under the given circumstances (e.g. classified as a matter of vascular internal medicine), and different activities improved the treatment of patients. Likewise, ALS was a disease that did not receive as much attention as other serious diseases do because it had no lobby.

Second, and this might be counterintuitive when we speak of *international* advocacy, both activities managed to grow after they were well embedded in a local community. We are aware that, *local* is an elastic term. While the first campaign was done on a meso-level, that is, it started locally and nationwide, the ice bucket challenge was done on Facebook. Despite being globally accessible, this platform can also be seen as a local community because members are interacting within clearly defined boundaries. Only by utilizing the strengths of this community (culture of sharing, use of videos, and so on), this campaign was able to gain momentum.

A reflection and own examples in advocacy campaigns

Although advocacy campaigns primarily address relevant target groups and stakeholders to create awareness and trigger actions, they may also reach people who are advocates themselves. In many cases, successful campaigns have an encouraging and inspiring effect on those who promote similar issues. In the following, we will reflect on how we tackled challenges in international advocacy, and report on personal experiences. While not all of us were involved in all cases, we report on them from a 'we' perspective.

Jumping on the ice bucket bandwagon?

Case description and learnings

In Austria, the news of the ice-bucket challenge spread quickly and before a strategy of participation could be defined, the first and most powerful wave of the campaign was already over. Press, news, and television asked for opinions in these advanced stages of the campaign and a few articles with little scientific impact appeared. The momentum to organize fundraising was lost. Despite the fact that several questions on how to possibly donate for the purpose of ALS research were received, no further progress was made and the fruits of labour could not be harvested.

Marginally benefitting from this campaign, the Austrian Society of Neurology approached the Austrian minister of social welfare to voice concern about the fate of patients with ALS and the lack of social institutions and especially the unacceptably long wait for social support after the diagnosis. As ALS progresses quickly, patient support is needed urgently to match the speed of the disease.

The minister assured his support and will for improvement and some civil servants were assigned to the tasks discussed. However, no progress was made. We approached the topic again, stressing the importance of our case but any attempt remained unsuccessful and we had to give up our idea.

Unfortunately, our project failed. Nevertheless, we believe that there are lessons to be learned from this experience.

Campaigns sometimes appear unexpectedly and need a quick decision to follow them and to take full advantage. In our case, we could not reach this decision quickly enough. When we finally approached the minister, the momentum had already gone. Furthermore, we did not consider what measures to take if it had been successful. We asked for funds because the time seemed right but we did not specify how that funding would be spent.

We experienced that bureaucracy needs to be avoided as much as possible, or at least taken into consideration that the pace of bureaucracy is different than the spirit of a campaign. In our case, the commitment ended with the expression of the will to change things but this will did not translate into a specific plan.

As an additional factor, we did not foresee that the administration of the ministry changed due to political shifts. Soon, our contacts were no longer available.

Leadership and advocacy: Reflecting on a setback

Case description

It is a merit of the American Academy of Neurology (AAN) to have created the 'Palatucci advocacy and leadership courses' (https://www.aan.com/conferences-community/leadership-programs/palatucci-advocacy-leadership/).

These were designed to give insight into the necessity of introducing the concept of advocacy on several levels to a selected group of neurologists. The courses increased awareness of individual responsibility to practice advocacy and also exposed the participants to many practical issues such as dealing with politicians and the press, and how to communicate crisply, succinctly, and effectively; see Chapter 17 for an in-depth analysis of the respective tools.

Participating in this course was 'eye opening', and we were fortunate to attend several other courses in different roles, also as advisors. The Palatucci courses also suggested that leadership was clearly involved in being able to advocate and to create, sustain, develop, and finalize advocacy projects. Without doubt, leadership is often underestimated and needs to be considered by medical doctors and neurologists at every stage.[13,14]

Returning from these short and fertile inspirations, we decided that the development of a European advocacy/leadership programme could be a feasible project that can possibly be a development or future joint development with the AAN. Being in charge of an education committee of a large European Society at the time, we were able to present this idea not only to the society's education committee but also to the executive committee.

However, things did not turn out as expected.

In both situations, but definitely more in the executive committee, we were not able to bring across our points well. Our idea was acknowledged, but clearly not appreciated. This could be due to an insufficient explanation from our side, an unprepared audience, or a combination of both. A clearer summary of content was requested and after a period of two years and two more executive meetings, the concept seemed more appreciated understood and we were asked to proceed.

Then the issue of financing came up. Back then, the society considered spending money on advocacy as irrelevant. At the same time, an unrestricted grant of a drug company could be secured and a financial plan involving all costs—venue, speakers, and organization—was developed; finally, the project seemed ready to go.

Then came the session where the executive committee should provide final approval. Having solved all issues, in particular the financial issue, we expected clearance and the directive to go ahead. Presenting the plan, we realized after a few minutes that the wind had changed. Members of the committee brought forth several unexpected arguments against this project, such as costs and overall need; it was even suggested that the participants should be selected for neuro-political reasons (instead of the quality of their application).

Finally, it was argued that it was not necessary for a scientific neurological society to invest in leadership as this could be potentially 'dangerous' for a society; it were not within the tasks of a scientific society to bring forward leaders and leadership. The concept of advocacy was new at the time, and it seemed that possibly the attachment to 'leadership' created irrational fears, as if the own position of the leadership was under threat. We were unprepared for this rejection, perhaps speechless. Although a compromise was finally offered, the project did not progress.

Both executive secretaries, who had actively worked with us on throughout the preparation, exposed a 'blank' face in this discussion. They provided no support. Additionally, remote members of the executive committee, who had never been involved in this project, added negative vibes and statements.

We invested a lot of time, effort, and energy into this project. However, after this meeting we were forced to cancel the project in the final stage.

Learnings

What can be learnt from this setback?

First and foremost, the project was new, and perhaps we did not do enough groundwork to communicate the aim of this project to others. In hindsight, we might have been overconfident that the project and its intended goals were supported by all members of the committee. We did not promote the project internally to engage and promote more potential supporters. Also, we should have prepared other strategies in the stage of preparation.

Furthermore, we missed the point that advocacy was not a trending topic at that time, and people involved did not understand what it really means. This issue might pertain today, and as this book is written, many questions on advocacy are still unsolved, such as the difference to lobbying.

As a further lesson learnt, we suggest that we should not have emphasized the term 'leadership' in the executive board. This may have caused fears to the members as it may have been interpreted as a threat to their present position. This highlights that a careful choice of wording, or if strong wording needs to be used, a level of clarification and additional explanation is necessary.

Such issues might have been detected through the eyes of others involved. However, we overestimated the bond and alliance with our close project co-workers. In particular, we felt comforted by some members who assured us that the project was on a good way and it would be only a matter of time until it was being realized.

Finally, we were not resilient enough. As suggested in Chapter 1, resilience is an important aspect to consider in all aspects of advocacy.[15] We did not have any exit strategy when we were confronted with a complete change of direction.

Organization-world-wide efforts: Advocacy in IFMSA

Case description

Although it becomes more widely accepted in the medical community that a physician's role includes being an advocate for his or her patients' health, they often do not engage in advocacy activities.[16,17] In order to live up to our profession's responsibilities and make our voices heard, we—future medical doctors of the International Federation of Medical Students' Associations (IFMSA)[iii]—decided to put an emphasis on advocacy within our work.

We did so by organizing widespread peer-to-peer training sessions on advocacy and focusing on advocacy campaigns as one of the federation's priorities.

The advocacy training sessions were held at international meetings, as well as national assemblies. Additionally, members were trained to train their fellow students, generating a snowball effect by passing on the skills to a large group of future medical doctors. The training was aimed at providing participants with the necessary knowledge and skills to set up advocacy campaigns. Through interactive exercises, students could gain confidence speaking up and learn how to approach stakeholders with their ideas. Furthermore, the training put a spotlight on advocacy and sparked discussions about its purpose and importance.

At the IFMSA's general assembly twice a year, policy statements, which summarize its stance on different issues such as climate change or breastfeeding, are discussed and adopted. These are important advocacy tools and are used when representing the federation towards its external partners and at international meetings, such as the World Health Assembly.[iv] The prioritizing of advocacy within IFMSA's work had seen a rise in proposed and adopted policy statements. Furthermore, efforts were made to improve and intensify external representation by strengthening ties to existing partners and establishing relations with new ones. A particular focus was set on ensuring that the federation is represented at important conferences and that the students representing it were well prepared.

The focus on both training and improving external representation led to the organization of the first Youth Pre- World Health Assembly by the IFMSA. This workshop, which was held just before the World Health Assembly, brought together students from different health-related disciplines such as medicine, dentistry, law, pharmacy, and public health. Over the course of a few days, the students listened to presentations by invited experts on key issues which were on the agenda for the World Health Assembly. Small working groups focused on these issues, and prepared briefing papers and interventions to use in interactions with stakeholders and presentations during the assembly. The students also underwent training in advocacy; for example, in simulation exercises, they were given the opportunity to enact WHO members to better understand the workings of decision-making processes and receive input and feedback on how to influence them.

[iii] The International Federation of Medical Students' Associations (IFMSA) is a student-run organization that was founded in May 1951 and represents medical students from 130 National Member Organizations in 122 countries (as of February 2017).

[iv] The World Health Assembly is the decision-making body of the World Health Organization (WHO). It is held annually and attended by delegations of all WHO member states. Key decisions concerning policies, WHO work programme, and budget are made at the World Health Assembly.

Although this concerted effort was made within the IFMSA, it is very difficult to tell how big its impact was. At international meetings, the opinion of medical students is listened to, but they are not given a seat at the table when it comes to decision-making. Sometimes professionals might even belittle the students' opinions for their naivety and argue that though their demands are aspirational, they are not realistic. This is a problem that non-professional organizations often face when it comes to advocacy. On the one hand, the students' notion of what is and what should be possible can be a necessary inspiration to change a practitioner's perception. On the other hand, they lack the experience to evaluate ideas in terms of what is necessary to achieve them.

The IFMSA is a federation encompassing more than a hundred national member organizations. Therefore, in order to pass a policy statement, students from very diverse cultural and ideological backgrounds have to agree on it. This often leads to the final statements being phrased in a quite general way lacking concrete suggestions for change, which diminishes their usefulness for advocacy purposes. More controversial ideas might even end up being rejected.

Learnings

Within our advocacy efforts we laid a lot of focus on changing big issues on an international level, which would have had a big impact but was very difficult to achieve, especially for students as mentioned earlier. Given the IFMSA's potential to reach a lot of medical students through its national member organizations, a strategy focusing on achieving small changes on the local level might have been more effective. It is important to consider the organization's strengths and reach when planning advocacy campaigns. Non-professional organizations such as the IFMSA often have less influence on the policy level but do have a lot of committed members who through awareness campaigns and consistent pressure on local stakeholders, can succeed in realizing changes.

It also might have been more effective to use the trainings to practice how participants could apply the taught skills on a particular issue and therefore already train them to advocate within a federation-wide campaign. But as there was no plan or concept for such a campaign, the training sessions were kept more general, aiming at providing skills without specifying their practical application.

Considering the aforementioned, the IFMSA's work on advocacy might not have led to big policy changes, but it nevertheless had a profound impact on the students involved. Discussions both on international and national level raised awareness among medical students for their responsibility as advocates for their patients and trainings gave them the skills to live up to this responsibility.

Although medical students might start medical school with an idealistic outlook, their idealism often declines throughout their training.[18,19] Besides other factors, this might be due to them being confronted with harsh realities of clinical practice, the rigidity of a system that is difficult to change and the attitude of senior colleagues that these limitations have to be accepted. Giving future doctors tools that enable them to work on changing things for the better might counteract this sense of powerlessness and complacency. Students pointing out flaws in the system and advocating for improvements can in turn inspire their colleagues to take action and create a positive momentum for change.

Even though the training on advocacy aimed at equipping participants with the skills to organize campaigns, its main benefit might have been that it reminded them that change is possible and encouraged them to work for it, thereby fostering the passion medical students feel for their patients' right to health. It is difficult to pinpoint where IFMSA's members thus empowered initiated small changes but we can assume that their exposure to advocacy trainings and campaigns impacted them and will influence their work well into their professional careers.

Prescriptions/lessons learnt

We started this chapter with advocacy campaigns that achieved international success for issues in neurology. What followed was a personal reflection on what has worked and what has failed when doing advocacy on an international level. Summarizing our learnings, we will now point to prescriptions and lessons learnt that can be helpful for anyone who is planning advocacy activities on an international level.

Prepare for the unexpected

An activity might be well planned through but there are always hidden threats that can turn events around quickly. Historians know this phenomenon as 'hinge factor',[20] stressing the possibility that wars can be lost due to very little and unforeseen changes. Advocates need to be prepared for the 'hinge factor' as well; we must cooperate with different stakeholders to realize our ideas (public, politicians, other organizations, and so on), which often leads to complex decision-making structures. They can bring about unexpected outcomes. In the second case, 'Leadership and advocacy', a compromise was offered, which suggested many significant changes from the concept, and was not acceptable at that time. Retrospectively, a further process of negotiation would have seemed reasonable.[21,22] Our experience shows that we should always have alternative plans at hand so that the advocacy mission can be executed despite some unexpected events.

Advocacy might change the status quo

In order to create a real difference for the well-being of our patients, we might often plan activities that require the organization to do things differently. For example, implementing advocacy activities might require new organizational structures or they might disrupt existing routines in the organization. This leads to resistance as people are generally reluctant to change. In that regard, scholars in the field of management and systems thinking point out that the harder one pushes a system the harder the system pushes back.[23] It is essential that ideas are not communicated as a 'too much at once' change. That might scare those who want to keep the status quo of the organization. For example, the section on 'Leadership and advocacy' suggests that we might have had more success if we would not have emphasized the leadership-aspect of our project.

Often times, when organizations have to make profound changes they require periods where they can *unlearn* their existing habits or mental models.[24,25] However, such processes take time and one has to be patient until such changes can be successfully realized.

Think locally, act globally

International advocacy campaigns must begin somewhere. It is important to keep that in mind when planning an advocacy campaign. The example of the ice bucket challenge illustrates that developments in social media require us to see the term 'local' from a new perspective. In the example of IFMSA, actively involving existing organizational structures on a local level allows us to share resources and have a faster impact. This might also mean that local actors are trained and empowered to realize ideas on their own. Top-down activities (i.e. planning and propagating our ideas to more local levels) is important but all bottom-up activities are important too, as some nationwide efforts are being recognized in other countries and contexts and sooner or later, similar ideas might connect. This becomes apparent in the example on how care of stroke patients evolved in Austria and was eventually backed up by international endeavours.

Be persistent and connect

Advocacy might sometimes face resistance and require resilience. The energy in invested in resilience must be carefully weighed against the expected results.

It is also advisable to seek exchange with other practitioners to see how they are dealing with such cases and how they work and manage their projects. Sharing experience is invaluable in international advocacy campaigns.

Conclusions

In this chapter, we focused on advocacy at an international level. Showing two different approaches to practising advocacy on an international level and reflecting on projects that we were involved in, we provided several lessons learnt that we find helpful when planning advocacy activities.

First, when planning advocacy, we should always prepare for the unexpected, having alternative plans and exit strategies ready. Second, we must consider that advocacy ideas change the status quo because they are incompatible with existing structures in an organization. This may trigger resistance by the system. Third, by thinking locally and acting globally, a campaign can grow and gain momentum within a clear and manageable environment. Fourth, we have to be persistent and connect with likeminded people to create strategic alliances.

While these lessons learnt result from our own subjective experience, we believe they have great relevance for anyone who is planning and implementing international advocacy activities.

References

1. **World Health Organization (WHO)** (2017) Fact Sheet: Noncommunicable diseases. Available at: http://www.who.int/mediacentre/factsheets/fs355/en/
2. **Indredavik, B., Bakke, F., Solberg, R., Rokseth, R., Haaheim LL, Holme, I.** (1991) Benefit of a stroke unit: a randomized controlled trial. *Stroke*, **22**(8), 1026–31.
3. **Dimyan, M. A., Cohen, L. G.** (2011) Neuroplasticity in the context of motor rehabilitation after stroke. *Nat Rev Neurol*, **7**(2), 76–85.
4. **Hartwigsen, G.** (2016) Adaptive plasticity in the healthy language network: implications for language recovery after stroke. *Neural Plast*, **2016**, e9674790.
5. **World Health Organization (WHO)** (2017) The 11th Revision of the International Classification of Diseases (ICD-11). Available at: http://www.who.int/classifications/icd/revision/en/
6. **Song, P.** (2014) The ice bucket challenge: the public sector should get ready to promptly promote the sustained development of a system of medical care for and research into rare diseases. *Intractable Rare Dis Res*, **3**(3), 94–6.
7. **Stampler, L.** (2014) This is how many ice bucket challenge videos people have posted on Facebook. Time. Available at: http://time.com/3117501/als-ice-bucket-challenge-videos-on-facebook/
8. **ALS Association** (2014) Ice bucket challenge donations reach $79.7 million—The ALS Association. Available at: http://web.alsa.org/site/PageNavigator/ibc_news_17.html
9. **Tracy, H. M.** (2016) The neuro funding rollercoaster. *Cerebrum Dana Forum Brain Sci*. Available at: http://www.ncbi.nlm.nih.gov/pmc/articles/PMC4938264/
10. **Broxton, T., Interian, Y., Vaver, J., Wattenhofer, M.** (2013) Catching a viral video. *J Intell Inf Syst*, **40**(2), 241–59.
11. **Hrastelj, J., Robertson, N. P.** (2016) Ice bucket challenge bears fruit for amyotrophic lateral sclerosis. *J Neurol*, **263**(11), 2355–7.
12. **Koohy, H., Koohy, B.** (2014) A lesson from the ice bucket challenge: using social networks to publicize science. *Front Genet*. Available at: http://www.ncbi.nlm.nih.gov/pmc/articles/PMC4266090/
13. **Aarons, G. A., Ehrhart, M. G., Farahnak, L. R., Hurlburt, M. S.** (2015) Leadership and organizational change for implementation (LOCI): a randomized mixed method pilot study of a leadership and organization development intervention for evidence-based practice implementation. *Implement Sci*, **10**, 11.
14. **Taichman, R. S., Parkinson, J. W., Nelson, B. A., Nordquist, B., Ferguson-Young, D. C., Thompson, J. F.** (2012) Program design considerations for leadership training for dental and dental hygiene students. *J Dent Educ*, **76**(2), 192–9.
15. **Olsson, L., Jerneck, A., Thoren, H., Persson, J., O'Byrne, D.** (2015) Why resilience is unappealing to social science: theoretical and empirical investigations of the scientific use of resilience. *Sci Adv*, **1**(4), e1400217.
16. **Gruen, R. L., Campbell, E. G., Blumenthal, D.** (2006) Public roles of US physicians: community participation, political involvement, and collective advocacy. *JAMA*, **296**(20) 2467–75.
17. **Campbell, E. G., Regan, S., Gruen, R. L., et al.** (2007) Professionalism in medicine: results of a national survey of physicians. *Ann Intern Med*, **147**(11), 795–802.
18. **Woloschuk, W., Harasym, P. H., Temple W.** (2004) Attitude change during medical school: a cohort study. *Med Educ*, **38**(5), 522–34.

19. **Griffith, C. H., Wilson, J. F.** (2003) The loss of idealism throughout internship. *Eval Health Prof*, **26**(4), 415–26.
20. **Durschmied, E.** (1999) *The Hinge Factor: How Chance and Stupidity Have Changed History*. London: Hodder & Stoughton.
21. **Brown, H., Simanowitz, A.** (1995) Alternative dispute resolution and mediation. *Qual Health Care*, **4**(2), 151–8.
22. **Klein, C. A., Klein, A. B.** (2008) Alternative dispute resolution part 2: mediation. *Nurse Pract*, **33**(2), 13–4.
23. **Senge, P. M.** (1990) *The Fifth Discipline: The Art and Practice of the Learning Organization*. New York: Doubleday.
24. **Brook, C. et al.** (2016). On stopping doing those things that are not getting us to where we want to be: Unlearning, wicked problems and critical action learning. *Hum Relat*, **69**(2), 369–89. http://journals.sagepub.com/doi/abs/10.1177/0018726715586243
25. **Tsang, E. W. K., Zahra, S. A.** (2008) Organizational unlearning. *Hum Relat*, **61**(10), 1435–62.

Chapter 19

Using PR tools for advocacy

Birgit Kofler

Introduction

Major awareness campaigns in the field of neurology—such as World Brain Day (https://www.wfneurology.org), World Stroke Day (https://www.worldstrokecampaign.org), World Parkinson's Day (https://www.worldparkinsonsday.com), World Alzheimer's Day and Month (http://www.alzinfo.org), International Epilepsy Day (https://www.epilepsy.org), to name just a few—include two components. They aim at educating (e.g. about symptoms, prevention, early detection, or available therapies) as well as advocating (e.g. with respect to access to therapies or resources for care).

Advocacy, public education, and public relations (PR) are tight-knit and closely interrelated. Awareness and public education efforts contribute to the spread of knowledge about diseases and conditions, prevention, diagnosis and treatments, and advocates mobilize for sufficient healthcare structures and funding. In order to reach the general public and decision-makers with their manifold messages, neurology advocates need to make use of PR instruments. Being aware of the major PR tools and using them in a professional way is a clear advantage for patient or medical advocates. In this chapter, PR instruments, particularly in the field of media relations, and their practical use will be described. However, some critical issues[1] with respect to the relationship between advocacy and efforts of the healthcare industry to integrate patients advocates and organizations of health professionals into their PR and lobbying strategies (see also Chapter 5) will also be discussed.

Advocacy and PR: Two sides of the same medal?

Whether advocacy may be seen as a subdiscipline of PR, or as an independent discipline in the broad field of targeted public communication, may be mainly of theoretical interest and of limited relevance for advocacy practitioners. These aspects include, for example, the discussion that PR is typically based on symmetrical, community-oriented communication, while advocacy is usually centred on persuasive communication and therefore cannot be symmetrical.[2,3]

But the question of how the instruments in the PR toolbox can be used for the purposes and aims of advocacy is of practical importance (see Box 19.1). As a matter of fact, advocacy activists are, in many instances, using PR instruments. PR tools play an important role in neurology advocacy. In some diseases, such as epilepsy, stroke,

> **Box 19.1 Definitions of PR**
>
> - 'The task of public relations is: To achieve mutual understanding and to establish beneficial relationships, between the organisation and its publics and environment, through two-way communication.' *European Public Relations Confederation*
> - 'Public relations serves a wide variety of institutions in society such as businesses, trade unions, government agencies, voluntary associations, foundations, hospitals, schools, colleges and religious institutions. To achieve their goals, these institutions must develop effective relationships with many different audiences or publics such as employees, members, customers, local communities, shareholders, and other institutions, and with society at large.' *Public Relations Society of America*

or dementia awareness campaigns, public information and education can make a big difference with respect to prevention, early diagnosis, or access to therapies.[4]

Advocacy—in whose interest?

There is also another important argument why advocacy activists should be familiar with the major PR instruments and should be able to use these expertly. Such skills enable them to act professionally, independently from other players, and in particular from the for-profit-sector.

Although there may be good reasons by patients or healthcare professionals to conduct advocacy efforts in alliances with members of the healthcare industry, advocates need to be aware of an important trend. It can be observed that parts of the industry tend to integrate advocacy efforts and the activities of patients or healthcare professional advocates into their PR strategies (this topic is discussed in more detail in Chapter 5.). The benefit for the for-profit-sector is obvious: patients or healthcare professionals can present issues such as the allocation of healthcare resources, or access to new therapies more credibly than a company with its obvious economic interest. 'Working with advocacy groups is one of the most accomplished means of raising awareness for a disease', as pharma executive Josh Weinstein puts it.[5] It is no wonder that efforts have also gone beyond mere cooperation, and the founding of advocacy groups itself is now often the result of industry initiatives.[6]

A recent survey study analysing the interrelations between patient advocacy organizations in the United States and the private sector found that 67% of the advocacy non-governmental organizations (NGOs) reported receiving funding from for-profit companies. Some 12% received more than 50% of their funding from the industry, with the pharmaceutical, device, and/or biotechnology industry being the most important promoters of advocacy activities. The authors call for increased transparency and clear conflict of interest policies and practices.[7]

Media relations—a core element of PR

While already about 10 years ago some in the PR field predicted the end of 'traditional PR' and anticipated that social media would 'reinvent' PR models,[8,9] 'classic' news media remain particularly important dialogue partners for PR and advocacy. In this context, 'classic' refers to the fact that the content of the media is produced by professional journalists, irrespective of the channel they use for distribution (print, radio, TV, online).

Even though PR is much broader than media relations, and without underestimating the growing importance of social media,[8] journalists remain very important multipliers, establishing contacts with relevant dialogue partners and bringing messages to the target groups. They can also reach different target groups at the same time—patients may watch TV or read the paper, just as politicians or social security officials do.

The fact that many media outlets are under economic pressure could ultimately even be helpful for healthcare advocates. With a view to reduced staff[10] and thus limited capacity for in-depth research, reporters need to rely on PR for story ideas, expert knowledge, and background information more than ever. Also, the trends towards involving 'citizen journalists' in the work of major news outlets may open the possibility for advocacy voices to be heard at different levels.

The benefit of media relations for healthcare advocates is obvious: media relations are still a powerful and cost-effective tool. It is still more powerful and credible if major news outlets report about your concerns than if you do the same on Facebook or Twitter (only). Therefore, it should be part of the skills of healthcare advocates to know how to provide journalists with interesting material or to be aware of the daily routines and working conditions of journalists.

As shown by the comprehensive report 'World Press Trends 2016',[11] more than 2.4 billion adults—the figure corresponds to around 40% of all adults—consume newspapers in print globally. The report estimates that at least 40% of Internet users read newspapers and news media online. The report states: ' . . . 2015 was a breakthrough year for their online and online revenues, as legacy news media often produced better journalism and higher subscription and advertising revenues than did their pure digital competitors'. As other surveys show, while there is a decline in the circulation of print newspaper titles, the newspapers' web traffic outpaces their circulation by a substantial margin.[10]

However, the important role of social media as amplifiers should not be underestimated.[12]

How journalists work

Whoever wants to engage in a successful dialogue with journalists should understand the specifics and logic of the media and of editorial departments. It is therefore important to be aware of the circumstances in which journalists work, such as, for example, information overload, heavy workload, time constraints, dependency on serious sources, and so on. The feasibility and the relevance of a story are other important aspects for editors. In order to be perceived against this background, the information offered to journalists must be significant, relevant, deviate from the usual and familiar, and affect the reader, listener, viewer, or user in any form.[13]

Experience shows that partnership-based collaboration, immediate availability for urgent questions, and support with background material are among the elements that journalists value most when they cooperate with PR professionals or advocacy activists.

Establishing media contacts—The media distribution list

As a rule, it will not be possible to be in constant personal contact with all relevant media representatives—even if this is very important for the major media for the respective topic.[14]

A tailor-made media distribution list is an important prerequisite for fruitful media contacts. This should not be a complete list of all journalists active in the target region. The target groups and the messages to be communicated will determine which media outlets and media representatives should be included in the distribution list. The establishment of a media distribution list is not a one-off act, on the contrary: it needs constant maintenance and updating.

Some basics on media messages

Before specific PR instruments such as media releases (see 'Media information and media release') are implemented, advocacy activists should have a very clear idea of the messages that should be conveyed.

As a general rule, messages need to be clear, easy to understand—it is always a good idea to stick to the 'KISS'-rule ('keep it simple and short'). Advocates should beware of professional jargon,[15] which doctors and other medical professionals tend to use. Replace 'medical'-ese by 'people-ese', as PR specialist Robin Cohn puts it in her *PR Crisis Bible*.[15]

For all dialogue groups, and especially for the media as multipliers, the following points should be considered while developing the messages:

- The information as such and the basic idea alone are not yet a message and certainly not a 'story'.
- If possible, the story and the message should be developed with a view to the following general rule: what is interesting in internal logic can be irrelevant from the outside—and vice versa.
- The message should bring the matter straight to the point. Long-winded speeches, in this context, usually result in a lack of success.
- Forget technical jargon—simple and clear statements are much better. Therefore PR experts like to refer to the 'KISS' rule: 'Keep it short and simple.'
- Good messages call for credibility.

Some important PR instruments

To make optimum use of PR tools for advocacy activities, some preliminary questions should be clarified (see also Chapter 17). These relate to the main content

> **Box 19.2 Before you start**
>
> What? (message)
> Who? (target group)
> Why now? (occasion)
> Through which channel? (medium)
> How? (method)
> With which objectives? (effect)

of the message, the target group, the occasion which triggers the actual PR activity, the communication channels, and the aims of the activity. The tools and communication channels used should be able to convey exactly the level and type of information that suits the expectations of and is easily accessible for the target audience (see Box 19.2).[16,17]

Media information and media releases

Among the most popular PR tools that permit the spread of messages and information to broad audiences through the media are press (media) releases. This describes a specifically designed piece of information which is distributed to a defined group of journalists and/or editorial offices.

At the same time, advocates using this powerful PR tool should also be aware of the fact that patients, their families, opinion leaders, decision-makers, and the public in general can also read their media releases online directly—unfiltered by the media.[8]

There are some important principles to consider when drafting press releases:

- Above all, something that might seem obvious but is often neglected: You should have something to communicate that is of general interest.
- Another key element for a successful media release: offer interesting facts and figures, not just views.
- 'Story, not history': The structure of a press release usually differs from the logic of other formats. Usually, you do not explain the chronology or the circumstances first and then come to the conclusion. On the contrary, the media release usually starts with the summary of what is the news, the main message or the major point, and then gets on with explaining the context and background. The paragraphs should be arranged in such a way that the text can be shortened from the back to the front without loss of core information.
- Just like a journalistic piece of information, a press release has to answer the usual 'W questions': Who? What? When? Where? Why? So what is special about my message/story?
- Quotes are indispensable in a press release.

- 'Write short—and they will read it. Write clearly—and they will understand it. Write graphically—and they will keep it in mind.' This was the advice for successful texts by Josef Pulitzer, the father of the famous prizes for journalists and authors. His recommendation probably holds true for any text, and most certainly for press releases.

Press kits

A press kit, sometimes also referred to as media kit, is a prefabricated set of information such as media releases or fact sheets, intended for distribution to media representatives. Electronic press kits, also known as EPKs, are the digital equivalent of the hard copy press or media kit.

Press kits are mainly created to accompany press conferences (see next section). In this context, the topics of the press conference are summarized for journalists present at the event as well as for others who are not able to attend. In this case, the press kit is only relevant for the specific occasion and therefore of limited topicality after the event.

However, in the context of advocacy activities it may also be appropriate to create a 'basic background press kit' with all the relevant aspects of the topic. This kind of press kit should be updated as needed when facts change or when new aspects arise. A basic press kit should consist of a collection of individual, journalistically designed 'stories' on the various topics which can be used independently from each other.

Press conference

A press conference is an event where media outlets are called together to cover a newsworthy message/occasion. A press conference can help publicize a message to many news outlets—at least in the specific region. It usually is a cost-effective tool to mobilize relevant media coverage, provided that the topic is suitable for this specific tool. Exclusive, unpublished news of relevance for the general public would certainly fit in this category, but also multifaceted topics that request comments by several experts.

Organizers should make sure that date and time of the press conference do not conflict with other important or revealing events in the same field that might draw attention away from the event. Morning press conferences are more popular with the media than afternoon meetings.

If possible, a press conference should be scheduled at least two weeks in advance to permit sufficient time to prepare press releases and to contact appropriate media. The invitation should include convincing arguments that describe why the event is worthy of reporting.

A representative of the organization should be appointed to welcome reporters as and to coordinate photo opportunities and interviews with speakers and representatives of the organization. In their presentations, speakers should be brief with remarks, highlight the key elements of the subject the press conference is about, and then open the floor for questions.

Letters to the editor/postings

Letters to the editor—and the same, of course, holds true for the 'web-based' version, online postings and comments—are a simple and effective way to publish comments relating to current topics, to place rectifications or dementias in an elegant manner, or to participate in controversial debates.

One of the advantages of this instrument is the fact that a variety of actors can spread particular messages. Letters to the editor and postings thus importantly raise public awareness and show the competence the sender's/poster's competence in the specific field and might be referenced for future purposes.

Creative tools in media relations

The term 'creative media relations' describes a set of tools aimed at communicating a cause to the media by other means than conventional press releases or press conferences. Networking and relationship management with reporters are important aspects with respect to these tools.

Some typical examples:

panel discussions with reporters as participants or audience

media workshops providing background information

actionism and 'photo opportunities'

media competitions and prizes for journalists in a specific area

appointment of reporters as members of a jury

Other PR tools: Platforms and spokespersons

The mobilization of support from third parties, the creation of platforms and alliances, and the mobilization of independent supporters and spokespersons play an important role in communicating advocacy concerns.

In this context, a specific format is the mobilization of VIPs as supporters or spokespersons for the cause. It seems that celebrities are credited with a particularly high credibility in many areas as has been shown by German research (see Table 19.1)[18]:

> 'Who do you think is particularly suited to influencing health attitudes of the public through the media?'

Table 19.1 A German survey among PR professionals and journalists shows who they think are best suited to influence the health attitudes of the public

Who	Opinion of PR professionals, %	Opinion of journalists, %
Experts, scientists	28.7	25.8
Non-experts	26.2	20.8
Celebrities	45.2	41.2
Others	2.9	9.3

Reproduced from Gottwald F, Gesundheitsöffentlichkeit. Entwicklung eines Netzwerkmodells für Journalismus und Public Relations, Copyright (2006), with permission from Halem Verlag.

Online PR

The Internet has enormously enriched the conventional PR toolkit and will continue to develop dynamically. Used in the proper way, it can support quick and easy communication with the relevant public(s), present an organization in a positive context, and help with crisis management.[19]

One of the main advantages of the Internet is its interactivity: it allows direct communication with relevant dialogue groups.

The website

A website should be a standard tool for organizations and/or advocacy projects. With respect to media relations, an online press area should be an important element. Surveys have shown that journalists have less time to conduct research today than they did five years ago. Search engines and specific websites relating to the topic are still gaining importance as research tools. Many reporters judge the 'round-the-clock' accessibility as particularly crucial.[20]

What makes advocacy organizations and activists interesting is a broad range of content available on the website. It is not only an interesting research tool for the media, but also a helpful resource for bloggers (see 'Online ('virtual') press conferences') and for other activists or advocates.[8]

An online press area ('virtual press office') is part of the website of the organization/campaign and should provide a great amount of information in different formats. This could include, inter alia, the following elements:

- fact sheets
- background information
- events
- media releases
- press kits
- contact information
- photos
- illustrations
- diagrams and charts
- audios, videos

Blogging and blogger relations

The boom of blogs and the extent to which bloggers have become important new multipliers can be useful in advocacy PR in two ways. On the one hand, your own blog as an advocate can help to comment on current topics very quickly, independently of the reception by conventional media, as well as in a more detailed and substantiated way than in social media posts. Advocates can support shaping discussions in their specific field of interest by writing their own blog.[8]

On the other hand, monitoring blogs in the advocacy activist's specific field of interest can help to understand what is particularly important to patients, families, or healthcare professionals in this area. And relations with bloggers being active in the specific area of interest should also be maintained[21,22] by commenting on their blogs and/or providing information to them.[8]

As journalists, bloggers can benefit from maintaining relations to PR professionals and make use of their information and know-how. Just as it goes for media relations, blogger relations are built on mutual respect and credibility of the information being provided for the public.[9] 'As you move forward with your campaigns, you should never be limited to either blogs or media', is the suggestion by PR expert Solis.[9]

It should, however, be noted that bloggers cannot be equated with journalists. They choose their themes according to personal preferences, which gives their reports a subjective character.[8] It is specifically that approach why bloggers, in many instances, enjoy the trust of specific target groups—and why, at the same time, they cannot be considered an independent or objective source.

Advocates should also be aware of the fact that there are many examples in the sphere of blogging—and interrelated social media accounts—that fake news are being used as an unethical, but nevertheless sustained strategy to motivate action. Factcheck.org and Snopes are popular verification sites that can be helpful in discovering hoaxes.

Online ('virtual') press conferences

Online press conferences gain popularity and are being held either in place of on-site press conferences, or in addition to these. In particular, in view of limited resources,[20] they offer a suitable opportunity for journalists to follow such an event without being present in person, and ideally to interact via chat.

To strengthen the element of interactivity for the remote participants of the online event, questions can be directed to the moderator or the presenters, depending on the technical platform, by email or via live chat.

After the event, a recording should be made available online to allow later viewings.[23]

The technical prerequisites for an online press conference are quite complex and therefore not within reach for every organization. A possible alternative, easier to implement, are pre-recorded video statements of the experts that are posted online. Interactivity is not possible in this format.

Social media

Nearly every organization or campaign is using social networks today. In particular, for activities of a mobilizing and motivating character, social media is an essential component of the communication toolkit. This is documented by current data: the number of users in social networks has risen worldwide from 0.97 billion in 2010 to 2.34 billion (2016). For the year 2020, experts expect a number of 2.95 billion users.[24]

The two most popular social media platforms in all areas are Facebook and Twitter. For advocacy activities, the operation of a YouTube channel or the use of Instagram may also be relevant, as may be to provide podcasts on a regular basis.[8]

The use of social media for advocacy and PR purposes contributes to new practices and forms of communication in this field and opens many possibilities of including activists in an interactive process.[25,26] A comprehensive content analysis of Facebook posts from major NGOs[27] showed that in particular dialogic and mobilizational messages are liked by fans, while they are more likely to share one-way informational messages with their own networks. This might show that in some respects social media communication might just be the continuation of traditional PR through different channels rather than a complete change in PR approaches.

In order to use these channels successfully, a social media strategy should be developed in order to define objectives, target groups, resources, and implementation measures as well as the selection of channels. It is also important to ensure that sufficient personnel resources are available. Regular dialogue-oriented communication on these platforms is essential. Tools to ensure this include questions to the community, stimulating the conversation, and quick responses to questions and comments. A crossmedial approach is recommended.[8,28]

Summary

Advocates in the field of neurology should be aware of the tools, the potential, and the limitations of PR with respect to their awareness, educational, and mobilization efforts. Although 'alternative' and social media have changed the possibilities and structures of communicating to different target audiences, news outlets and journalistic sources still play an important role for PR purposes. Apart from using PR tools in a professional way, people involved in neurology advocacy should also be aware of the fact that their efforts may be part of PR strategies of for-profit organizations.

Acknowledgements

The author wishes to thank Eva Maria Freitag, Wolfsberg, Austria, and Anna Maria Comina, Ebreichsdorf, Austria, for their important and valuable inputs and contributions to this text.

References

1. **Fischer, C.** (2011) Advocacy und Lobby im Gesundheitswesen. In: Hensen P., Kölzer C. (eds). *Die gesunde Gesellschaft*. Wiesbaden: VS Verlag für Sozialwissenschaften.
2. **Baker, S.** (1999) Five baselines for justification in persuasion. *Journal of Mass Media Ethics*, **14**(2), 69–81.
3. **Leeper, K. A.** (1999) Public relations ethics and communitarianism: a preliminary investigation. *Public Relations Review*, **22**(2), 163–79.
4. **Caron R. M.** (2015) *Health Communication: Advocacy Strategies, Effectiveness and Emerging Challenges*. New York: Nova Science Publishing.
5. **Weinstein, J.** (2004) Public relations: why advocacy beats DTC. *PharmExec.com*. Available at: http://static1.1.sqspcdn.com/static/f/1072889/16030499/1326503960260/ Pharma+marketing+newsletter+2004.pdf?token=46XgkbjQSAISRDUf3MNFWymGK8 A%3D

6. **Krüger-Brand, H. E.** (2012) Patientenpartizipation: informiert entscheiden können. *Deutsches Ärzteblatt*, **109**(13), A632
7. **Rose, S. L**, **Highland, J.**, **Karafa, M. T.**, **Joffe, S.** (2017) Patient advocacy organizations, industry funding, and conflicts of interest. *JAMA Intern Med*, **177**(3), 344–50.
8. **Scott, D. M.** (2009) *The New Rules of Marketing & PR*. New York: Gildan Media Corporation.
9. **Solis, B.**, **Breakenridge, D.** (2009) *Putting the Public Back in Public Relations: How Social Media is Reinventing the Ageing Business of PR*. Upper Saddle River, NJ: Pearson Education.
10. **Barthel, M.** (2016) Newspapers: Fact Sheet; Pew Research Center. Available at: http://www.journalism.org/2016/06/15/newspapers-fact-sheet/
11. **Milosevic, M.** (2016) World Press Trends 2016. Available at: http://www.wan-ifra.org/microsites/world-press-trends
12. **Smith, R.** (2013) *Public Relations: The Basics*. New York: Routledge.
13. **Köhler, T.**, **Schaffranietz, A.** (2005) *Public Relations—Perspektiven und Potenziale im 21. Jahrhundert*. Wiesbaden: Springer Publishing.
14. **Deg, R.** (2006) *Basiswissen Public Relations. Professionelle Press- und Öffentlichkeitsarbeit*. Berlin and Heidelberg: Springer Publishing,
15. **Cohn, R.** (2000) *The PR Crisis Bible: How to Take Charge of the Media When All Hell Breaks Loose*. New York: Truman Talley Books/St. Martin's Press.
16. **Young, E.**, **Quinn, L.** (2012) *Making Research Evidence Matter: A Guide to Policy Advocacy in Transition Countries* (Online Publication–International Centre for Policy Advocacy). Available at: http://advocacyguide.icpolicyadvocacy.org
17. **Breitwieser, J.**, **Neu, H.** (2005) *Public Relations: Die besten Tricks der Medienprofis*. Göttingen: BusinessVillage.
18. **Gottwald, F.** (2006) *Gesundheitsöffentlichkeit. Entwicklung eines Netzwerkmodells für Journalismus und Public Relations*. Konstanz: UVK Verlagsgesellschaft.
19. **Bogula, W.** (2007) *Leitfaden Online-PR. PR Praxis: Bd. 10*. Konstanz: UVK.
20. **Rennhak, C.** (2015) *Recherchieren 2015. Eine Studie zum Rechercheverhalten deutscher Journalisten*. Available at: https://www.recherchescout.com/wp-content/uploads/2015/12/Recherchieren-2015.pdf
21. **Baric-Gaspar, I.** (2015) Was ist Online PR heute? Available at: https://keen-communication.com/was-ist-online-pr-heute/
22. **Liechtenecker** (2013) 10 wichtige Punkte zu Blogger-Relations. Available at: https://liechtenecker.at/10-wichtige-punkte-zu-blogger-relations/
23. **Ruisinger, D.** (2011) *Online Relations*. Stuttgart: Schäffer Poeschel.
24. **Statista**. Prognose zur Anzahl der Nutzer sozialer Netzwerke weltweit bis 2020; 2016. Available at: https://de.statista.com/statistik/daten/studie/219903/umfrage/prognose-zur-anzahl-der-weltweiten-nutzer-sozialer-netzwerke/
25. **Guo, C.**, **Saxton, G. D.** (2013) Tweeting social change. how social media are changing nonprofit advocacy. *Nonprofit and Voluntary Sector Quarterly*, **43**(1), 57–79.
26. **Cho, M.**, **Schweickart, T.**, **Haase, C.** (2014) Public engagement with non-profit organizations on Facebook. *Public Relations Review*, **40**(3), 565–7.
27. **Saxton, G. D.**, **Waters, R. D.** (2014) What do stakeholders like on Facebook? Examining public reactions to nonprofit organizations' informational, promotional, and community-building messages. *Journal of Public Relations Research*, **26**(3), 280–99.
28. **Huber, M.** (2013). *Kommunikation und Social Media*, 3rd edition. München: UVK.

Section 4

Advocacy in different neurological diseases

Chapter 20

Advocacy for stroke

Tissa Wijeratne, Sheila Crewther, and David Crewther

Introduction

Stroke is the second commonest cause of death for people over 60 worldwide,[1] and is a leading cause of adult disability.[2,3] It is estimated that each year, 16 million people worldwide suffer a stroke with approximately six million dying and another five million being left permanently disabled. Recent research also suggests that nearly 90% of all such stroke cases are preventable[4] and treatable[5] if seen rapidly.

The Framingham Heart Study is the largest running prospective study, in operation for more than 60 years.[6] The study found stroke and dementia to be the main neurological causes of morbidity and mortality in 1997.[6] Members of the studied population had a 1 in 3 chance to be affected by stroke or dementia during their lives.[6] Strokes change the lives of almost all patients, families, and friends.

In 2011 the first World Stroke Campaign was launched to fight against stroke.[7] suggesting that advocacy via practitioners skilled in education, clinical service development and translational clinical research, are important components required to provide the best care for all stroke patients and associated families irrespective of the social backgrounds and disparities in healthcare globally.[8,9] Such optimization of services requires a team of clinicians, administrators, funders and, most importantly, patients and families.

Advocacy can be defined as acting on behalf of a disadvantaged person or group to promote their welfare and bring about change in policies, practices, and attitudes of organizations and institutions about stroke.[10,11] Examples of stroke advocacy include setting up a stroke service, advocating a stroke awareness campaign in the local region or country, advising national policies in stroke prevention, and management of acute stroke and related complications.

Thus, the question arises as to how can physicians become the best advocate for their patients and lead with rationale authenticity given the complex environment wherein they are facing challenges from every direction.[12,13] Physicians are ideally placed to observe and address social determinants of health and disparities in healthcare and traditionally the public have trusted physicians with the belief that their Hippocratic Oath will see them do what is best for the patient as opposed to themselves.

The need for better stroke advocacy in political and medical circles is largely driven by the recent significant advances in scientific and clinical stroke care, ranging from prevention to acute and subacute intervention. Stroke advocates are in an ideal position to translate these advances and promote better brain health through effective advocacy now. Hence the next section will highlight selected case studies where some of these advocacy efforts have been successful (Case studies 20.1–20.8).

Case study 20.1 Stroke advocacy at Western Health, Melbourne, Australia

This illustrates a real-life story of a stroke service development with limited resources in a metropolitan Melbourne, Australia.

Western Health[i] is the local metropolitan provider of health services in the Western Region of Melbourne, Victoria, Australia that caters for a rapidly growing population of one million. The key feature of the western suburbs of Melbourne's population is its unique cultural diversity which clearly sets it apart from other areas of Victoria's health services while providing additional challenges in service delivery. Nearly 33% of Western Health catchment area's patient population are from a non-English speaking background and speak more than 100 languages. The most commonly requested interpreting services at Western Health are Vietnamese, Greek, Italian, Cantonese, Macedonian, Croatian, Serbian, Arabic, and Spanish.

In 2007, Western Health treated approximately 570 patients with a diagnosis of stroke and 260 patients with a diagnosis of transient ischaemic attack (TIA). At the same time, 30% of the patients from Western Health bypassed the catchment region and presented to other health services for treatment. Such decisions were presumably due to the ambulance service's awareness of Western Health's lack of a dedicated stroke unit, absence of computed tomography (CT) brain imaging, and treatment options such as thrombolytic therapy for acute ischaemic stroke at Western Health.

Stroke thrombolysis was not offered despite the availability of the medication in the hospital, presumably due to a lack of specialized stroke physicians and nurses with expertise and confidence. Many patients stayed in the hospital far too long, with the discharge destination a nursing home, and large numbers of patients died. There was no opportunity for training in stroke medicine. The standard stroke care was non-existent and opportunities for stroke research were nil.

The following clinical vignette shows the sorry in stroke care at Western Health in 2006. A 22-year-old woman, a recent immigrant to Melbourne suffered a left hemisphere stroke and was admitted to one of the affiliated emergency centres in Footscray. Given that there was no stroke thrombolysis service in the hospital, the patient was managed in the neurology ward with classic antiplatelet therapy and post-stroke care and was eventually discharged to a nursing home with severe disability. Following 2006, a young neurologist with stroke expertise was appointed to champion improvement in stroke services at Western Health by better utilizing the available minimum resources. A dedicated stroke unit was established within the allocated beds to the neurology ward at Western Health where close to 90% of the acute workload related to stroke. At the same time, a new Victorian State stroke care strategies protocol was implemented with eight stroke network facilitators being appointed in selected hospitals, to enable the establishment of stroke units, develop thrombolysis services. Concurrently a dedicated stroke advocacy team was also established at Western Health between the part time stroke network facilitator and the part time stroke champion neurologist.

---

[i] Western Health manages three acute public hospitals: Footscray Hospital at Footscray; Sunshine Hospital at St Albans; and the Williamstown Hospital. Services are provided to the western region of Melbourne which has a population of approximately 1,000,000 people.

ADVOCACY FOR STROKE | 221

The team noted the gaps in stroke care at Western Health, including:

1. Absence of an ambulance prenotification system for cases of strokes.
2. Lack of adequate triage of patients with stroke symptoms in the emergency department. Stroke patients were generally the last patients to be seen unless their pulse, blood pressure, and/or level of consciousness were impaired.
3. CT brain scans were not high priority and were seldom done immediately. Some patients did not even have a CT brain.
4. Absence of a formal standard operating procedure for stroke care pathway.
5. Absence of a stroke thrombolysis protocol.
6. Absence of a subacute stroke care pathway.
7. No end-of-life care pathway for disabling stroke patients.
8. There was no formal head of stroke services.
9. There was no formally organized acute stroke service despite the large population catchment of the health organization.
10. No formal referral relationships between other health services.
11. No high-quality written information about stroke.
12. No formal care coordination throughout continuum of care.
13. No formal pathway for stroke patients to return to the community.
14. No formal stroke care workforce training and education.
15. No formal stroke fellowship for doctors in training.
16. No stroke nurse coordinator or stroke nurse practitioner.
17. No clinical neuropsychologist for stroke service.
18. No formal stroke research programme.
19. No formal stroke education programme for patients.
20. No formal stroke education programme for primary care physicians despite the 600 primary care physician practices linked with Western Health in 2006.
21. No formal stroke clinic or TIA clinic for organized ambulatory care.

There was a strong need to bring change to the organization to fill these gaps, with a view to providing better stroke care for patients.

Advocacy for better stroke care at Western Health, beyond 2007

A clinical practice guideline for the management of acute stroke was formulated in 2007, and the Stroke Research Unit was established to bring clinical research activities in acute stroke care, as it was noted to be a key component of high-quality acute stroke service. Further a subcommittee was developed for education, aimed at arranging a full educational training day to cover all aspects of acute stroke management and to organize monthly one-hour ongoing medical education sessions in stroke medicine for doctors, nurses, and allied health colleagues. The guidelines were established in plain and simple language with bullet points, with regular updates as new knowledge became available. These guidelines were subsequently endorsed by the Western Health Policy & Guidelines Committee and inserted to the Intranet. The stroke guidelines outlined:

- General stroke treatment.
- Prevention and treatment of complications of stroke.
- Early secondary prevention.
- Discharge planning.

♦ Speech and language, visual, motor, sensory, other high cortical functions and rehabilitation throughput, stroke classification, post-stroke complications, stroke risk factors, stroke mimics followed by a dedicated section of management of acute stroke addressing diagnosis, other considerations, examinations, investigations, and a section on medical therapy.

A dedicated four-bed acute stroke unit was established and the delivery of thrombolysis was established as a first-line treatment in the emergency department. The initial performance target within the first six months of the establishment of clinical practice guidelines was to have 3% of the patients presenting to Western Health with acute ischaemic stroke within the then accepted 3 hours of onset, to undergo thrombolysis. In April 2009, this was finally implemented in full force, after several educational sessions for the emergency department, the newly established stroke team (head of the stroke service, stroke coordinator, stroke fellow), and for Ambulance Victoria (who are responsible for prehospital care for most stroke patients). By July 2009, after the implementation of the clinical practice guidelines, six patients were treated with thrombolysis. We achieved thrombolysis rates of 4% in April 8% in May and 4% in June 2009. Patient outcomes post-thrombolysis was measured relative to improvement of NH Stroke Scale (NIHSS) over a 24-hour period and all six patients statistically significant improvement was seen.

By July 2009, data collection revealed better compliance with the clinical practice guidelines and acute stroke treatment protocol with

♦ 100% of stroke patients being triaged at Category 2 (Category 2 patients in the emergency department must be seeing within ten minutes of their arrival in Victoria, Australia)
♦ and required blood tests and electrocardiogram (ECG) being administered to all.

Among the thrombolysed patients, no patients had haemorrhagic complications and no patients died. Our discharge rate to home was 50% and among the surviving patients 50% were discharged to rehabilitation services compared to less than 40% discharge home during the previous year. It was evident that within the first 3 months of the establishment of clinical practice guidelines of acute stroke care there had been a strong uptake for the change of clinical practice. However, the absence of a dedicated acute stroke nurse was still resulting in significant delays making it obvious that there was a strong case for this to occur.

Since 2007, the advocacy efforts in acute stroke medicine at Western Health have made significant advances in the treatment and management of acute strokes. The START-EXTEND IA collaborative research study (2015) showcases how our efforts have contributed to better patient outcomes. The START-EXTEND IA study combined two types of stroke treatment (the traditional clot busting medication and mechanical removal of the clot with new stent technology) and nearly doubled the numbers of surviving severe stroke patients. The study also used advanced brain imaging to identify which parts of the brain were irreversibly damaged and which parts were salvageable. Patients with enough salvageable brain tissues were first treated with traditional clot-busting medications at Western Health. Then we worked with our collaborators at Melbourne Health, Victoria, Australia (www.mh.org.au) to remove the clot, using new stent technology. When we combined the two treatments, the number of patients who did not sustain a disability after the stroke went from 40% to 70%.[14,15] As of today, Western Health provides a comprehensive stroke care programme in collaboration with RMH for selected patients for thrombectomy at present.

The Western Health stroke research programme has trained 17 Australian neurologists to date, while 9 overseas neurologists have completed stroke fellowships with the organization. At present, there are 5 PhD students working on several pioneering stroke research programmes.

Case study 20.2 Heart and Stroke Foundation of Canada

Working with key stake holders and government is a key towards the successful advocacy in stroke. Heart and Stroke Foundation of Canada is a good example for this.

Ontario is the most populous of the Canadian provinces with 13.6 million residents. It is regarded as one of the most culturally diverse province in the world with nearly half of its population born outside Canada. Stroke was a neglected disease in Canada in the mid-1990s. Only 4% of acute hospitals had dedicated stroke units at that time. A tireless group of stroke advocates, led by the Heart and Stroke Foundation and the Ontario Government came up with a ground breaking strategy that reorganized stroke care across the province ensuring that all Ontarians had access to quality stroke care which revealed a 32.4% reduction in stroke incidence rates in Ontario between 2002 and 2013.[10]

The new policy stated that:

1. It was necessary to build public awareness to recognize the signs of stroke and understand it as a medical emergency.
2. They had to improve systems and services through professional education and implementing system changes across the continuum of stroke care.
3. They had to convince the government to obtain funding and support stating that investing in stroke care would improve health of their citizens.
4. It was necessary to build a coalition as many stakeholders needed to be involved including healthcare system, hospitals, healthcare providers, healthcare consumers (stroke survivors and caregivers) to convince the government of the importance of stroke care improvement.
5. Four hospitals came up as leaders by testing a model of coordinated stroke care regionally. They tested a three-year pilot as a coordinated stroke strategy. These pilots became critical as they built credibility by show casing the success. One hospital which ran a public awareness campaign resulted in 12% of stroke patients receiving clot buster treatment.

The Ontario Stroke System a great success story in stroke advocacy. This was due to a combination of stroke champions (many stroke leaders made a significant commitment of time and leadership across the continuum of stroke advocacy from participation in working groups and panels, participation in educational activities, meetings with the government, participation in steering committees, overseeing pilot projects, teaching and training), strategic decisions, evidence-based practice, involving key stakeholders, telling the right stories to right people, hard work, good timing, perseverance, and luck.[10]

Source: data from World Stroke Organization, WSO Advocacy Toolkit: Advocacy & Awareness Case Study Submissions, Copyright (2016), World Stroke Organization, Available at: http://www.worldstrokecampaign.org/images/wso_advocacy_toolkit/2016-06_-_Advocacy_Case_Studies_Collated_v3.pdf

Case study 20.3 The Stroke Alliance for Europe

During the sixth World Congress of Neurology (WCN) in Vienna, Austria (2013), the Stroke Patient Organization, SAFE, launched the first ever manifesto for better stroke care prevention and care across Europe with the overall aim of reducing the effects of strokes across Europe and with the vision for all people affected /touched by stroke to receive the support, help, and rehabilitation they need.[16]

In 2003, there was only small number of stroke support organizations in Europe and patients with stroke were very badly served at the time. The SAFE was commenced by a top down mechanism, with members of the European Parliament holding a strategic workshop in stroke prevention in 2003 with formal launch of SAFE in October 2004 with participation from seven stroke support organizations (SSOs).

SAFE involved creating educational opportunities in European areas without SSOs (Eastern Europe) and paying travel and accommodation costs for people who were interested in organizing and establishing SSOs in these countries. There are now more than 30 SSOs in Europe and SAFE has recently coordinated a 250,000-Euro research project examining the burden of stroke in Europe. The WSO/SAFE toolkit on how to form a SSO is a great resource for readers who are interested in SSOs.[10]

Source: data from World Stroke Organization, WSO Advocacy Toolkit: Advocacy & Awareness Case Study Submissions, Copyright (2016), World Stroke Organization, Available at: http://www.worldstrokecampaign.org/images/wso_advocacy_toolkit/2016-06_-_Advocacy_Case_Studies_Collated_v3.pdf

Case study 20.4 Latin America Summit for Stroke; a further example of successful stroke advocacy

On Thursday 29 October 2015, World Stroke Day, the American Heart Association/American Stroke Association convened a three-day Latin American Summit in Santiago, Chile. Dr Salvador Cruz-Flores, University of El Paso led this important meeting which was represented by 22 organizations, 42 stroke leaders, and ministry of health. It was the first such summit in the region, where stroke is among the leading causes of death.

Representatives from leading health organizations and government agencies from Argentina, Brazil, Chile, Colombia, Mexico, and Peru met to discuss how to integrate stroke prevention and care into programmes and health plans that address non-communicable diseases.

World Health Organization has named stroke as the number 1 cause of death in Chile, the number 2 cause of death in Argentina and Brazil, and number 3 in Colombia and Mexico. These countries were the focus of the summit, with health insurance, lifestyle factors, and quality of stroke care among the topics that were discussed.

Leaders aimed to create a common vision and commitment for the region to prevent and treat stroke with the help of the AHA/ASA, the Pan American Health Organization (PAHO), the Ibero-American Stroke Society, Stroke Network leaders, and each country's government representatives.

One of the key results of this meeting was the Carta de Santiago, a road map for the region to improve stroke prevention, treatment, and measures to advance public policies in stroke with commitment to uptake policy and systems changes necessary to impact stroke care and outcomes.[10]

Source: data from World Stroke Organization, WSO Advocacy Toolkit: Advocacy & Awareness Case Study Submissions, Copyright (2016), World Stroke Organization, Available at: http://www.worldstrokecampaign.org/images/wso_advocacy_toolkit/2016-06_-_Advocacy_Case_Studies_Collated_v3.pdf

Case study 20.5 Stroke support organization in Nigeria

This case illustrates how one SSO is improving stroke awareness in local communities in Nigeria.[10]

Case vignette

Macdonald who pioneered the Acha Memorial Foundation in Nigeria lost his father from stroke in Nigeria in 2015. He noticed the gaps in stroke care in Nigeria in this tragic situation and decided to commence a project with the goal of improving stroke awareness in Nigeria.[17] He managed to gather a few other people with a similar goal and managed to set up a non-profit, Acha Memorial Foundation (in memory of his father) and the team commenced a project called 'Master Stroke' targeting 10 million Nigerians or Africans about stroke awareness in five years.

The SSO partnered with the World Stroke Organization, local hospitals, and universities (more than 15 universities), hospitals and health organizations, local churches and mosques, with a wide variety of educational activities throughout Nigeria.

1. Within the first two months, the SSO managed to educate about 10,000 Nigerians.[10]

Source: data from World Stroke Organization, WSO Advocacy Toolkit: Advocacy & Awareness Case Study Submissions, Copyright (2016), World Stroke Organization, Available at: http://www.worldstrokecampaign.org/images/wso_advocacy_toolkit/2016-06_-_Advocacy_Case_Studies_Collated_v3.pdf

Case study 20.6 StrokeCare.sg: Online resources for stroke survivors, caregivers, and healthcare workers in Singapore

Singapore is (a well-developed urban nation in Southeast Asia) with a population close to 5.5 million. Singapore boasts first class, accessible health services for all. In October 2016 on its twentieth birthday, the Singapore National Stroke Association launched a one-stop online portal (http://www.stokecare.org.sg) strokecare for stroke survivors, caregivers, families, healthcare workers with the mission of provision of easily digestible information to stroke survivors and families and to raise awareness also to be a public advocate for stroke survivors and families.

Readers who visit this web portal will be convinced that it is indeed a very useful website which does live up to the mission statement. The web portal is a comprehensive educational resource for the stroke patients, caregivers, and staff alike.

Source: data from World Stroke Organization, WSO Advocacy Toolkit: Advocacy & Awareness Case Study Submissions, Copyright (2016), World Stroke Organization, Available at: http://www.worldstrokecampaign.org/images/wso_advocacy_toolkit/2016-06_-_Advocacy_Case_Studies_Collated_v3.pdf

Case study 20.7 The Chinese Stroke Association

The Chinese Stroke Association (CSA) Chinese Stroke Association was established in 2015. The mission of CSA is to improve the stroke care in China by providing medical education to healthcare professionals and public, implementing the state science, technology, and health policy. CSA partner with other stake holders covering about 1,000 hospitals to promote World Stroke Day activities regularly.

In 2015, a major stroke education campaign was launched in line with World Stroke Day across China. More than 1,000 education campaigns were conducted with the help of over

10,000 medical staff coming from the 861 hospitals in the 123 cities of 32 province during the World Stroke Day activities in 2015.[10]

Source: data from World Stroke Organization, WSO Advocacy Toolkit: Advocacy & Awareness Case Study Submissions, Copyright (2016), World Stroke Organization, Available at: http://www.worldstrokecampaign.org/images/wso_advocacy_toolkit/2016-06_-_Advocacy_Case_Studies_Collated_v3.pdf

Case study 20.8 Stroke advocacy in Sri Lanka

Sri Lanka is a small island in the Indian Ocean off the south-eastern coast of India. Sri Lanka has an ageing population with an impending epidemic of stroke at hand.[18] The first stroke unit in Sri Lanka was established in 2000 and SSO the National Stroke Association of Sri Lanka (NSASL) was established in 2001.

In November 2008, at the Association of Sri Lankan Neurologists (ASN) Annual Meeting in Colombo, Sri Lanka hosted the first ever International Stroke Conference (ISC) on state-of-the-art stroke care. On the eve of the ISC, a panel of leading national and international figures in health and stroke care held a press conference and make the strong argument for better stroke care in front of the federal minister of health, Sri Lanka and other key dignitaries of the Department of Health, Sri Lanka.

The ISC was a huge success, with more than one hundred attendees, and a diverse faculty representing Australia, United Kingdom, United States, India, Canada, and Pakistan. There were four Palatucci Forum graduates at the ISC in Sri Lanka, lending their advocacy efforts to the project.[12]

This ISC led to the establishment of additional stroke units across number of major hospitals across Sri Lanka (Badulla, Anuradhapuraya, and Diyathalawa).

In 2009, NSASL came up with a massive World Stroke Day educational campaign throughout Sri Lanka. There was a well-organized media conference with 100 media personnel covering all major media outlets with a view to spread the message of need for better stroke care throughout Sri Lanka at that time. A 20-minute video documentary covering stroke symptoms, risk factors, and treatment was telecasted on prime-time TV throughout Sri Lanka. The team went on to win the first ever gold award for World Stroke Day activities in 2009.[19,20]

Case studies 20.1–20.8 demonstrate the breadth and power of effective advocacy from setting up a stroke service, setting up SSOs, educational activities, policy changes, and the global impact. Stroke advocacy encompasses continuum of stroke care from prevention, acute treatment, subacute care, stroke research, fundraising, and policy changes leading towards better stroke care.[21,22]

Advocacy toolkit: World Stroke Organization

Stroke advocacy is the key to developing the best possible stroke care globally. Last year, the advocacy toolkit was launched by the World Stroke Organization as a guide to improving awareness and understanding of stroke[10] or potentially any cause. It also describes the tactics and tools that are important in successful advocacy. The toolkit is full of good ideas and advice on how to become a successful stroke advocate and how to assist in developing a stroke advocacy action plan. These are the critical steps towards development of an effective advocacy strategy, which the authors adopted from the Democracy Center (www.democracyctr.org).

The nine steps to achieve change are as follows:

1. Goals and objectives (what do the advocates want to achieve?)
2. Key decision-makers (who can give it to the advocates?)

3. Messages (what do the decision-makers must know?)
4. Influencers, alliances, coalitions (who do the decision-makers need to hear it from?)
5. Delivery of the messages (how does the advocate get the decision-makers to hear the message?)
6. Strengths and resources (what have the advocates got as effective resources and strengths?)
7. Gaps and challenges (what do the advocates need to build/develop further?)
8. Baby steps (where to begin, how to begin?)
9. Evaluation (how will the advocates know their strategy is working or not?)[10]

Conclusion

Stroke is the leading neurological disorder with a huge threat to better brain health globally. Clearly, there is a strong need for good stroke advocates from neurologists, other healthcare workers, patients, and caregivers globally. The World Stroke Organization advocacy tool kit is highly recommended as a practical roadmap aimed at enabling prospective stroke advocates. Being an effective stroke advocate is enormously rewarding. We cordially invite the readers to get in to the mix and combat stroke whether in prevention, acute treatment, or rehabilitation with a view to promote better brain health globally.

References

1. **Murray, C. J., Lopez, A. D.** (1996) Evidence-based health policy—lessons from the Global Burden of Disease Study. *Science*, **274**(5288), 740–3.
2. **Feigin, V. L., Krishnamurthi, R. V., Parmar, P., et al.** (2015) Update on the global burden of ischemic and hemorrhagic stroke in 1990–2013: the GBD 2013 study. *Neuroepidemiology*, **45**(3), 161–76.
3. **Feigin, V. L., Mensah, G. A., Norrving, B., Murray, C. J., Roth, G. A., Group GBDSPE** (2015) Atlas of the global burden of stroke (1990–2013): The GBD 2013 study. *Neuroepidemiology*, **45**(3), 230–6.
4. **Feigin, V. L., Krishnamurthi, R., Bhattacharjee, R., et al.** (2015) New strategy to reduce the global burden of stroke. *Stroke*, **46**(6), 1740–7.
5. **Wijeratne, T., Gamage, R., Pathirana, G., et al.** (2011) Stroke care development in Sri Lanka: the urgent need for neurorehabilitation services. *Neurology Asia*, **16**(2), 149–51.
6. **Seshadri, S., Wolf, P. A., Beiser, A., et al.** (1997) Lifetime risk of dementia and Alzheimer's disease. The impact of mortality on risk estimates in the Framingham Study. *Neurology*, **49**(6), 1498–504.
7. **Shehadah, A., Franklin, G. M., Benson, R. T.** (2016) Global disparities in stroke and why we should care. *Neurology*, **87**(5), 450–1.
8. **Mendis, S., Abegunde, D., Yusuf, S., et al.** (2005) WHO study on Prevention of REcurrences of Myocardial Infarction and StrokE (WHO-PREMISE). *Bull World Health Organ*, **83**(11), 820–9.
9. **Langhorne, P., de Villiers, L., Pandian, J. D.** (2012) Applicability of stroke-unit care to low-income and middle-income countries. *Lancet Neurol*, **11**(4), 341–8.
10. **World Stroke Organization** (1997) **WSO Advocacy Toolkit**. Available at: http://www.worldstrokecampaign.org/get-involved/wso-advocacy-toolkit.html

11. **World Stroke Organization.** Advocacy activities. Available at: https://world-stroke.org/membership/renewal/membership-renewal-for-societies/15-news/104-advocacy
12. **Wijeratne, T., DePold Hohler, A.** (2013) Residency training: advocacy training in neurology: lessons from the Palatucci Advocacy Leadership Forum. *Neurology*, **80**(1), e1–3.
13. **Gill, P. J., Gill, H. S., Marrie, T. J.** (2010) Health advocacy training: now is the time to develop physician leaders. *Acad Med*, **85**(1), 5.
14. **Campbell, B. C., Mitchell, P. J., Kleinig, T. J., et al.** (2015) Endovascular therapy for ischemic stroke with perfusion-imaging selection. *N Engl J Med*, **372**(11), 1009–18.
15. **Campbell, B. C., Mitchell, P. J., Yan, B., et al.** (2014) A multicenter, randomized, controlled study to investigate EXtending the time for Thrombolysis in Emergency Neurological Deficits with Intra-Arterial therapy (EXTEND-IA). *Int J Stroke*, **9**(1), 126–32.
16. **Levy, S.** (2010) SAFE: the Stroke Alliance for Europe. *Int J Stroke*, **5**(6), 483.
17. **MasterStroke.** Available at: https://www.facebook.com/GoMasterStroke
18. **Wijeratne, T.** (2012) Neurorehabilitation in Sri Lanka: an emerging sub-specialty for neurology trainees. *Int J Stroke*, **7**(2), 163–4.
19. **Gunaratne, P. S.** (2009) A step forward in stroke care in Sri Lanka. *Int J Stroke*, **4**(4), 293.
20. **Gunaratne, P. S., Jeevatharan, H.** (2010) World Stroke Day 2009, gold award winner. *Int J Stroke*, **5**(4), 323–4.
21. **Krishnamurthi, R. V., Feigin, V. L., Forouzanfar, M. H., et al.** (2013) Global and regional burden of first-ever ischaemic and haemorrhagic stroke during 1990–2010: findings from the Global Burden of Disease Study 2010. *Lancet Glob Health*, **1**(5), e259–81.
22. **Krishnamurthi, R. V., Moran, A. E., Forouzanfar, M. H., et al.** (2014) The global burden of hemorrhagic stroke: a summary of findings from the GBD 2010 study. *Glob Heart*, **9**(1), 101–6.

Chapter 21

Two decades of patient advocacy in multiple sclerosis: The success story of the European Multiple Sclerosis Platform

Christoph Thalheim

Patient advocacy in MS—how did it start?

As in most, if not all patient advocacy groups, there is a patient, a family member, or a doctor at the beginning of the story, who personally experiences an 'unmet need'—no advice and support for the newly diagnosed, no information material (or not the right sort), no one with any real interest to exchange personal stories with, no one who understands, who cares, and who tries to help.[1-4] To match this 'unmet need', this situation calls for a 'self-help group' defined as a group of people being affected by the same disease, unified by the wish to help each other. If all goes well and a 'critical mass' of affected patients and a 'visionary person thinking beyond his/her own needs' find each other, then the question of 'How can we not only help each other, but influence our healthcare and social environment?' might mark the birth of a patient advocacy group. In the case of multiple sclerosis (MS), the honour of being the first person who created a sustainable self-help- and advocacy movement goes to American lawyer Sylvia Lawry, who founded first the National Multiple Sclerosis Society in the United States in 1947 and co-founded the global Multiple Sclerosis International Federation (MSIF) a bit later in the same year.[5] As in many similar stories, the nucleus for a disease-specific advocacy- and research support group was coming through a personal experience within the own family; in Sylvia Lawry's case it was the diagnosis with MS for her brother Bernard. She rightfully can be regarded as the most impactful advocate for people with MS ever, as transformed the idea of self-help and personal stories to the level of a political influencer, as her picture of 1955 with Ralph Glock, president of the US National MS Society and senator Everett M. Dirksen as key speaker of the Society's Annual National Conference suggests (Fig. 21.1).

While Lawry died in 2001, her idea was kept alive worldwide and remains so until today, with the globally acting Multiple Sclerosis International Federation and the regionally focused European MS Platform working hand in hand on Lawry's vision of a world without multiple sclerosis.

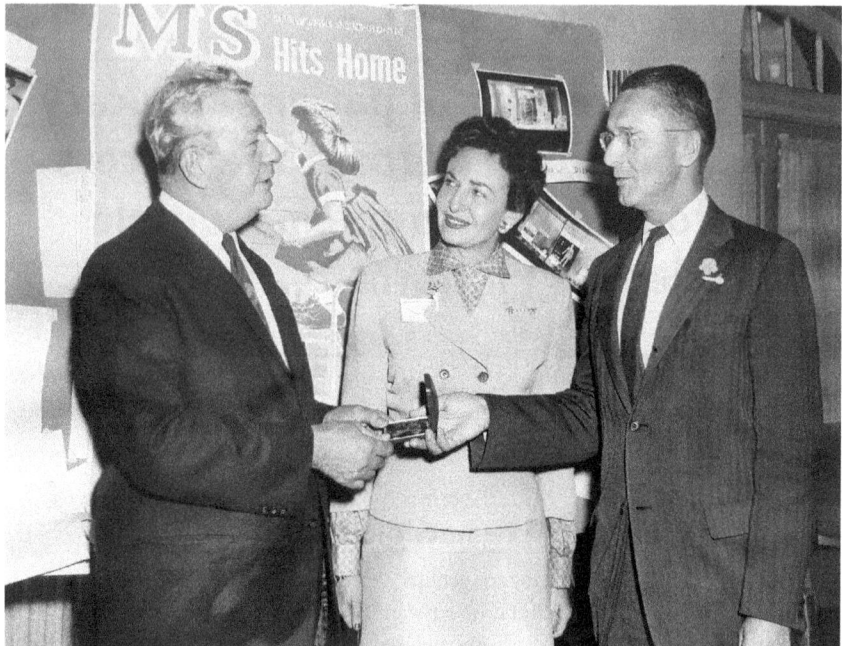

Fig. 21.1 Sylvia Lawry, director of the National Multiple Sclerosis Society (US), in 1955.

When 27 national MS patient organizations decided in 1989 that a European umbrella organization was needed, there were mainly three points which encouraged those European Multiple Sclerosis Platform (EMSP) founders to act together. It is probably fair to say that the envisaged European identity for the MS communities in Europe was the overarching vision, while the practical need for funds through EU-(co-) funded projects and the wish to strengthen the first goal through capacity building for the less developed MS patient organizations were the real key drivers for the creation of the platform.

First, the founding members installed a 'moving virtual office' driven by the volunteer EMSP President and a local assistant with a commitment of one day per week.

Some basic cross-border projects arose from this structure, but it took more than a decade for the EMSP members to realize that 'you'll get peanuts if you pay for peanuts'. The installation of a small, but permanent liaison office in Brussels was the logical consequence—replacing the dysfunctional mix of national and European responsibilities shared between the EMSP President and his assistant over the past ten years.

Starting in 2000 and strongly supported by both Board and members, EMSP's first paid staff person in Brussels now added one brick to the next to build a well-respected European voice for the 27 national MS societies and its hundreds of thousands of people with MS being represented by them.

Soon funds were approved by the European Commission towards a multistakeholder project. This, in addition to the organization of regular annual European membership conferences and the progression towards a sustainable network of industry partners, attracted a growing number of national MS societies to the EMSP.

Major EMSP projects—and their value for people with MS and their families

A very early story of success and a good example for a patient advocacy area, in which a cross-border approach was the best way forward to start national lobby initiatives, was a major EMSP conference on Intimacy and Sexuality by People with MS, held in the year 2000 in Oslo, Norway.

Why were participants still speaking about this specific conference even years later? Because for many of them this subject had been a major problem in their home countries, but also a 'taboo' subject for discussion in public. In the international environment of a Nordic capital, it suddenly become possible to openly share experiences, explain problems, and identify needs for support through experts and therapies back home. Today, intimacy, sexuality and pregnancy in MS are no longer 'taboo' subjects; instead, they form a major part of the abundant information- and guidance materials on offer, even in predominant Catholic countries such as Ireland, Spain, and Poland.

Another key subject for almost every patient organization is the question of sustainable funding for their activities. As mentioned earlier, EMSP identified the huge interest shown by most of its member organizations in becoming part of EU-(co-)funded projects. EMSP partnered early on with experts in EU funding, such as the European Citizen Action Service. By doing so, it was possible to act as multiplier and mediator for MS patient organizations in Central-and Eastern Europe long before they became part of the EU. If you wish, you can regard EMSP as a kind of political actor in this context, because our member organizations in Central and Eastern European (CEE) countries were addressing healthcare and social issues which their governments had not (yet) even thought of.

There was almost always a need to come up with other additional funding sources in the early days of EU project funding. EMSP guidance in multinational projects for people with MS (such as the intercultural and intergenerational learning in a 'MS Cybercafé') allowed a transnational approach, not only in the project content, but also in its funding methods. Being one of EMSP's first EU co-funded projects, the impact on the solidarity between East and West, young and old, disabled patient and healthy IT-specialist in 'MS Cybercafés' was not only remarkable because of its multifacet approach, it also created sustainability for the project beyond its period of financial support by the European Commission. Several MS societies identified alternative funding for 'their MS Cybercafé'—in some places it does exist until today.

A true milestone in EMSP's lobbying and awareness raising was the approval of the very first MS Report signed by 240 Members of the European Parliament (Petition 842/2001),[3] concerning the effects of discriminatory treatment towards persons with MS, within the European Union.

> '... persons with Multiple Sclerosis, and many other chronic long-term illnesses, are subject to varying levels of medical and therapeutic care depending on their place of residence and . . . insufficient priority has been accorded by Member States of the Union . . . to remedying this fact.'

It is worth mentioning in this context that one single European citizen, who did not accept the inequalities in access to therapies and care in her country, initiated the change of this situation for her and many others with the help of engaged Members and Staff of the European Parliament and the facilitation provided by the European MS Platform.

Many new advocacy tools and initiatives were developed by EMSP and its members thanks to this first success in the European Parliament, some of which are still in use today (2019):

At the request of the European Parliament, EMSP developed a European Code of Good Practice in MS,[6] with regular updates and connected thematic consensus papers.

Annual European MS conferences for member organizations and stakeholders, focusing on varying subjects such as 'Sexuality and Intimacy in MS', 'Cognitive Dysfunctions and Care for Care Givers', and 'Rehabilitation in MS', used as awareness raising, capacity building, and networking events.

Studies and surveys on FACTS & FIGURES in MS (e.g. the MS ATLAS),[7] developed under the leadership of MSIF and therefore providing a global picture, are used for public awareness raising combined with the demand for more efforts by public services until today.

The European MS Nurse Survey (MS-NEED), to understand the varying roles of MS nurses in European countries, identifying best practice for education, certification, training and additional tasks of MS nurses in order to improve patient quality of life and provide incentives to the MS nurses. The results of the survey inspired EMSP's MS Nurse PRO,[8] an online training programme for MS nurses, beating in its reach out all expectations.

As a biannual tool, the MS Barometer[9] is a comparative survey based on key MS data being collected by the national MS societies. First launched in 2008, the MS Barometer raises awareness on the geographical divide that underpins the difference in MS management across Europe. It also serves as a benchmarking tool outlining improvements and actions that can be adopted by national MS societies in order to influence their political decision makers. The MS Barometer targets healthcare stakeholders at all levels, including MS patients; healthcare professionals; governmental institutions; insurers and other payers; politicians and financial supporters.

Disease management varies considerably from one country to another. The Barometer provides an overview of the weaknesses and challenges to be addressed in each country covered. It enables EMSP as well as individual MS societies to actively engage with the relevant stakeholders and work together to improve the quality of life for people with MS. Now marking its fifth edition, the MS Barometer has built up a strong track-record in supporting MS advocacy at both European and national level.

How does the MS Barometer work? The MS Barometer is a questionnaire with points scored based on the responses. The goal is for each national administration to score maximum points through the implementation of effective policies which optimize the situation for people with MS. The higher the score, the better the disease management, level of support, and quality of life for people with MS. The questionnaire is structured around the priority policy areas defined in EMSP's Code of Good Practice and covers four key areas of patient relevance and concern (Table 21.1):

Table 21.1 Four key areas of patient relevance as defined in EMSP's Code of Good Practice

1. Access to healthcare	2. MS research and data
3. Participation in society of people with MS	4. Empowerment of people with MS

For the future, EMSP expects to obtain most of the data via MS Data Alliance, the planned European Network of National Patient Registries in Multiple Sclerosis.[10]

Another prominent example of our advocacy tools for both our members and for our work on European level is a ground-breaking multimedia project, called 'Under Pressure',[11] our answer to the question whether it is possible to reduce health inequalities through visualized cross-border comparison and benchmarking. Our answer was 'Yes!'—so we bundled our forces with a team of five top-class photographers who accompanied people with MS and their families in 12 different countries.

EMSP's project website[11] tells the stunning stories of those people, hosts an impressive photo gallery of six hundred photos accompanied by informative country profiles and a collection of short video documentaries. The focus of this valuable footage centres on story-telling and awareness raising.

The combination of the MS Barometer data and a selection of Under Pressure photos and videos has proven to be most effective in both national and European level patient advocacy, because it tells true stories of patient journeys backed up by recent survey data.

Job retention or access to employment are major issues for many people with MS. EMSP is determined to open new paths to employment for people with MS and other neurodegenerative conditions. How? By running two flagship projects—Paving the Path to Participation (PPP)[12] and Believe & Achieve (B&A)[13]—with both projects aiming at the implementation of support plans to help people with MS and their employers to cope with their condition while at work.

Paving the Path to Participation (PPP) aims to promote policy change that will support maximum participation of people with MS in the labour market in Europe. Pact PPP relies on a multistakeholder network in its efforts to promote a European Employment Pact. People with MS, employers, healthcare providers, and policymakers are all taking part.

Believe & Achieve (B&A) aims to provide young people with MS with opportunities to work in supportive environments by partnering through paid internships with businesses across Europe, while MS@Work addresses other labour related questions for any person with MS.

Beyond traditional advocacy: Can patients influence the education of healthcare professionals?

MS nurses play an integral role in providing support and advice on everyday issues for people with MS and coordinate a collaborative approach to management. However, as the responsibilities of the MS Nurse continue to expand, the findings of the largest survey of MS nurses across Europe—MS-NEED: European Survey (2010)—highlighted that there are significant disparities in the provision and quality of service provided by MS nurses. Therefore, there is a need not only to raise awareness of the role of the MS Nurse, but also to standardize their training in order to underpin their position in the management of MS and to optimize care for people with MS.

The mission of MS Nurse Professional,[8] developed by the MS-NEED Study Group, is:

- To provide a modular, online training curriculum to support the evolving role of European MS nurses, in line with the recently published MS Nurse Consensus Paper entitled 'Moving towards the pan-European unification and recognition of MS nurses'.
- To increase the competency of MS nurses in patient/family advocacy and brokerage, health education, symptom and treatment management.
- To develop leadership skills for the advancement of patient care.

Meanwhile, over 6,000 multiple sclerosis (MS) nurses enrolled for MS Nurse PRO between 2012 and the end of 2018 and so far more than 1,000 of them finished the online education course successfully.

This ongoing project is led by the EMSP in collaboration with the International Organization of Multiple Sclerosis Nurses (IOMSN) and Rehabilitation in MS (RIMS). Collectively, this group is known as the Multiple Sclerosis-Nurse Empowering Education (MS-NEED). The project's latest success was an acknowledgement and reinforcement of the support agreement between MS Nurse PRO with the European Committee for Treatment and Research in MS (ECTRIMS).

Big data for better outcomes—patient data collection in registries

Multiple Sclerosis—Information Dividend

As the title of the project suggests, Multiple Sclerosis—Information Dividend (MS-ID) concerns information about MS and the benefits to be gained from such information. In Europe, very limited data are gathered about MS, its incidence, who is taking which drugs as treatment, how MS impacts on the lives of those who are affected, and what additional support the state provides and needs to provide. However, in order to better understand the impact of MS, we have to know the effects it has on society in general. In essence, the MS-ID project consisted of two priorities:

1. The development and piloting of a European register on MS. This register will gather data on people with MS from organizations participating in the project. The advantage of developing this tool on a European level means that the information will be comparative across borders. For example, one can assert that a treatment accessed by 40% of those with MS in one country may only be accessed by 5% of the MS population in another country. Without this information, no light can be shed on the situation of people with MS in Europe.

2. Activation of the European Code of Good Practice in MS across the participating organizations, with eventual roll-out to all EMSP members.

Which were the expected achievements?

- To raise awareness across the EU about MS, enabling stakeholders both at European level and in the member states to better understand the condition and share information on the positive impact of early diagnosis coupled with high-quality treatments, choice of therapies, sufficient social support, and the benefits of good MS management.
- To identify and address the major inequalities in MS treatment and care across the EU and within member states through the development of new and effective strategies and indicators to measure performance; this will enhance the quality, comparability, applicability, and transfer of statistical and factual data and qualitative information on MS across EU member states.
- To use high-quality comparable data at EU and transnational levels to positively impact on EU/national MS policy and programmes; ultimately, this will empower those EU citizens directly and indirectly affected by MS.

In short, the MS-ID project was aiming high for an improved, better managed, and more equitable approach to the treatment of MS in Europe, enabling people with MS to contribute and rightfully participate as full and equal citizens in society.

While the three objectives just listed were achieved only in part, MS-ID delivered an unplanned and unexpected result of the highest value: it paved the path as feasibility study to the European Registry for MS (EUReMS).[14]

As a vital step towards better exploitation of real-world evidence outcome data. Collecting standardized data in national patient registries for temporary pooling and central analysis on European level was the ambitious aim of five national MS registers and six other project partners which gathered in 2011. The fact that by the end of the project in 2014 the number of participating registries had grown from originally five to thirteen is an indirect indicator for success, but it certainly had not made negotiations easier on core data sets, substudy protocols, and data handling routines for the harmonization of the heterogeneous data of the different registers into comparable study data sets.

As often being the case in long-term projects, promised deliverables such as a functioning network of MS registries had to be adapted to the more feasible proof of concept for such a network. The agreement by previously non-connected 13 registries to standard parameters in collection and temporary pooling of vital patient data for the purpose of central analysis of those data on European level!

The most important achievement from the patient advocate's point of view was (and still is) the movement towards inclusion of more patient-relevant and patient-reported outcomes data,[15] coupled by a raised awareness of the cost of illness and burden of disease data as vital factors for the sustainability of our healthcare systems.

Until 2007, very limited data was gathered about MS, its incidence, treatments, and impact on social life and employment. With the MS Information Dividend (MS-ID) project being set up in 2007 and the EUReMS project following in 2011, EMSP become a 'frontrunner' on data sharing by independent patient registries and the importance of real-world evidence data[16] for healthcare decisions.

Briefly after the first positive interim results of EUReMS work became known, the five biggest MS registries accepted a proposal by industry to develop their own collaboration structure, being identical in part to the one with in EUReMS and using a similar methodology for temporary pooling.

EU bodies and initiatives—targets or partner for patient advocacy?

With the PARENT Joint Action (cross-border patient registries initiative)[17] of the European Commission and 17 member states on interoperability questions of patient registries an effort was started in 2013 to give a response to poor cross-border availability of health data for public health and research. PARENT brought added value by providing member states with recommendations and tools for implementation of interoperable and cross-border enabled patient registries—and the EUReMS group was proud to contribute to those recommendations and tools from its own experiences gathered within their project.

The European Medicines Agency (EMA),[18] as 'gate keeper' for many therapies on the European market, is probably one of the best examples for the seemingly unsolvable 'friend or foe' dilemma of patient advocacy groups. I say seemingly, because it is only a very superficial glance which would bring EMA and patient advocacy groups in the opposite corners of the healthcare boxing ring. In reality, they have been working well together for more than a decade and this collaboration is regarded as success story by both sides. Within the MS field, there are plenty of examples where the opinions of EMA and EMSP were initially diverging, but ultimately agreements were reached in all those cases, whether it was on benefit-risk assessments, the value for patients of a new treatment or any other question. Of great help for building trust and mutual understanding is EMSP's membership in the 'Patient and Consumer Working Party' (PCWP),[19] which recently celebrated its tenth anniversary. Four to five times a year, EMA representatives and delegates from European patient or consumer organizations meet as PCWP members to discuss questions of mutual relevance.

A great example of how patience and persistence can lead to win-win situations is the 'Cross-Committee Working Party on Patient Registries' of the EMA,[20] in which EMSP has tried to promote its concept of common core data sets for disease-specific national registries to allow temporary pooling and central analysis for cases, in which single registry data do not provide a sufficient base. After 18 months of discussion, EMA agreed to organize a workshop for MS registries, the regulators, the payers and the market authorization holders (industry) to discuss this concept as pilot for MS and other diseases. As next steps, EMA has started qualification processes for the first few

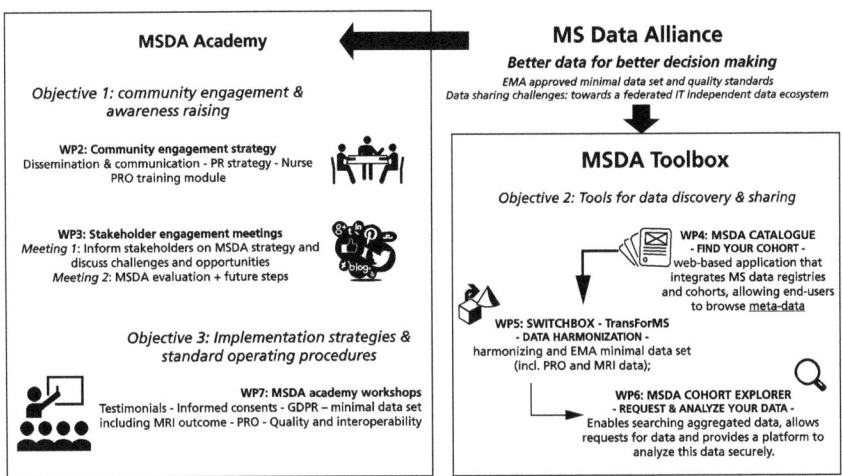

Fig. 21.2 MS Data Alliance graphic.

European disease specific registry networks and presented a draft proposal for the use of patient registries for regulatory purposes in December 2018 (Fig. 21.2).

EUnetHTA[21] stands for 'European Network of Health Technology Assessment'; its EUnetHTA Joint Action 3 aims to define and implement a sustainable model for the scientific and technical cooperation on Health Technology Assessment (HTA) in Europe.[22] EUnetHTA will support evidence-based, sustainable, and equitable choices in healthcare and health technologies and support re-use in regional and national HTA reports and activities. To develop a voluntary, sustainable European Collaboration on HTA, the model focuses on supporting Members States in receiving HTA relevant information that is objective, reliable, timely, and comparable. It goes without saying, that the (future) role of patients and patient advocacy groups in this process cannot be overestimated; especially in ensuring the integration of patient relevant outcomes data into HTA recommendations leading to payer decisions. Consequently, EMSP is one of six patient or consumer organizations actively pushing for a more meaningful and sustainable involvement of patients in HTA processes.

For a quarter of a century, European Committee for Treatment and Research in Multiple Sclerosis (ECTRIMS)[23] has served as Europe's and the world's largest professional organization dedicated to the understanding and treatment of MS. ECTRIMS works with researchers and clinicians from its member countries and with other organizations that share similar missions and objectives on a worldwide scale, creating networking and collaboration opportunities. The ultimate goal of ECTRIMS is to improve basic and clinical research and clinical outcomes in MS. With the mission to 'facilitate communication, create synergies, and promote and enhance research and learning among professionals for the ultimate benefit of people affected by MS', it was a logical, although overdue step by ECTRIMS and EMSP to join forces and formally agree on areas of collaboration in a Memorandum of Understanding as of mid-2016.

What were/are the key challenges and how did EMSP address them?

Lack of financial support by public institutions for costs being necessary to run a European patient advocacy group professionally is the second biggest challenge, this being true not only for EMSP, but for almost all comparable organizations. As a result of several years of patient organizations' active lobbying, the European Commission finally introduced a support scheme for European patient organizations in 2012 called the 'Operating Grant'. EMSP was among the first 10 successful applicants and was able to repeat this success twice, until in 2015 new rules were introduced by the Commission. With the collaboration between patient organizations and healthcare industry always being an area of concern for the EU institutions, a limit of 20% had been fixed for industry contribution to patient organization's core funding, which was manageable somehow as long as the 20% rule was applied for the year in which the Operating Grant was paid. By a simple change of the 20% rule's application to the year *before* the payment of the Operating Grant the Commission not only made many of the patient organizations ineligible, but also achieved the opposite of its intention for the change of the rule: Many patient organizations were forced into even closer collaboration with industry instead of the previous healthy diversification between public and private funding sources.

Collaboration with industry is a story of success for EMSP and a permanent challenge at the same time. More precisely: there is an ongoing need to establish case by case, and again and again the right balance between mutually beneficial collaboration and industry's (understandable) wish to widely promote their products.

Outside of commercial considerations, there are naturally overlapping areas of mutual interest for industry and patients, such as pharmacovigilance, drug efficacy, and more.

Within and beside those overlapping interests, many of EMSP's awareness raising, capacity building, and advocacy projects have been developed with unconditional grants by pharmaceutical firms and other companies.

To avoid any impression of bias, EMSP has put a major effort into continuously enlarging its network of industry partners in combination with a maximum of transparency, fostering a kind of 'natural mutual control by competitors'. Mutual respect for the aims and integrity of each party, good understanding of each other's structures and key representatives, ethical standards as regulated by the EMA requests for transparency, the European Federation of Pharmaceutical Industries and Associations (EFPIA) Code, ABPI Code of Practice, and patient organizations' own ethical rules—all this helps to manage the working relation as win-win ultimately, but has not been a guarantee of problem-free collaboration in the past and will not be in the future.

EMSP's work as European voice of people with MS in Europe—what comes next?

According to Wikipedia, there are 50 internationally recognized sovereign states with territory located within the common definition of Europe and/or membership in

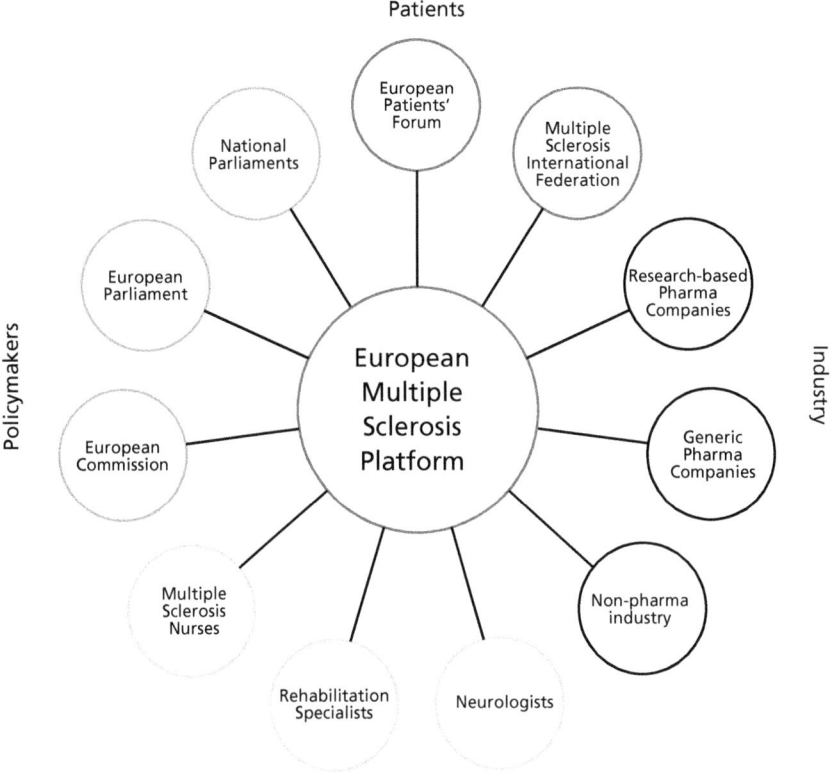

Fig. 21.3 The European Multiple Sclerosis Platform in its professional context.

international European organizations, 36 of which have an MS patient organization with EMSP membership, while in 5 of those countries a second MS patient organization exists. EMSP is therefore seen as the one and only voice of more than 700.000 people with MS in Europe and widely recognized among stakeholders on European and national level. The key stakeholders for our work can be best summarized by Fig. 21.3.

EMSP will continue to fight for a better quality of life for all people with MS until in the hopefully not too distant future our work as patient advocates will become obsolete—by a cure for multiple sclerosis!

In the meantime, we see one key area of direct or indirect relevance for people with MS, in which more advocacy efforts on both the national and the European level could have a substantial impact:

Patient-relevant and patient-reported outcomes data[15] should be standardized as vital part of real-world evidence,[16] required for all kind of healthcare related decisions. This could be done either by the regulator (e.g. for pharmacovigilance aspects), by HTA agencies (e.g. for cost-efficiency questions), or by the healthcare professional. The findings can then be used to improve quality of care.

The importance of a standardized approach to the collection and interpretation of those patient-reported outcomes data (not only in MS) becomes obvious by looking at their potential:

1. They can help as next step towards more personalized medicines, because they demonstrate more or less impact of a therapy to patient relevant symptoms and consequences of the disease.
2. They can help to improve cost-efficiency of a therapy by separating those patients with low outcomes (no need to continue with the therapy in question) from those with high outcomes (therapy to be continued).
3. If standardized patient-reported outcomes data from rehabilitation activities are added to the patient registries, evidence-based recommendations for rehabilitation effectiveness can be given—for potential combination approaches of drug and rehabilitation included.
4. On 'cost of illness and burden of disease' questions, making such registry networks fit for purpose could cooperate with large relevant studies, such as EMSP's recent 17,000-patient survey in 16 European countries.[24] This would allow a cost-and time-efficient minimum Central Office of Information (COI) data set to be completed every five years with a much smaller and shorter control survey.
5. Once minimum data sets for patient-reported outcomes (and clinical) data will be implemented into all disease-specific registries of a European (or even global) network of MS registries and those minimum data sets will be approved for the use by regulators, HTA bodies, and payers, the concept of patient advocacy will move to a completely different and much more effective level.

References

1. **European Multiple Sclerosis Platform**. Available at: http://www.emsp.org/
2. **MS International Federation**. Available at: https://www.msif.org/
3. **Aaltonen, U.** (2003) Report on petition 842/2001 concerning the effects of discriminatory treatment afforded to persons with Multiple Sclerosis, within the European Union, Committee on Petitions, European Parliament, 2003. Available at: http://www.europarl.europa.eu/sides/getDoc.do?pubRef=-//EP//TEXT+REPORT+A5-2003-0451+0+DOC+XML+V0//EN&language=en
4. **European Patients Forum**. Available at: http://www.eu-patient.eu/
5. **Sylvia Lawry** (15 March 2017, last edit). In: *Wikipedia*. Available at: https://en.wikipedia.org/wiki/Sylvia_Lawry
6. **Willet, A.** (2014) *Defeating MS Together: the European Code of Good Practice in MS, European MS Platform*. Available at: http://www.emsp.org/wp-content/uploads/2015/06/140824-Revised-Code-of-Good-Practice.pdf
7. **MS International Federation** (2013) Atlas of MS. Available at: https://www.msif.org/about-us/advocacy/atlas/?gclid=Cj0KEQjwn_3GBRDc8rCnup-1x8wBEiQAdw3OAWcA9s7mrfpWTchQ5kI9BHEBmGE2LyRHZoZTQI3soNUaAura8P8HAQ
8. **European MS Platform** (2012) MS Nurse PRO, 2012–ongoing. Available at: http://www.msnursepro.org/

9. **European MS Platform** (2009) MS Barometer, 2009–ongoing. Available at: http://www.emsp.org/projects/ms-barometer/
10. **European MS Platform** (2018) Opportunities and challenges for the European Network of MS Data Alliance. Available at: http://www.emsp.org/wp-content/uploads/2018/12/summary-proposal-nov-2018-ms-data-alliance.pdf
11. **European MS Platform** (2013) Under Pressure—Living with MS in Europe. Available at: http://www.underpressureproject.eu/web
12. **European MS Platform** (2015) Paving the Path to Participation. Available at: http://www.emsp.org/projects/paving-the-path-to-participation/
13. **European MS Platform** (2015) Believe and Achieve. Available at: http://www.emsp.org/projects/believe-and-achieve/
14. **European MS Platform** (2011–2014) The European Register for Multiple Sclerosis (EUReMS). Available at: http://www.emsp.org/projects/eurems/
15. **Klose, K.**, **Kreimeier, S.**, **Tangermann, U.**, **et al.** (2016) Patient- and person-reports on healthcare: preferences, outcomes, experiences, and satisfaction—an essay. *Health Econ Rev*, **6**, 18.
16. **Annemans, L.**, **Aristides, M.**, **Kubin, M.** (2007) Real-life data: a growing need. *ISPOR Connections*, **13**, 8–12.
17. **PARENT, Cross Border Patient Registries Initiative (PARENT), EUnetHTA group**, **et al.** (2008–2013) Available at: http://www.eunethta.eu/parent
18. **European Medicines Agency**. Available at: http://www.ema.europa.eu/ema/
19. **Patients' and Consumers' Working Party, European Medicines Agency** (2005) Available at: http://www.ema.europa.eu/ema/index.jsp?curl=pages/partners_and_networks/general/general_content_000708.jsp&mid=WC0b01ac05809e2d8c
20. **European Medicines Agency** (2016) Patient Registries Workshop–Observations and recommendations arising from the workshop, 28 October 2016. Available at: http://www.ema.europa.eu/docs/en_GB/document_library/Report/2017/02/WC500221618.pdf
21. **European Network of Health Technology Assessment (EUnetHTA)**. Available at: http://www.eunethta.eu/
22. **EUnetHTA Joint Action 3 (2016–2020)** Available at: https://5026.makemeweb.net/activities/joint-action-3/jointaction31/eunethta-joint-action-3-2016-2020
23. **European Committee for Treatment and Research in Multiple Sclerosis (ECTRIMS)**. Available at: https://www.ectrims.eu/
24. **Kobelt, G.**, **Thompson, A**. (2016) Cost of Illness study: New insight into cost and burden of MS. Available at: http://www.emsp.org/news-messages/new-insight-into-cost-and-burden-of-ms/

Chapter 22

Advocacy in amyotrophic lateral sclerosis

Albert C. Ludolph

Amyotrophic lateral sclerosis

Amyotrophic lateral sclerosis (ALS) is one of the most severe neurodegenerative diseases.[1] Although it affects many neuronal populations of the central nervous system,[2] it clinically concerns predominantly the motor system in a progressive manner.[3] It leads to generalized paresis and immobilization and after a short disease course leaves the individual in a 'differentiated' state: the patient becomes unable to communicate by speech, writing, mimics, gesture, and posture. Since ALS is a multisystem degenerative disease affecting also frontal and in a few patients also temporal structures,[2] in up to 50% of the patients clinically minor cognitive, behavioural, and language deficits can also be observed.[4] However, these are mild in about 95% of ALS patients, and judgement and decision skills are practically not impaired.[5] However, because of the loss of efferent pathways of the brain alone, ALS patients obviously need to be supported by communication skills from the outside—advocacy—to express voices and opinions in a pluralistic world. This is partially done by modern communication devices,[6,7] but also needs support from healthy professionals and laypersons.

It is widely unknown that the incidence of ALS in parts of the world which have undergone the demographic change is steadily rising. Currently the incidence rate is 3.1/100,000 in a comprehensive register in Southern Germany, meaning that 1:400 of the population of an industrialized country will be affected by and will eventually die from the disease.[8,9] These numbers are consistent with areas of the world underlying demographic change,[10,11] while in other parts of the world incidence and prevalence rates are much lower. Until very recently when the 'ice bucket challenge' increased public interest in ALS worldwide, the disease was virtually ignored by the public and its political representatives. It is a hope for the future that the ice bucket challenge has the long-term effect that sustained support for ALS patients can be developed, which—by the nature of the disease—must include external advocacy.

The need for advocacy in ALS

How does the nature of the disease make advocacy a pressing need and challenge?

In the early phase of ALS, when the patient is confronted with the diagnosis in a comparatively healthy state, the clinical picture is complicated by a reactive depression, especially in the first year after diagnosis.[12] This depression is regularly seen at disease onset when the patients and their relatives are confronted with the diagnosis and the threat of fast physical deterioration and eventually death.[12] Ironically, in this state the motor ('efferent') abilities are still comparatively intact and often permit communication, but the patient is in a transitory affective state which does not permit expressive action. Later in the disease there is a decline in depression[13] and the frequency of clinically significant depressions is only mildly increased from a healthy population.[14] Only those patients suffering from rapid deterioration[15] often experience an affective disorder beyond the reactive depression at disease onset, and some may experience end-of-life despair in the final months of life with increased anxiety.[16,17]

Because they anticipate disease-associated loss, unfortunately the relatives and carers also suffer from initial depressive reactions and after they have overcome it—during the malignant course of the disease—they are most often completely occupied by the daily care for the patient with negative impact on their affective state.[18] Often they are unable to raise their voice.

Therefore, the *last phase* of the disease is characterized by the complete loss of the patient's communication skills and the overwhelming burden of care for the relatives. So, also in this stage of the disease advocacy is not possible either for patients or for carers.

In addition, it is a common clinical experience that *after the patient has died*, relatives are often physically and psychologically exhausted and focus on an adaptation to the loss with the consequence that they are no longer an advocate for this group of patients.

Ideal advocates for ALS

In practice, the strongest advocates for ALS are therefore those patients who suffer from slowly evolving disease (about 5% of the entire population live longer than 10 years) and relatives who survive the patient and still have the energy to engage themselves for ALS patients. *These small groups are strong allies in advocacy for ALS.*

For all of these reasons, it is an important and natural task of ALS scientists and physicians to raise their voice for their patients and play—beyond their normal role—the role of advocates for their patients. However, this role cannot be done naively and requires profound knowledge.

It does not only need a compassionate approach, but also needs a deep understanding of the psychological well-being of patients and their relatives in order not to raise one's own voice and opinions, but to understand the principles of differences of views between healthy, unaffected laypersons and politicians, carers and patients themselves.[15,19] It is well-known that during the disease course, outside views of the disease and the associated suffering of laypeople and carers greatly differs from the view of the patient.[15] For example, the public grossly underestimates the subjective quality of life and overestimates the patients' depressiveness and wish to hasten death.[15] Also, the influence of cultural and religious factors is often underestimated by the public in parts of the world where individualism and the wish for autonomy has largely replaced traditional social and religious bonds.[20]

Quality of life in ALS is often comparable to less severe and not life-threatening disease states[14] even in locked-in state,[21] which may come as a surprise to the outside world.[15] In reality, patients are rarely suicidal and during the course of the disease increasingly prefer to rely on established social bonds and subsequently focus on them.[4,22] Indeed, if these bonds are not present, patients are in danger to wish hastened death. Also, if laypeople from the outside world (which may include physicians) who do not have contact with ALS patients for obvious reasons, like general practitioners[19] try to participate in the decision-making process of ALS patients, catastrophic consequences may result. In my view, physicians who are not familiar with the disease and the rules for the associated psychological state should not be part of the decision process in patients which cannot communicate. This is particularly true, if a social system even runs euthanasia programmes. Here, compliance with the general rule is important— that a healthy person should not decide about the fate of a sick or disabled person without communicating thoroughly with the individual.

It is a major task for advocates of ALS patients to communicate this established knowledge, since the patients themselves are unable to do so and the relatives are burdened with the patient's fate.

Dangers of advocacy in ALS

The dangers of uncritical advocacy are even more important since the confrontation with the devastating disease ALS often leads to emotional overreactions, which may lead to motivated, but also over motivated advocacy. For obvious reasons, the effect of overmotivation is often not sustained and therefore it might end up as being counterproductive and nihilistic. Eventually, these 'honest' reactions lead to a non-realistic underestimation of the clinical and scientific challenges inherent in the disease and finally frustration. Overmotivated laypeople often invest time and money to find a 'therapy' or 'cure' but do not develop a deeper understanding of the biology of the disease. This is also the background of unjustified approaches to 'miracle cures' such as 'stem cell treatment' and may lead to non-scrupulous medical business all over the world which further exploit the patients and their families and often add to their fate. In the past, these reactions have often discredited the entire field, further adding to the problem and production of nihilism.

Therefore, it is easy to conclude that advocacy for ALS patients and the disease is needed without any doubt and on different levels:

- the level of the affected families
- the level of semi-professionals and professionals
- the level of laypersons/the public/patient support groups

- the level of health politics
- the level of science politics

Social aspects and support

Advocacy in families

As a general rule, chronically sick and disabled patients tend to restrict their social bonds to the network they are most familiar with—their family and closest friends.[14,23] Therefore, each attempt to influence the social environment in a favourable manner for the patient must start in the close vicinity of the patient.

Advocacy in families must start with an attempt to understand the disease and its prognosis rationally. This is not easy since it is an often-heard argument that it is cruel and non-sensible to tell the patient 'the entire truth'. It is interesting to note that this argument is often raised by the relatives, but not by the patient themselves. The latter most often want to be informed, but certainly in a sensible and responsible manner.[24]

It is comparatively easy to lead the patients and their families to a better understanding of the patients and their psychological reaction. This includes consideration of the initial depression, but also of the relatively high well-being of the sick person—to an astonishing degree for the naive layperson. This also includes understanding of the phenomenon of 'pathological crying and laughing'; for example, that the internal life of a patient does not necessarily correspond to the uncontrolled emotional outbursts is a relief for the patients and the relatives—even though initially it hardly seems credible for the family. It is also hardly believed that coping mechanisms even exist in such a severe disease.

Also, a layperson often cannot understand that a patient suffering from such a severe disease develops coping mechanisms enabling him or her to organize their limited lifespan autonomously.

It is an important aspect of our individualistic, anonymous society that autonomous behaviour is politically supported by most voters. Therefore, it is an important task to advise the patient how to handle—the often politically glorified—advance directives. It is important not to accept the 'politically beaten path', which reflects the opinion of the healthy environment, but rather to insist on a dynamic procedure. Only a dynamic view of advice directives takes the patients changing affective states and their coping mechanisms into account. In the extreme, a tragedy is provoked if the differentiated patient's fate is decided by a healthy lay environment, because of an advance directive by a previously healthy individual—the patient.

In the same way, it is also important not to rely on non-experienced professionals ('physicians', 'psychologists', 'social workers') who are not familiar with the psychological mechanisms associated with the disease. The experience with the patient and the disease makes the difference, not the professional background.

Advocacy in the family also includes the way how to approach the problem of miracle cures and the non-scrupulous business often surrounding it. Many blue-eyed, non- or half-educated individuals are so desperate that they grasp myths which are not only beyond any medical insights, but also financially detrimental to the family such as highly expensive stem cell therapy.

It is even more difficult how to approach the discussion on physician-assisted suicide and euthanasia in a transparent manner. It is a 'modern' view in the industrialized world that these approaches to diseases should be legalized. However, most programmes consider the fact that nobody (which includes—of course—physicians) should kill patients when they are depressed and/or cannot express their thoughts—because of differentiation. It is the 'arrogance of the healthy' which ignores these medically and psychologically well-known facts.

Advocacy on the level of the professionals and semi-professionals confronted with the disease

It is a major task of an advocate for ALS and the affected patients to provide views for professionals and semi-professionals what can be realistically done and cannot be done. This is true for simple procedures such as the application of immunoglobulins for 'multifocal motor neuropathies'; an entity which is extremely rare and very often diagnosed even when diagnostic criteria are not met. In the author's opinion, most patients treated after getting this diagnosis are ALS patients. We should try to reduce the number of patients wrongly diagnosed and treated.

On the other hand, realistic procedures increasing the quality of life and lifespan of the patient are still underused[25-27] and meet with scepticism by many.[28] Non-invasive ventilation (NIV) can reliably reduce suffering from the initial stages of CO_2 narcosis, such as sleep disturbances, cognitive deficits, headache, and emotional instability. NIV is also a reliable intervention to prolong the lifespan of the patient, in patients with thoracic onset this procedure may increase lifespan for up to 3 years. It is more difficult to make a decision to treat the inevitable respiratory deficiency by a tracheostomy. Although this procedure is technically no major challenge anymore, the burden of patients having a tracheostomy to their environment (practically their family) cannot be overestimated. The introduction of such a life-prolonging intervention is handled very differently in the world; the highest number of patients ventilated by a tracheostomy seem to be present in Japan[29] whereas the other extreme are the Netherlands where a large number of ALS patients seem to be treated by physician-assisted suicide.[30] This indicates that social factors and beliefs influence the decision-making process. For the sake of the patient (and the medical profession) it is important that dynamic advance directives should be used, affective states of the—differentiated!—patient should be considered and in the end—the patient her-/himself takes the decision. It is a well-recognized ethical dilemma that in most cases of decisions in favour of a tracheostomy the social environment is a critical issue of this individual decision-making process.

The decision for physical and orthopaedic support should not be influenced by social interactions. The support a patient experiences through the use of a wheel chair and other orthopaedic aids cannot be overestimated. However, there are several confounding factors which need to be considered.

First, it is the patient her-/himself who often considers the use of an orthopaedic device as a 'defeat' against the disease. It is the task of health professionals to point out the positive aspects of such devices. Second, the painful discussion on supportive devices must be done in advance of an immediate need. This is often difficult because the patient does not only hope to avoid such a support (and the associated disease state), but even shows a hopeless 'fight against disease' attitude. It is the task of professionals to introduce realistic views without reducing hope.

The explanation and introduction of the percutaneous endoscopic gastrostomy (PEG) procedure is also an important task for the professional caring for ALS patients. Also, introduction of a PEG is often seen as a 'defeat' in the fight against the disease by the patient. The professional view that aspiration pneumonia and its consequences is a risk which can be avoided by PEG insertion and that catabolism is a strong negative predictor of survival must be communicated. On the positive side, it should be communicated that patients are able to eat orally as long as the disease permits.

As already mentioned, it is mandatory to improve the understanding of the patients and their psychological reactions. Reactive depressions and the phenomenon of 'pathological crying and laughing' have already been mentioned. But it is also important to make laypeople aware of coping mechanisms, including the patient's tendency—during the disease course—to restrict their activities to their social environment which includes that they want to avoid long stays in hospitals. It is a modern saying that there is 'frontal involvement',[31] meaning that many ALS patients lack empathy and critical insight into their disease. This might be true for a few, but is not a practical issue in 95% of patients as these mild cognitive impairment do not interfere with patient's decision-making capacity.[25]

It is also an important task of healthcare professionals to help to avoid exploitation of the patients and their families ('miracle cures', 'stem cell therapy' as mentioned earlier) and to realize that care for the exhausted relatives is necessary for the majority. The latter can often only be realized if the relatives are actively approached and the unjustified shame about the 'weakness' not to be able to provide care for 24 hours is actively addressed.

Advocacy on the level of the general public (laypersons)

Advocacy on the level of the general public and laypersons has similar themes as those discussed previously. However, the level of communication is often journalistic, often in the worst sense: it must sell.

It is an obvious task to avoid high expectations and hype ('cure'). The public should be sceptical of organizations that promise 'cure'. A socially interesting example is the European organization ENCALS (European Network for the Cure of ALS)—the name obviously seems to promise cure. I suggest that the naming of this group—which as an organization is certainly a major step forward—should be thoroughly discussed.

It is a major and often non-realistic task to make laypeople and the general public understand the patients and their psychological reactions. The fact that these reactions are not similar to the reaction of a healthy person and the change of scope are counterintuitive for many. One has to be aware of the fact that arguments against emotionally entertained 'intuitions' require time and efforts which may often not be realistic. In the boulevard press non-realistic and overreaction or hype are commonplace—this of course partially mirrors human nature—since this may be the easiest way to neglect reality.

However, whenever a chance of hope for cure exists, for example, the public should be informed in a fast and professional manner. Older aged laypersons have experience with a relative who suffered from a deadly disease but each patient has his own personal course. Therefore, the task to inform the public in general is often challenging; however, with the background of an individual experience it is quiet easy. It follows that public education should be based on realistic individual experiences, not on stories. The success of individuals writing up their experiences on deadly diseases (such as cancer and ALS) shows clearly that this option exists—beyond views from the boulevard. Also, realistic movies on the fate of ALS patients can have a sustained impact on attitudes of the public.

Advocacy on the level of health politics

It is a fact that health politics tends to ignore ALS because in many countries no strong lobby for this disease exists. However, we have also made the experience that the fate of a single patient can change this attitude immediately. These changes may, however, not be sustained, because—as on the individual level—the fate of ALS patients is as fast forgotten as it impresses people.

It is the task of responsible health politics

1. To support fast non-bureaucratic responses with foresight by health organizations. Since ALS is a fast progressing disease, it is a permanent challenge for an administrative process working in the framework of a legal system. In this regard, political and administrative courage is needed to even foster decisions which seem to be risky for a layperson. However, evidence-based medicine supports many decisions—and on this basis they can be made. On the other hand gaps will remain in the grey zone not supported by evidence-based medicine leading to uncertainties in the decision process. In the author's experience, a visit of an administrative decision-maker to the patient can often be the basis of a right decision.
2. To accept that small steps in symptomatic care efficiently supports the patient (and families). The current goal of ALS therapy is not a cure; it is the insight that small steps (wheel chair, PEG, NIV) are a major support to the patient. This attitude was often counterintuitive and difficult to sell. However, acceptance of this view is increasing. In particular, it is the political will in many countries to improve palliative care, to improve access to hospices for ALS patients and there is wide acceptance of the view that multiprofessional ALS centres improve the patient's prognosis.
3. Not to play down current pharmaceutical approaches to treatment. For example, it is not uncommon to state that 'riluzole prolongs life by only 3 months'. It should not be ignored that riluzole still remains the only drug which has been repeatedly shown to influence the natural history of a degenerative brain disease, that this effect has been shown in a cohort which had an average life expectancy of 12 months only and that the drug has no side effects—in comparison to many cancer drugs with similar efficacy. In the end, the patient needs transparent information about all of these facts—to make his own individual decision on treatment.

Advocacy on the level of science politics

In the past, ALS was not in the centre of interest for science politics. This has considerably changed because interesting mechanistic aspects of the pathogenesis have been shown[2,32,33] which parallel and are of interest also for other neurodegenerative diseases of the brain. The view that ALS is a rare disease has been replaced by a more differentiated view: the prevalence of ALS suggests that we deal with an orphan disease but the incidence of ALS is too high to fulfil the official criteria for an orphan disease. Still, ALS has been given an orphan disease status.

It is also realistically acknowledged that rapid success is not in sight and basic descriptive and mechanistic scientific approaches are urgently needed. Most colleagues understand that it is a mistake to react to or even induce public overreactions; most have learned that these public reactions come and go—but are not of any help neither for the patients nor for a deeper understanding of the disease.

For science politics, it is important to understand that ALS is a disease which severely limits lifespan with little time to react for those who are affected. Sustained investments—beyond the fate of an individual—are the basis of any scientific approach. In practice this means to finance the build-up of patients' registries and cohorts, biorepositories, and banking systems.

Most colleagues agree that it is a mistake in ALS to make unjustified promises, but also to avoid ignorant reactions such as 'an investment is not justified, since no cure is in sight'. ALS science must be sustained.

Summary and conclusions

Advocacy for ALS patients and their disease must be part of the concerns of each physician and scientist concerned with the disease. This is not easy, since compassion alone does not lead to the necessary consequences and actions, and might even be counterproductive because it may lead to non-productive overreactions. Many resources have been wasted in the field of ALS research when half-informed semi-professionals jumped to conclusions, which also potentially led to financial exploitation of the patient. Only a realistic approach can be the common ground on which advocacy for ALS can be based, and enable the beginning of a sustained development serving the patient and leading to more efficient, realistic therapeutic approaches.

References

1. **Charcot, J.** (1874) De la sclérose latérale amyotrophique. *Prog Med*, **2**, 341–453.
2. **Braak, H., Brettschneider, J., Ludolph, A. C., Lee, V. M., Trojanowski, J. Q., Del Tredici, K.** (2013) Amyotrophic lateral sclerosis—a model of corticofugal axonal spread. *Nat Rev Neurol*, **9**, 708–14.
3. **Brooks, B. R., Miller, R. G., Swash, M., Munsat, T. L.; World Federation of Neurology Research Group on Motor Neuron Diseases** (2000) El Escorial revisited: revised criteria for the diagnosis of amyotrophic lateral sclerosis. *Amyotroph Lateral Scler Other Motor Neuron Disord*, **1**, 293–9.
4. **Lulé, D., Nonnenmacher, S., Sorg, S., et al.** (2014) Live and let die: existential decision processes in a fatal disease. *J Neurol*, **261**(3), 518–25.
5. **Böhm, S., Aho-Özhan, H. E., Keller, J., et al.** (2016) Medical decisions are independent of cognitive impairment in amyotrophic lateral sclerosis. *Neurology*, **87**(16), 1737–8.
6. **Keller, J., Gorges, M., Aho-Özhan, H. E., et al.** (2016) Eye-tracking control to assess cognitive functions in patients with amyotrophic lateral sclerosis. *J Vis Exp*, (116). doi: 10.3791/54634.

7. **Chaudhary, U., Xia, B., Silvoni, S., Cohen, L. G., Birbaumer, N.** (2017) Brain-computer interface-based communication in the completely locked-in state. *PLoS Biol*, **15**(1), e1002593.
8. **Uenal, H., Rosenbohm, A., Kufeldt, J., et al.** (2014) Incidence and geographical variation of amyotrophic lateral sclerosis (ALS) in Southern Germany—completeness of the ALS registry Swabia. *PLoS One*, **9**(4), e93932.
9. **Rosenbohm, A., Peter, R. S., Erhardt, S., et al.** (2017) Epidemiology of amyotrophic lateral sclerosis in Southern Germany. *J Neurol*, **264**(4), 749–57.
10. **Seljeseth, Y. M., Vollset, S. E., Tysnes, O. B.** (2000) Increasing mortality from amyotrophic lateral sclerosis in Norway? *Neurology*, **55**(9), 1262–6.
11. **Abhinav, K., Stanton, B., Johnston, C., et al.** (2007) Amyotrophic lateral sclerosis in South-East England: a population-based study. The South-East England register for amyotrophic lateral sclerosis (SEALS Registry). *Neuroepidemiology*, **29**(1–2), 44–8.
12. **Roos, E., Mariosa, D., Ingre, C., et al.** (2016) Depression in amyotrophic lateral sclerosis. *Neurology*, **86**, 2271–7.
13. **Kübler, A., Winter, S., Ludolph, A. C., Hautzinger, M., Birbaumer, N.** (2005) Severity of depressive symptoms and quality of life in patients with amyotrophic lateral sclerosis. *Neurorehabil Neural Repair*, **19**(3), 182–93.
14. **Lulé, D., Häcker, S., Ludolph, A., Birbaumer, N., Kübler, A.** (2008) Depression and quality of life in patients with amyotrophic lateral sclerosis [Depression und Lebensqualität bei Patienten mit amyotropher Lateralsklerose]. *Dtsch Arztebl Int*, **105**(23), 397–403.
15. **Lulé, D., Ehlich, B., Lang, D., et al.** (2013) Quality of life in fatal disease: the flawed judgement of the social environment. *J Neurol*, **260**(11), 2836–43.
16. **Neudert, C., Oliver, D., Wasner, M., Borasio, G. D.** (2001) The course of the terminal phase in patients with amyotrophic lateral sclerosis. *J Neurol*, **248**(7), 612–6.
17. **Ganzini, L., Johnston, W. S., Silveira, M. J.** (2002) The final month of life in patients with ALS. *Neurology*, **59**(3), 428–31.
18. **Gauthier, A., Vignola, A., Calvo, A., et al.** (2007) A longitudinal study on quality of life and depression in ALS patient–caregiver couples. *Neurology*, **68**, 923–6.
19. **Aho-Özhan, H., Böhm, S., Keller, J., et al.** (2017) Experience matters: neurologists' perspectives on ALS patients' well-being. *J Neurol*, **264**(4), 639–46.
20. **Andersen, P. M., Kuzma-Kozakiewicz, M., Keller, J., et al.** (2018) Therapeutic decisions in ALS patients—cross-cultural differences and clinical implications. *J Neurol*, **265**(7), 1600–6.
21. **Lulé, D., Zickler, C., Häcker, S., et al.** (2009) Life may be worth living in locked-in syndrome. Coma science: clinical and ethical implications. *Prog Brain Res*, **177**, 339–51.
22. **Matuz, T., Birbaumer, N., Hautzinger, M., Kübler, A.** (2010) Coping with amyotrophic lateral sclerosis: an integrative view. *J Neurol Neurosurg Psychiatry*, **81**(8), 893–8.
23. **Lulé, D., Pauli, S., Altintas, E., et al.** (2012) Emotional adjustment in amyotrophic lateral sclerosis (ALS). *J Neurol*, **259**(2), 334–41.
24. **Pizzimenti, A., Gori, M. C., Onesti, E., John, B., Inghilleri, M.** (2015) Communication of diagnosis in amyotrophic lateral sclerosis: stratification of patients for the estimation of the individual needs. *Front Psychol*, **6**, 745.
25. **Böhm, S., Ludolph, A. C., Lulé, D.** (2015) Lebensverlängernde oder—verkürzende Maßnahmen bei ALS-Patienten. *Neurotransmitter*, **26**(9), 38–41.

26. **Martin, N. H., Lawrence, V., Murray, J., et al.** (2016) Decision making about gastrostomy and noninvasive ventilation in amyotrophic lateral sclerosis. *Qual Health Res*, **26**(10), 1366–81.
27. **Kurt, A., Nijboer, F., Matuz, T., Kübler, A.** (2007) Depression and anxiety in individuals with amyotrophic lateral sclerosis: epidemiology and management. *CNS Drugs*, **21**(4), 279–91.
28. **Greenaway, L. P., Martin, N. H., Lawrence, V., et al.** (2015) Accepting or declining non-invasive ventilation or gastrostomy in amyotrophic lateral sclerosis: patients' perspectives. *J Neurol*, **262**(4), 1002–13.
29. **Kimura, F.** (2016) Tracheostomy and invasive mechanical ventilation in amyotrophic lateral sclerosis: decision-making factors and survival analysis. *Rinsho Shinkeigaku*, **56**(4), 241–7.
30. **Veldink, J. H., Wokke, J. H., van der Wal, G., Vianney de Jong, J. M., van den Berg, L. H.** (2002) Euthanasia and physician-assisted suicide among patients with amyotrophic lateral sclerosis in the Netherlands. *N Engl J Med*, **346**(21), 1638–44.
31. **Goldstein, L. H., Abrahams, S.** (2013) Changes in cognition and behaviour in amyotrophic lateral sclerosis: nature of impairment and implications for assessment. *Lancet Neurol*, **12**, 368–80.
32. **Ludolph, A. C., Brettschneider, J.** (2015) TDP-43 in amyotrophic lateral sclerosis–is it a prion disease? *Eur J Neurol*, **22**(5), 753–61.
33. **Jucker, M., Walker, L. C.** (2013) Self-propagation of pathogenic protein aggregates in neurodegenerative diseases. *Nature*, **501**(7465), 45–51.

Chapter 23

Neuromuscular disorders and advocacy

Elaine C. Jones and John D. England

An overview of neuromuscular disorders

Incidence/Prevalence

Patients with neuromuscular disorders can be difficult to diagnose. They require access to good neurological evaluation including professionals trained in the diagnosis and treatment of nervous system disorders.[1] While it is difficult to obtain data on access to neurological care around the world, it is estimated that hundreds of millions of people worldwide are affected by neurological disorders. More than 6 million people die because of stroke each year; over 80% of these deaths take place in low- and middle-income countries. More than 50 million people have epilepsy worldwide. It is estimated that there are globally 47.5 million people with dementia with 7.7 million new cases every year—Alzheimer's disease is the most common cause of dementia and may contribute to 60–70% of cases. The prevalence of migraine is more than 10% worldwide.[2,3]

The incidence of neuromuscular diseases is more difficult to determine and is usually broken down into the specific disorders. The incidence of amyotrophic lateral sclerosis (ALS) in North America (United States and Canada) is 1.7–2.2/100,000; while in Europe it ranges from 1.1–3.6/100,000 and in Asia (Japan, China, Iran) it is 1.4–3.3/100,000.[4] The prevalence of all muscular dystrophies (MD) is estimated at 19.8–25.1/100,000 with wide variability between countries. The most common forms are Duchenne and Fascioscapulohumoral (FSH) at 1.7–4.2 and 3.2–4.6, respectively.[5] The prevalence of myasthenia gravis in Europe is 1.2/10,000 (with the highest in England/Sweden and lowest in Greece/Denmark).[6] Spinal muscular atrophies occur with a prevalence of 1/6,000–10,000.[7] According to the World Health Organization (WHO) the prevalence of leprosy (which affects peripheral nerves) declined in 2015 with 176,176 cases reported, and poliomyelitis had a reported 74 new cases in 2015; however, syphilis which can cause neurological complications such as *tabes dorsalis* had a prevalence of 5.6 million cases in 2015. The WHO has a global strategy for a leprosy-free world by 2020.[8]

One of the more common neuromuscular disorders is peripheral neuropathy, but the causes are numerous, and so the reporting of this category is done in different ways for different countries. A recent report looking at the incidence of neuropathic pain as a marker for neuropathy noted that in the United Kingdom, 26% of people with diabetes were found to have peripheral neuropathic pain.[9] Another study found the incidence of diabetic neuropathy is 29% of patients with type 2 diabetes in Northern India.[10] Approximately 20% (18.7–21.4%) of people with cancer have cancer-related neuropathic pain, as a result of either the disease or its treatment.[9] The lifetime incidence of herpes zoster (shingles) is around 25%. Studies in the United States and the Netherlands found that 2.6% and 10%, respectively, will develop chronic post-herpetic neuralgia.[9] Of the 33 million people infected with HIV across the world, around 35% have neuropathic pain, which does not respond well to standard treatments.[9]

Barriers

In 2010 a joint study by the WHO and World Federation of Neurology (WFN) surveyed 102 countries (representing 90% of the world's population) about neurologic conditions and access to care. In terms of the population covered, 25% have access to more than one neurologist per 100,000 population. 10.4% of the countries have a separate budget within the country's health budget for care of neurological illnesses.[11]

In the primary care setting they found:

- No emergency care for neurological disorders at primary care level was available in 34.1% of countries in the WHO/WFN study in Europe; 25% in Africa; 23.5% in the Eastern Mediterranean; 22.2% in the Western Pacific; 16.7% in Southeast Asia; and 7.7% in the Americas.
- Follow-up treatment facilities for neurological disorders at primary care level are not available in 33.3% of the responding countries in the Western Pacific; 31.2% in Africa; 26.8% in Europe; 23.5% in the Eastern Mediterranean; and 7.7% in the Americas.
- Regarding access to medications, at least one anti-epileptic drug (mainly phenobarbitone) is available through the primary healthcare system in 84.4% of responding countries. But in 24.1% of low-income countries, no anti-epileptic drugs are available through the primary healthcare system.
- There is large variation in the availability of anti-Parkinsonian drugs based on income groups: 17.2% of the low-income countries reported the availability of at least one anti-Parkinsonian drug, while 84.4% of the high-income countries reported that at least one anti-Parkinsonian drug was available through the primary healthcare system.[11]

In the specialty care setting:

- Neuropathies accounted for 35.8% of the diseases encountered.
- Only 8.8% of people have access to more than one neurological bed per 10,000 population; however, the median number of neurological beds per 10,000 varies widely across regions: 0.03 in Africa and Southeast Asia; 0.15 in the Eastern Mediterranean; 0.17 in the Americas; 0.26 in the Western Pacific; and 1.71 in Europe.
- Access to neurological rehabilitation service is present in 73.2% of responding countries, but in low-income countries 60.7% have no neurological rehabilitation

services, and in 81.2% of African countries no neurological rehabilitation services are present.
- Access to subspecialty neurological care (neuropediatric, neuroradiology, and stroke units) were even less available worldwide.
- Of the responding countries, 71% have access to less than one neurological nurse per 100,000 population; 39% have no neurological nurses.
- Postgraduate training facilities in neurology are available in 76.2% of the responding countries. No facility for postgraduate training in neurology exists in 51.7% of low-income countries.[11]

Recognition of the needs of disabled people:
- Of the responding countries, 70.5% reported the availability of some form of disability benefit for patients with neurological disorders.
- Of the low-income countries, 67.9% reported non-availability of any kind of disability benefit for neurological disorders, compared with 3.2% of high-income countries.
- Regarding the types of disability benefits reported by countries, monetary benefits (75.7%) and rehabilitation and health benefits (64.9%) are the most commonly reported, followed by other benefits including housing, transport, education, and special discounts (45.9%) and benefits at the workplace (37.8%).
- A national neurological association exists in 87% of the responding countries.
- There is a health reporting system for neurological disorders in 78.1% of the responding countries.[11]

Attention must be given to some of the physical needs and barriers of patients with neuromuscular conditions. The patients frequently have limitations of movement and require aids to walk or function. Consideration needs to be given to infrastructure within a location to allow access for these patients. For example, if someone lives in a town/city without paved sidewalks or where buildings do not have handicap access entries or bathrooms then these patients will face many challenges. Employment opportunities may be limited as well. The European Union (EU) laid out a strategy to empower people with disabilities so they can experience a 'Barrier-Free Europe'. This encourages accessibility, equality, employment, education/training, social protection, and health access. It also works to raise awareness of disability-related issues, increase funding, and improve data collection.[12]

In 2011, the WHO and the World Bank published a document entitled the World Report on Disability. It suggests that barriers for people with disabilities include such things as inadequate policies and standards, negative attitudes towards people with disabilities, lack of available services and problems with service delivery and accessibility for people with disabilities, inadequate funding for services and support needs, lack of consultation and involvement in care and planning needs from people with disabilities, and lack of data and evidence on the needs for those with disabilities.[13]

It concluded that what was needed to aid people with disabilities includes better support through peer support groups, training needs, information on services and resources, and advice at the point of care. The rights of persons with disabilities need to be promoted within their local communities. Examples of this include conducting access audits, delivering disability equality training, and campaigning for human rights in the communities. There needs to be awareness-raising and social marketing campaigns to educate others on the needs of disabled people. There should be a focus on forums (international, national, local) to determine priorities for change, to influence policy, and to shape service delivery within their countries and regions. Finally, there needs to be participation in research projects to aid in better understanding the needs of disabled persons and to explore what solutions work.[13]

These are the areas to focus on for advocacy needs in patients with neuromuscular disorders.

Advocacy needs and neuromuscular patients

Access to care and medicine

As discussed previously, patients with neuromuscular disorders will have special needs with regard to diagnosis and treatment. Let's look at some case studies as examples (Case studies 23.1—23.4)

Case study 23.1 Peripheral neuropathy

A 74-year-old male presented to the clinic with six months of progressive right hand and arm weakness. For the past year he has noticed twitching in his muscles. He denies numbness or tingling. Lately he is noticing that he trips over his left foot a lot.

Discussion

This presentation could reflect a lot of disorders including cervical radiculopathy, focal neuropathy, motor neuron disease, multifocal motor neuropathy, and even non-neurological problems. Thorough neurological exam and evaluation with nerve conduction testing could clarify a diagnosis of multifocal motor neuropathy (MMN) by demonstrating motor conduction block. Obtaining the correct diagnosis for this patient early on could prevent inappropriate treatments (such as surgery for cervical radiculopathy) or delayed treatment. Correctly diagnosing this patient with MMN and then instituting treatment with intravenous immunoglobulin (IVIg) could prevent the development of permanent disability.

Barriers in this case include issues with lack of access. This would include access to neurological evaluation, to appropriate testing, to appropriate treatments, and to physical/occupational therapy for improving weakness and preventing further injuries.

Case study 23.2 Neurofibromatosis and spinal cord injury

A 23-year-old male tripped and fell while playing soccer. He developed immediate midthoracic back pain, weakness, and numbness in his legs. After this accident he was unable to walk. For six months prior to this accident he had noticed his walking was a bit clumsy. He had been tripping and stumbling. He lives in a remote location where there are no medical services. One year later he is visiting family in the city and presents to the clinic in a wheelchair. On exam he has atrophy and increased tone in his legs bilaterally. He is hyper-reflexic in his legs. He has decreased sensation from a T8 level to his toes. Imaging of his spine shows a mass deforming the spine/cord at T6. Further examination reveals small nodules under the skin in his scalp, arms, and legs, patches of skin discoloration, and freckles in his armpits and groin.

Discussion

At this point the patient is diagnosed with neurofibromatosis (NF1). The spinal compression is chronic and surgery is unlikely to aid in functional recovery. Had the patient had access to neurologic evaluation as a child his diagnosis might have been identified earlier in life. Additionally, if the spinal cord injury had been identified at the time of his accident, then immediate treatment might have prevented permanent disability. For the past year the patient had been limited in activities due to his inability to ambulate. In the clinic the patient was supplied with a wheelchair to aid mobility and the patient/family were taught how to do stretching exercises to prevent worsening contractures and discomfort.

> Barriers in this case include lack of access to appropriate medical care including paediatrics, neurological, neurosurgical interventions, lack of access to diagnostic testing, and lack of access to physical/occupational therapy or to aids to assist his functioning.

Research

For neuromuscular disorders, the pathophysiology and approaches to treatment may not be known. This is why it is so important to study these disorders and learn how to prevent them or to better treat them. It is also important to study diseases and treatments in a wide array of patient populations due to genetic variabilities. Many studies are done in first world countries with homogenous populations. However genetic and racial variations can play a significant role.

Case study 23.3 Genetic variability and treatments

A 34-year-old Asian female presented to the clinic with three days of severe right facial pain. It was described as a sharp, electrical shock in her right cheek and jaw. Exam demonstrated no rashes, oral abnormalities, or injuries in the face or head. The remainder of her exam was normal. She was diagnosed with trigeminal neuralgia and started on carbamazepine for pain management.

Two days later she returned to the clinic complaining of a diffuse rash and sores in her mouth. She is immediately diagnosed with toxic epidermal necrolysis related to the carbamazepine and admitted to the hospital.

In 2008 the United States Food and Drug Administration (FDA) changed labelling on carbamazepine to recommend genotyping all Asians for the *HLA allele B*1502* for the risk of Stevens–Johnson syndrome and toxic epidermal necrolysis. This was as a result of reports showing an increased risk of these potentially deadly reactions in Han Chinese patients. It has since been found that there is an increased risk in many Asian populations. Current final recommendations are to use alternative treatments in these populations or if there are not alternatives, to perform genetic testing to assess the risk.[14]

> Barriers in this case include lack of research in specific populations, lack of expertise in neurological medications and their risks, and lack of testing options for genetic mutations.

Trials

There are many ways for patients and physicians to get involved in research trials locally or internationally. The WHO has an International Clinical Trials Registry Platform and states that '[t]he registration of all international trials is a scientific, ethical, and moral responsibility'.[15] Other sources for international studies include UNICEF[16] and Medicins Sans Frontiers[17] as well as local and national governmental agencies. Despite these resources, research opportunities may be limited in many areas. Patients, caregivers, and healthcare providers can use their advocacy skills to bring these trials to their area. Reaching out to organizations participating in trials can be a very important step.

Physical needs and support

Patients with neuromuscular diseases can have physical limitations which can impact their lives and may exclude them from mainstream activities including employment, activities of daily living, and social activities. The United Nations produced an overview of international legal frameworks for disability legislation that provides useful background information for countries to improve support for people with disabilities. It is important for countries to have comprehensive legislation to ensure the rights of disabled persons in all aspects—political, civil, economic, social, and cultural rights—on an equal basis with persons without disabilities. If the infrastructure in a town is not set up for people with physical limitations simple activities such as going to the market can be difficult or impossible. Translation from an international convention, standard, or norm to national law and then to local implementation is slow and complex but fundamental.[18]

Case study 23.4 United States Americans with Disabilities Act

The Americans with Disabilities Act (ADA) was signed into law on 26 July 1990, but the history of this monumental legislation started in movements decades before. In 1973 Congress passed Section 504 of the 1973 Rehabilitation Act which banned discrimination based on disability for recipients of federal funds. Over the next almost two decades, advocates for this community worked with legislators and courts to craft laws and regulations that prevented discrimination of disabled people.[19] While there are still barriers, this landmark legislation has transformed access for disabled Americans and is the direct result of advocacy work by disabled people, their families, and healthcare professionals.

Advocacy focus

As stated earlier in this book, advocacy is considered an activity to support or promote a person, a group, or a cause. It can be performed by a variety of people for a variety of reasons. The patient or caregiver can advocate for themselves or their needs. A healthcare provider can advocate for their patient's needs. Administrators or public officials can advocate for the needs of a population. The focus can be at the local level to improve a patient's access to work, support services, treatments, and so on. Advocacy can focus on national changes in legislative or regulatory areas to help a group with a specific need. Finally, there can be international advocacy to help patients in other countries or to help a group of patients with similar needs across countries. No matter what the issue or target audience, there are certain approaches to advocacy projects that can be followed to help achieve the desired goals.

Action planning

Once an issue has been identified, it is important to set up an action plan (Case study 23.5). This is an organized, stepwise approach to accomplishing the goal. It can help identify steps along the way, resources needed, and barriers that will need to be overcome. The first step is to state the ultimate goal, then to list the smaller goals along the way that will lead to the ultimate goal. What smaller steps will be needed and how will these be performed? How will you know you have succeeded at these? What time frame do you expect each step to take? What resources will you need to complete the tasks? Writing all this out

Case study 23.5 Action plan

Table 23.1 is an example of an action plan developed to improve access to neurological care at a clinic in Port Au Prince, Haiti. Currently there is limited specialty training for providers in Haiti and so developing a clinic that focuses on neurological issues would improve care to these patients. This included neuromuscular patients who currently may have no specialty care or access. The template can be used for any advocacy goal whether related to access to medications, testing, or support services for neuromuscular patients. Action plans should be approached as a fluid document that you check into periodically to keep the project moving forward but also can be adjusted as new issues or barriers arise.

Conclusions

Advocating for our patients is as important as appropriately diagnosing and treating them. Patients with neuromuscular diseases need access to good diagnostic and therapeutic care—educated providers, diagnostic testing, medications, and so on. They also have a unique set of needs regarding management of the sequelae of the disease—handicap access, educational support, nutritional support, and so on. Recently it has become obvious that genetic differences can influence treatment risks and outcomes. It is therefore imperative that a global approach to neuromuscular research be pursued and that these patients are encouraged and allowed to participate. No matter where in the world they live, barriers exist to meeting these needs of patients with neuromuscular diseases. Healthcare providers can apply advocacy techniques using focused action planning and these barriers can be overcome and a successful goal reached. With focused effort and the right resources, much can be achieved (Table 23.2).

Table 23.1 Example of an action plan. Issue: to improve access to outpatient neurological care at St. Luke Hospital, Haiti

Objectives	Reason	Actions	Target audience	Resources/Needs	Success measures	Timeline
Organize volunteers	Allows better coverage and avoids overlap. Identifies gaps	1. Collect contact information on people already involved 2. Develop a calendar for travel 3. Identify gaps volunteer needs 4. Develop recruitment tools	Neurologists/healthcare providers	– Learn Excel – Email lists – Research on recruiting medical volunteers	– Using Excel – Email lists completed – Monthly coverage of clinic	3 months 3 months Next year
Identify resources in Haiti	Clarifies needs and who to go to. Prevents miscommunications	1. Identify services already available 2. dentify key contacts 3. Develop resource lists	St Luke staff and Medical director	– Meet with Haiti team – Excel – Review prior materials developed by others	– List of services/needs – Contact list developed	3 months 3 months
Develop communications	Prevent overlap travel. Continuity of care. Organizes teaching	1. Develop general access calendar for travel 2. Develop process for patient record-keeping 3. Develop teaching programme	Volunteers and St Luke staff	– Research doc sharing websites – Review HER options – Meet with local MDs – Review teaching materials available	– Shared calendar available – Record keeping in place – Teaching programme identified	3 months 3 months 6 months
Develop participant packets	Aid participation. Improve experience	1. Develop packing list 2. General information on legal/ethical/immunization needs 3. Identify language learning opportunities	Volunteers	– Review current materials – Travel websites and guides – Review language learning opportunities	– Packet available	6 months

Table 23.2 Advocacy resources

	Organization	Jurisdiction	Focus	Electronic contact/Link
International	Disability rights Education and Defense Fund (DREDF)	United States	Database of country-based laws protecting rights of disabled people	https://dredf.org/legal-advocacy/international-disability-rights/international-laws/
	United Nations Enable	United Nations	Provides standards for people with disabilities and promotes human rights equality	http://www.un.org/esa/socdev/enable/comp001.htm
	Unicef World Report on Disability	WHO report (PDF)	Suggests steps for all stakeholders to benefit lives of disabled people	http://www.unicef.org/protection/World_report_on_disability_eng.pdf
	International Alliance of ALS/MND Association	England	Coordinate ALS/MND associations from around the world to advance awareness and support of people with ALS/MND	http://www.alsmndalliance.org/
	International Congress on Neuromuscular Diseases	Varies every two years	Organized by the Applied Research Group of WFN: Present a wide spectrum of neuromuscular diseases from the perspective of advances in research, diagnosis, and treatment	https://www.wfneurology.org/icnmd2018 https://www.wfneurology.org/calendar
Personal	American Academy of Neurology Palatucci Advocacy Leadership Forum	United States	Annual training programme sponsored by the AAN to teach advocacy skills	https://www.youtube.com/watch?v=Zb3PYL--UKE
	World Congress of Neurology Advocacy Leadership Programme	United Kingdom	Annual meeting of WFN that incorporates advocacy training opportunities	https://www.wfneurology.org/
	ALS Association Become an advocate	United States	Organizing advocates to draw awareness and resources to the needs of ALS patients	http://www.alsa.org/advocacy/get-involved/

References

1. **Katirji, B., Kaminski, H. J., Preston, D. C., Ruff, R. L., Shapiro, B. E.** (2014) *Neuromuscular Disorders in Clinical Practice.* Oxford: Butterworth-Heinmann, pp. 3–10.
2. **World Health Organization** (2016) What are neurological diseases? Online Q&A. Geneva: World Health Organization [updated May 2016]. Available at: http://www.who.int/features/qa/55/en/
3. **World Health Organization** (2016) WHO Global Health Workforce Statistics database. Geneva: World Health Organization. Available at: http://www.who.int/hrh/statistics/hwfstats/
4. **Chio, A., Logroscino, G., Traynor, B. J., et al.** (2013) Global epidemiology of amyotrophic lateral sclerosis: a systemic review of the published literature. *Neuroepidemiology*, **41**(2), 118–30.
5. **Theadom, A., Rodrigues, M., Roxburgh, R., et al.** (2014) Prevalence of muscular dystrophies: a systemic literature review. *Neuroepidemiology*, **43**(3–4), 259–68.
6. **Epidemiology of myasthenia gravis**. Available at: http://www.iss.it/binary/neph/cont/Report%20on%20the%20descriptive%20epidemiology%20of%20Myasthenia%20Gravis.1183558284.pdf
7. **D'Amico, A., Mercuri, E., Tiziano, F. D., Bertini, E.** (2011) Spinal muscular atrophy. *Orphanet Journal of Rare Diseases*, **6**, 71.
8. **World Health Organization** (2016) Fact sheet: Leprosy. Geneva: World Health Organization [updated October 2016]. Available at: http://www.who.int/mediacentre/factsheets/fs101/en/
9. **Smith, B. H., Torrance, N.** (2011) Neuropathic pain. In: Croft, P. (ed.). *Chronic Pain Epidemiology: From Aetiology to Public Health.* Oxford: Oxford University Press, pp. 209–33.
10. **Bansal, D., Gudala, K., Muthyala, H., et al.** (2014) Prevalence and risk factors of development of peripheral diabetic neuropathy in type 2 diabetes mellitus in a tertiary care setting. *J Diabetes Invesig*, **5**(6), 714–21.
11. **WHO Library Cataloguing-in-Publication Data** (2004) *Atlas: Country Resources for Neurological Disorders.* Geneva: World Health Organization.
12. **EUR-Lex** (2010) Communication from the Commission to the European Parliament, the Council, the European Economic and Social Committee and the Committee of the Regions: European Disability Strategy 2010–2020: A Renewed Commitment to a Barrier-Free Europe. Available at: http://eur-lex.europa.eu/legal-content/EN/TXT/?uri=celex%3A52010DC0636
13. **Unicef** (2011) World Report on Disability. Available at: https://www.unicef.org/protection/World_report_on_disability_eng.pdf
14. **Ferrell, P. B., McLeod, H. L.** (2008) Carbamazepine, HLA-B*1502 and risk of Stevens–Johnson syndrome and toxic epidermal necrolysis: US FDA Recommendations. *Pharmacogenomcs*, **9**(10), 1543–6.
15. **World Health Organization**. WHO International Clinical Trials Registry Platform. Available at: http://www.who.int/ictrp/en/
16. **Unicef**. Office of Research-Innocenti. Available at: https://www.unicef-irc.org/

17. **MSF Field Research** (2017) Fieldresearch.msf.org. Available at: http://fieldresearch.msf.org/msf/
18. **United Nations** (2007) Overview of International Legal Frameworks for Disability Legislation. Available at: http://www.un.org/esa/socdev/enable/disovlf.htm
19. **Mayerson, A.** (1992) The History of the Americans with Disabilities Act. Disability Rights Education & Defense Fund. Available at: https://dredf.org/news/publications/the-history-of-the-ada/

Chapter 24

Advocacy for movement disorders

Francesca Mancini and Carlo Colosimo

Introduction

Advocacy for movement disorders: Global overview

This topic is addressed first, starting from what a patient or caregiver would do when looking for advocacy: use the search engines on the Internet and then ask for more information from physicians and acquaintances.

The search engines on the Internet were used as a starting point, being the only globally shared way to obtain information.

There are several organizations around the world that aim to advocate for patients and caregivers impacted by diseases labelled as 'movement disorders'.

In the following paragraphs, the most representative organizations for each disease are listed, describing the ones with original characteristics and distinguishing, when possible, advocacy for *patients* from advocacy for *research* focusing on the specific disease. This differentiation is possible for more frequent diseases (i.e. Parkinson's disease) while for a less common disease (i.e. atypical parkinsonism), both forms of advocacy are promoted by the same association.

Moreover, movement disorders include a miscellaneous group of diseases, which differ in grade and type of functional disability, availability of treatments, and age range of affected patients. Accordingly, different diseases define different needs for patients, underlining the uniqueness of movement disorders as regards advocacy.

In general, advocacy for movement disorder diseases is performed with a 'meso' level of action, with the aim of supporting patients and caregivers and/or promoting research. Associations or organizations are mainly based in the United States or northern Europe; typically they are created by patients and/or neurologists.

As an initial reference, we suggest starting from the web page 'Links to International Organizations & Foundations' of the website of the International Parkinson and Movement Disorder Society,[1] where organizations are listed according to the advocated condition: ataxic disorders, choric disorders, dystonic disorders, general movement disorders, and general neurology (these categories include both patients' associations as well as groups for physicians and nurses), other parkinsonian disorders, and Parkinson's disease.

As a result of the heterogeneity of movement disorders conditions, each disease requires a specific advocacy, but it is helpful to mention the European Federation of Neurological Associations (EFNA),[2] an organization that operates at a 'meso' level, with a pyramidal structure, with the objective of serving advocates of neurological diseases and to encourage and support all groups of patients with a neurological disease.

EFNA aims to improve access to information and to promote awareness and understanding of different neurological conditions to the public, the authorities, and healthcare workers. The final purpose is to increase the priority given to neurology by policy and decision makers and by healthcare providers.

Members of EFNA are made up of European patient support organizations; it also cooperates closely with the European Academy of Neurology (EAN), constituted by clinicians and researchers.

Members or associated partners of EFNA are NeuroPozytywni[3] and Neuroalianza,[4] which is also made up of several patients' associations, among which the FEP (Spanish Parkinson Federation).

Every year, EFNA holds its Neurology Advocacy Awards. These awards recognize the contribution of an individual or group, patient, or clinician, to the development and promotion of advocacy for people with neurological disorders in Europe. Within the field of movement disorders, in 2015, the Media Category of the EFNA Advocacy Award winner was Jeroen de Schepper, the candidate put forward by the European Huntington Association (EHA), and in 2016 the EFNA Neurology Advocacy Award for Health Professional was won by Professor Paola Giunti, for her work in in advocating for ataxia patients.

Another interesting activity of EFNA is its Patient Advocate Workshops at the London School of Economics (LSE), one of the most advanced and useful implications of advocacy, to train patient groups on health technology assessment (HTA), pharmaceutical pricing, access and reimbursement, and the most salient regulations addressing coverage/access and how these affect patient access.

Looking on a global level for advocacy dedicated to research in movement disorders, mention should be made on the Patient-Centered Outcomes Research Institute (PCORI), an independent non-profit, non-governmental organization created in 2010 and located in Washington, DC.[5] PCORI's mandate is to improve the quality and relevance of evidence available to make informed health decisions, funding comparative clinical effectiveness research as well as support work that will improve the methods used to conduct such studies.

Regarding movement disorders, in 2015 PCORI funded two Research Projects: 'Improving the Quality of care for the Wyoming Parkinson's Disease Community' (Cheyenne Wyoming Parkinson's Disease Support Group), and 'Using technology to deliver multidisciplinary care to individuals with Parkinson's Disease in their homes'. (University of Rochester).

Parkinson's disease

Parkinson's disease (PD) is the most common cause of parkinsonism and is characterized by neurodegenerative changes in the basal ganglia, mainly in the substantia nigra.

PD begins between the ages of 40 and 80 years, with peak onset between the ages of 55 and 60 years. The prevalence of PD is approximately 160 cases per 100,000 populations, and the incidence is about 20 cases per 100,000 populations.[6] The cause of PD is multifactorial, including hereditary predisposition, environmental toxins, and ageing. PD is more common among relatives of index cases.[7]

The primary lesion of PD is degeneration of neurons in the pars compacta of the substantia nigra. Akinesia, rigidity, resting tremor, and impairment of postural reflexes are the principal clinical motor signs and symptoms of PD, with a slow progression. The diagnosis remains clinical, on the basis of the presence of characteristic features and response to levodopa therapy; definitive PD is diagnosed only at autopsy by the presence of Lewy bodies and specific neuropathological findings.[8] The main treatment of PD is pharmacologic and symptomatic, focusing on controlling the functional disability. While levodopa remains the most efficacious drug available for the relief of symptoms in PD, its chronic administration associated with disease progression causes motor complications within a few years.[9] Motor fluctuations, involuntary movements, non-motor symptoms, psychotic and behavioural disorders can highly impact on quality of life. To prevent and/or treat these symptoms, additional pharmacologic developments have been generated: dopamine agonists, inhibitors of catechol-0-methyltransferase (COMT), monoamine oxidase type B (MAO-B) inhibitors. More recently, device mediated treatments have become available for select patients with a complicated disease stage: neurosurgical operations (chronic deep-brain stimulation of the subthalamic nucleus and globus pallidus internus using an implantable pulse generator), administration of a gel suspension of levodopa/carbidopa using an infusion pump that delivers the medication directly into the small intestine through a gastrostomy, and subcutaneous continuous infusion of apomorphine by a dedicated pump.[10]

Advocacy for Parkinson's disease

Patients' associations (meso level, among others)

The National Parkinson Foundation[11] founded in the United States in 1957, states that its purpose is to make life better for people with PD through expert care and research, '. . .until there is a tomorrow without PD'.

The European Parkinson's Disease Association (EPDA),[12] is the only European Parkinson's umbrella organization, with nearly 25 years' experience working with the European PD community.

These associations enable communications and discussions between Parkinson's stakeholders to implement collaborations and partnerships that directly benefit people with Parkinson's and their families. The common aim is to bring together national Parkinson's organizations that in turn gather local associations, to learn from each other and share good practices and to raise awareness of the impact of Parkinson's across respective countries.

Advocate for research in Parkinson's disease

The Parkinson's Disease Foundation (PDF),[13] is a United States-based presence in Parkinson's disease research, education, and public advocacy that, since 1975, is a division of the National Parkinson Foundation. PDF funds promising scientific research while supporting people living with PD through educational programmes and services, with the objective of finding a cure for the disease and ensuring the best possible quality of life for patients.

The Michael J. Fox Foundation (MJFF)

Michael J. Fox, born in 1961 in Canada, has been since the 1970s an international film and television star. Though he didn't share the news with the public for seven years, Fox was diagnosed with young-onset PD in 1991. Upon disclosing his condition in 1998, he committed himself to the campaign for increased Parkinson's research. Fox announced his retirement from acting in January 2000 and later that year launched The Michael J. Fox Foundation (MJFF) for Parkinson's Research.[14]

From its creation, MJFF is dedicated to finding a cure for Parkinson's disease through an aggressively funded research agenda and to ensuring the development of improved therapies for those living with PD today. The team works with the goal of accelerating breakthroughs patients can feel in their everyday lives.

Speed treatments that can slow, stop or reverse the progression of PD, treat the currently unaddressed or symptoms of the disease and the debilitating side effects of current PD drugs are the foundation's commitments.

MJFF has invested in high-risk, high-reward research targets and has created an in-house team of formally trained PhDs and business-trained project managers.

Atypical parkinsonism

Apart from PD, the most common cause of parkinsonism, Multiple system atrophy (MSA), progressive supranuclear palsy (PSP), and corticobasal degeneration (CBD) has to be considered in the differential diagnosis of parkinsonism due to a degenerative condition.

Known as 'atypical parkinsonism', these disorders are mainly characterized by a poor response to levodopa treatment and have a more rapid and worse progression compared to idiopathic PD.[15-18]

Forms of symptomatic parkinsonism following vascular, drug-related, infectious, toxic, structural, and other known secondary causes are frequent. Drug-induced parkinsonism is the most common secondary form of parkinsonism and arises via the intake of agents that block post-synaptic dopamine D2 receptors with high affinity. Vascular parkinsonism tends to have a lower body emphasis where gait disturbance and concomitant cognitive impairment are predominant.[19]

Advocacy for patients and research in atypical parkinsonism

CURE PSP[20] is a worldwide organization that promotes research in a spectrum of relatively rare degenerative diseases like PSP, corticobasal degeneration (CBD), frontotemporal dementia (FTD), and others that often afflict individuals during their productive and active years, leading to debilitating symptoms and early death.

Moreover, since there is currently no treatment and no cure for these disorders, this organization provides support for patients, families, and caregivers.

The Multiple System Atrophy (MSA) Coalition®[21] is a charitable organization dedicated to supporting patients and caregivers affected by MSA, to financing research toward identifying a cause and finding a cure for MSA and to advocating for issues important to the MSA community, including greater awareness.

Other associations that advocate atypical parkinsonism around the world are the PSP Association,[22] PSP Australia,[23] and PSP Germany.[24]

Essential tremor

Essential tremor (ET) is the most common cause of tremor, characterized by postural and action tremor of hands, head, and voice, rarely in the legs, trunk, and face, with a frequency of 4–7 Hz. Frequently with a familial incidence, ET is more frequent at an old age but can also onset early in life, increasing in severity over the years. When disabling, ET impairs the activities of daily life and the execution of specific tasks. ET is exacerbated by stress, fatigue, caffeine, smoking, and certain medications but it has been found that at times it improves with relaxation and alcohol. Task or position specific tremor, isolated voice or chin tremor, and orthostatic tremor are considered variants of ET.

The most common treatments for ET include primidone, beta-blockers such as propranolol and benzodiazepines, and chronic deep-brain stimulation of the thalamus in select patients.[25]

Advocacy for essential tremor

The International Essential Tremor Foundation (IETF),[26] was founded in 1988 as a non-profit membership organization, made up of patients, physicians, educators, healthcare workers, parents, relatives, friends, and volunteers.

Its mission is to provide global educational information, services, and support to children and adults challenged by ET, to their families and healthcare providers, as well as to promote and fund ET research. Moreover, this association promotes Brain Tissue Donation in order to further essential tremor research.

The National Tremor Foundation (NTF),[27] founded in 1992 in United Kingdom, is an organization that aims to provide help, support and advice to all those living with any form of tremors, irrespective of age.

Advocacy for research in essential tremor

The Tremor Action Network (TAN, tremoraction.org) is dedicated to advocating for patients with ET, building a network of advocates to inform the public, government agencies, and the healthcare industry on the universal needs of the tremor population. TAN promotes innovative surveys, clinical trials, studies, diagnostic, therapeutic, and assistive technology products.

The Tremor Research Group (TRG),[28] founded in 2001, is organized as an independent, non-profit organization of scientific investigators who conduct research in institutions committed to cooperative planning, implementation, analysis as well as reporting of controlled clinical trials and of other research for tremor disorders.

Chorea and Huntington's disease

Chorea is a motor symptom characterized by the presence of involuntary brief, abrupt, irregular, unpredictable, non-stereotyped movements that can affect various body parts, and interfere with speech, swallowing, posture, and gait.

When occurring with athetosis (a distal, slower, writhing, abnormal movement) chorea is known as choreoathetosis. Ballism consists in more severe choreiform movements, wild, violent, and involving flinging of a body part. Chorea may also occur with other abnormal movements such as dystonia.[29]

Causes of chorea are of several origins: pregnancy (chorea gravidarum); inherited forms such as Huntington's disease and benign hereditary chorea; infection/immune-related such as Sydenham's chorea and systemic lupus erythematosus; focal vascular lesions in the basal ganglia; drugs such as levodopa, neuroleptics, and oral contraception; various metabolic and endocrinological disorders such as hyperthyroidism, hypo/hyperparathyroidism, and hypo/hyperglycaemia.[30] A functional dysregulation of the basal ganglia motor circuit, with increase of the final thalamo-cortical output is its common pathophysiology.[31]

Treatment of chorea usually implies its aetiology, when possible, but symptomatic treatments are often used: atypical neuroleptic agents or other dopamine depleters and benzodiazepines.[32]

Huntington's disease (HD) is an autosomal dominant neurodegenerative disorder caused by the abnormal expansion of IT-15 gene on chromosome 4, encoding for the protein Huntington. It usually appears in individuals between 30 and 54 years of age but can manifest as early as 4 years old and as late as 80 years.

HD is characterized by motor, cognitive, and psychiatric symptoms. Motor features include: presence of choric movements; reduced manual dexterity, dysarthria, dysphagia, balance impairment, and falls. The Westphal variant, typical of young onset, may also present with parkinsonism and dystonia. Global cognitive impairment progressively develops over years. Psychiatric features include: depression (most common), mania, obsessive-compulsive disorder, irritability, anxiety, agitation, impulsivity, apathy, and social withdrawal.[33]

A definitive diagnosis of HD is made by genetic testing and previous genetic counselling.

Other genetic causes of chorea are neuroacanthocytosis, dentatorubro–pallidolusyian atrophy, Huntington's disease like-syndromes, some of the spinocerebellar ataxias, benign hereditary chorea, Wilson's disease, and mitochondrial disorders.

Advocacy for chorea and Huntington's disease

The International Huntington Association (IHA),[34] is a federation made up of national voluntary health agencies. It promotes lay and professional education; individual and family support; psycho-social, clinical and biomedical research; and ethical and legal considerations related to HD in the various countries where national agencies are active.

Since 1974 IHA organizes meetings to promote international collaboration in the search for a cure for HD, maintains close liaison with research scientists in developing and sharing information and resources among member countries (to avoid duplication of effort), and assists in organizing and developing new or existing national HD organizations.

Jeroen de Schepper, the winner of the Media Category of the EFNA Advocacy Award in 2015, relative of some HD patients. He has succeeded in raising awareness of HD in the media with his 'crosscountry4huntington' initiative; travelling throughout Europe by bike, he visited families affected by HD and called on nursing homes and local Huntington Associations).[35]

An example of virtual advocacy

Since April 2000 the mission of the HDlighthouse Families Web Site[36] is to present and explain the latest research findings so that families affected by HD can become proactive in the care of their family members and make good decisions. The name of this project is inspired by the Huntington Harbor Lighthouse (located north of Long Island) where Dr George Huntington observed and wrote about his patients with HD.

HDLF.org provides an active chat board/forum where it is possible to actively participate, helping others or getting answers to questions you might have about HD and associated issues.

Advocacy for research in Huntington's disease

The mission of the Hereditary Disease Foundation[37] is to fund innovative research focused on curing HD and impacting other brain disorders. In 1983, the Hereditary Disease Foundation was the first to use DNA markers to discover the neighbourhood of the HD gene. This breakthrough helped launch the Human Genome Project. Following this discovery, the Hereditary Disease Foundation pioneered many technologies for mapping and finding genes as well as identifying the specific HD gene, its defect, and the protein that encodes it. This research has helped in unlocking some of the critical knowledge needed to find a cure. The Scientific Advisory Board of the Hereditary Disease Foundation is composed of distinguished scientists from around the world.

Dystonia

Dystonia is a motor symptom characterized by sustained or intermittent muscle contractions causing abnormal postures, often associated with repetitive movements or tremor. Dystonia can be present at rest and is often worsened by voluntary action and associated with overflow muscle activation.

At first, the diagnosis is clinical, based on the observation of dystonic postures and movements and their variability in different conditions. A typical sign is the presence of a specific voluntary gesture (known as 'geste antagoniste') that can reduce the involuntary movement or posture.

The pathophysiology of dystonia resides in the basal ganglia, cerebellum, supplementary motor areas, and sensorimotor cortex, affected by an impaired inhibition, abnormal plasticity, and sensorimotor dysfunction.

Dystonia syndromes are classified in order of: age at onset, body distribution (focal, segmental, and generalized forms) and temporal pattern (disease course and diurnal fluctuations). Dystonia can be isolated or present in other movement disorder syndromes, such as parkinsonism or myoclonus. The aetiology of dystonias can be differentiated in two different lines: the presence of a nervous system pathology and inheritance or acquired condition. Dystonic cerebral palsy following perinatal brain injury is a frequent form caused by a structural lesion. Inherited dystonias can have different sorts of transmission patterns. Acquired dystonias recognize a variety of causes such as infection, drugs, toxic, vascular, and so on.

In many cases of isolated dystonia there is no evidence of degeneration or structural lesion (e.g. DYT1, DYT6) while idiopathic dystonias (whether sporadic or familial) are genetically unclassified forms.[38]

Dystonia is the third most common movement disorder (annual incidence: 15–25 per 100,000) after PD and tremor.[39] The most frequent forms of dystonia are the focal/segmental syndromes: blepharospasm, cervical dystonia, or torticollis; spasmodic dysphonia; oromandibular dystonia; task-specific dystonia. The treatment of first choice is botulinum toxin, a neurotoxin that blocks the neuromuscular signal transmission.[40]

Advocacy for dystonia

The Dystonia Advocacy Network (DAN),[41] is a grassroots organization in the United States that brings dystonia-affected individuals together and is constituted by a group of dystonia organizations (Table 24.1), each dedicated to a specific form of dystonia.

DAN continuously works to adopt and advance a legislative agenda, aimed at raising awareness of dystonia, educating policymakers, addressing issues about patient care, and moving research forward.

Advocacy in dystonia and social networks

Patients with dystonia are very active in social networks, offering an alternative and effective form of advocacy. Here are some examples and relative links:

Table 24.1 List of organizations focusing on dystonia

Type of dystonia	Organization	Website
Blepharospasm	Benign Essential Blepharospasm Research Foundation (BEBRF)	http://www.blepharospasm.org
Spasmodic torticollis	DySTonia, Inc National Spasmodic Torticollis Association (NSTA)	http://www.spasmodictorticollis.org http://www.torticollis.org
Dysphonia	National Spasmodic Dysphonia Association (NSDA)	https://www.dysphonia.org
All	Dystonia Medical Research Foundation (DMRF)	https://www.dystonia-foundation.org

An example of BLOG advocacy: dystonia blog from around the word[42]
An example of YOUTUBE advocacy
Bionic Dystonic: How I Advocate for Dystonia Awareness
Posted by David Novotny, September 23, 2016[43]
An example of FACEBOOK advocacy: down with dystonia[44]

Advocacy for research in dystonia

The Dystonia Medical Research Foundation (DMRF),[45] is an organization based in the United States and dedicated to serving all people with dystonia and their families.

Since 1976, DMRF has grown from a small family-based foundation into a membership-driven organization led by a Board of Directors and network of volunteers with personal connections to dystonia. Its leadership is motivated by a drive to find a cure and an unwavering commitment to serving people affected by dystonia. In addition, DMRF aims to improve society's recognition and understanding of dystonia, to increase awareness and to fundraise for research. Moreover, DMRF aims to educate and influence legislators and government officials who make decisions, for example, about how much money is allocated to medical research year, who will have access to treatments, and other issues that impact people with dystonia.

Tics and Tourette's syndrome

A tic is defined as an involuntary movement or vocalization that is usually of sudden onset, brief, repetitive, stereotyped but occurring out of a background of normal activity. The onset of a tic is often associated with a sensation of urgency to perform the specific movement, and usually is associated with a sense of relief once performed.

Tics are classified as motor (movement) or vocal (sound), and simple or complex. Simple motor tics involve only a specific body part and can appear as clonic, tonic, or dystonic movements. Simple vocal tics consist of sounds that do not form words but noises or rattles.[46]

Tic disorders are classified by the DSM-IV in three main categories: transient tic disorders, chronic motor or vocal tic disorder, and Tourette disorder.

The diagnosis of Tourette syndrome (TS) is clinical and implies the presence of both multiple motor and one or more vocal tics, not necessarily concurrently; the tics occur numerous times during the day and over a period of at least a year. The onset of TS is usually before age 18 and substance abuse or other medical conditions should be excluded.[47]

Pharmacological treatment is required only when the intensity and or frequency of the tics disables daily living and social interaction. Education and psychological counselling can be satisfactory for most patients with mild symptoms. When necessary, the treatment of tics is centred on the dopamine receptor blocking agent, both typical and atypical antipsychotics. Other treatments reported to be beneficial are botulinum toxin for (focal tics) and clonidine and chronic deep-brain stimulation of the globus pallidus internus and thalamus.[48]

Advocacy for patients and research for tics and Tourette's syndrome

Founded in 1972, the Tourette Association of America (formerly known as the Tourette Syndrome Association)[49] has emerged as the leading national non-profit organization in the United States that's working to make life better for anyone affected by Tourette's syndrome and tic disorders. The Association's objectives are to raise public awareness and foster social acceptance, to advance scientific understanding, treatment options, and care and to educate professionals to better serve the needs of children, adults, and families challenged by Tourette's and tic disorders. Moreover, the association aims to advocate for public policies and services that promote positive school, work, and social environments.

The Tourette Association has taken the lead in developing the Tourette Syndrome Caucus made up of members of Congress to promote (at a government level) patients' needs. Developing a caucus can be an important form of advocacy. In the States, a caucus is a meeting of supporters or members of a specific political party or movement with the purpose of coordinating members' actions, choosing group policy, or nominating candidates for various offices.

Tourette's Action (TA)[50] works in England, Wales, and Northern Ireland, and is a support and research charity for people with Tourette's syndrome and their families. Tourette's Action has launched a Research Participant Registry, a voluntary database of individuals willing to consider participating in research studies. This allows TA to contact patients about ongoing studies.

Ataxia

Ataxia is defined as a deficiency of coordination during voluntary movements, in particular during gait. Hemiataxia is the condition limited to one side of the body while dystaxia is the mild degree form of ataxia.

Ataxia is a non-specific clinical manifestation that can be present, and caused, by several possible aetiologies, in any case implying a dysfunction of the cerebellum.

The diagnosis of ataxic syndromes requires a complete personal and family history, physical examination, neuroimaging, extensive laboratory evaluation, and frequently its aetiology remains indeterminate.

Several chronic cerebellar ataxias are familial and genetically determined, or caused by nutritional abnormalities, mitochondrial disease, or autoimmune syndromes. Ataxia may also occur sporadically in different neurological disorders (Multiple Sclerosis, multisystem atrophy, brain tumours) or general pathological conditions (vitamin B12 deficiency); infectious, vascular, structural, or metabolic lesions can cause acute forms of ataxic syndromes.[51]

In recent years, it has become easier to identify the genetic causes of ataxia. Recessive forms are related to forms of GM2 gangliosidoses, sulfatide lipidoses, and other syndromes involving deposition of abnormal metabolic intermediates. Friedreich's ataxia, hereditary ataxia with vitamin E deficiency, and abetalipoproteinemia are other causes of recessive ataxia.

Causes of autosomal dominant ataxia include SCA1, SCA2, SCA3, SCA6, SCA7, SCA17, DRPLA (caused by CAG repeats encoding a polyglutamine protein domain) and SCA8, associated with a CTG expansion.

A rare form of dominantly inherited genetic entity is episodic ataxia, types 1 and 2.[52]

The correction of symptomatic causes is the first approach to symptomatic forms, while acetazolamide may be a useful therapy of episodic ataxia.

Treatment of other forms of ataxia is supportive and includes physical, occupational, and speech therapy.

Advocacy for ataxia

The Friedreich's Ataxia Research Alliance (FARA)[53] advocates on behalf of the patient community, academic investigators, industry partners and government agencies such as the National Institutes of Health (NIH) and the Food and Drug Administration (FDA).

Moreover, FARA supports awareness campaigns, budgets of the NIH and the FDA, newborn screening, and patient-focused drug development.

One of the peculiarities of this association is the development of an Ambassador programme. FARA Ambassadors is a united team of patient volunteers living with FA who are committed to supporting FARA in the search for a treatment and cure, speaking at events to volunteers, potential donors, scientific groups, pharma industry partners, media interviews, and others to raise awareness and search for fundraising opportunities.

Other associations include the Friedreich's Ataxia Parents Group (an online support organization), the National Ataxia Foundation (NAF), the National Organization for Rare Disorders (NORD), and the Muscular Dystrophy Association (MDA).

Advocacy for research in ataxia

Professor Paola Giunti, the winner of the EFNA Neurology Advocacy Award for Health Professional in 2016, established the Specialist Ataxia Centre in London (54) as a way to concentrate research and expertise in this group of rare diseases and to create a translational service made up of multidisciplinary and multiprofessional teams. A unique feature of the Centre is the involvement of the Ataxia UK patients' support group (55), volunteers with direct personal experience of ataxia who are available to talk to patients.

Conclusions

Advocacy in movement disorders currently offers a heterogeneous and abundant variety of options focusing primarily on the most frequent movement disorders. For example, PD is represented by organizations of different kinds—from patients' associations that take care of quality of life to scientific foundations promoting and funding research.

Disorders that are less common, such as atypical parkinsonisms, can count on a smaller variety of organizations. Generally speaking, a single association promotes both for support oriented to patients and their caregivers as well as research funding.

The availability of several forms of advocacy for a single disease can lead to the dispersal of energy and resources. But it can also signify a way to better develop and differentiate skills, in particular in research funding or advocacy opportunities.

In conclusion, through a global overview of the various advocacies for movement disorders that are available, the best solution seems to be the existence (for each pathology) of a national association for patients and their caregivers that collects and coordinates more local levels of activity combined with a foundation dedicated to scientific research funding and execution. The latter should collaborate closely with the patients' association.

Another important role of advocacy in movement disorders is the possibility to represent the totality of affected individuals together to pronounce—with a common, powerful voice—on legislative and public policy issues.

Moreover, legislative and public policy health issues are can be very different from country to country, so a meso level of intervention could be more suitable to realize proper projects in relation to the specific needs of patients in that peculiar background.

A suggestion for the right structure of an advocacy group can be the presence of two types of institutions (organized on a national level with local branches and international collaborations) which work, respectively, on the quality of life in daily living for patients and on scientific research sponsorship.

Local, regional branches could better facilitate the access to local resources (medical, welfare, rules, and regulations for financial assistance) while international collaborations can focus on helping patients gain access to the best available treatments and on fundraising.

Although there are many associations that advocate for movement disorders patients, covering various aspects and problems of the diseases, some issues are not fully developed. In Table 24.2, some unmet needs as regards advocacy for movement disorders are listed. In particular, for diseases such as PD, parkinsonisms, and Huntington disease, 'end of life' issues are rarely faced in many countries. Patients with

Table 24.2 Missing in advocacy for movement disorders

Issue	Shortcoming
End of life	Help in management, availability of adequate institutions (in particular for Parkinson's disease, parkinsonisms, and Huntington disease)
Alternative treatments	Advice in selecting proper time and type
Communication	Training courses for physicians and health professionals
Scientific information	Facilitation to accessing understandable scientific information
Research	Strengthen the link between patient associations and research centres, promoting the establishment of Research Participant Registry
Public health policy	Strengthen presence in legislative and public policy health topics

a chronic disease and scarce availability of symptomatic and effective treatments often look for palliative and alternative self-prescribed treatments, with the risk of searching out inappropriate therapies. Patients' associations can provide appropriate counselling and connect physicians and patients.

Physician-patient communications is not yet the subject of medical school courses. In several chronic and progressive neurological diseases, such as most of the Movements Disorders, good communications between the patient and his or her clinician accounts for 50% of the therapy. An important role of advocacy can be promoting specific training courses that help medical personnel to become more effective communicators.

Advocates should both facilitate patients' access to scientific information as well as their participation in clinical trials and research databases.

References

1. **International Parkinson and Movement Disorder Society**. Links to International Organizations & Foundations. Available at: http://www.movementdisorders.org/MDS/Resources/Helpful-Links.htm
2. **European Federation of Neurological Associations**. Available at: http://efna.net
3. **The NeuroPositive Foundation**. Available at: http://neuropozytywni.pl
4. **Neuroalianza**. Available at: http://neuroalianza.org
5. **Patient-Centered Outcomes Research Institute**. Available at: http://www.pcori.org
6. **Driver, J. A., Logroscino, G., Gaziano, J. M., Kurth, T.** (2009) Incidence and remaining lifetime risk of Parkinson disease in advanced age. *Neurology*, **72**, 432–8.
7. **Lee, A. J., Hardy, J., Revesz, T.** (2009) Parkinson's disease. *Lancet*, **373**(9680), 2055–66.
8. **Hoehn, M. M., Yahr, M. D.** (1967) Parkinsonism: onset, progression and mortality. *Neurology*, **17**(5), 427–42.
9. **Cilia, R., Akpalu, A., Sarfo, F. S., et al.** (2014) The modern pre-levodopa era of Parkinson's disease: insights into motor complications from sub-Saharan Africa. *Brain*, **137**(Pt 10), 2731–42.
10. **Giugni, J. C., Okun, M. S.** (2014) Treatment of advanced Parkinson's disease. *Curr Opin Neurol*, **27**(4), 450–60.
11. **Parkinson's Foundation**. Available at: http://www.parkinson.org
12. **European Parkinson's Disease Association**. Available at: http://www.epda.eu.com/en/
13. **Parkinson's Disease Foundation**. Available at: http://www.pdf.org
14. **The Michael J. Fox Foundation for Parkinson's Research**. Available at: https://www.michaeljfox.org
15. **Gilman, S., Wenning, G. K., Low, P. A., et al.** (2008) Second consensus statement on the diagnosis of multiple system atrophy. *Neurology*, **71**, 670–6.
16. **Stamelou, M., Bhatia, K. P.** (2015) Atypical parkinsonism: diagnosis and treatment. *Neurol Clin*, **33**, 39–56.
17. **Colosimo, C., Bak, T. H., Bologna, M., Berardelli, A.** (2014) Fifty years of progressive supranuclear palsy. *J Neurol Neurosurg Psychiatry*, **85**(8), 938–44.
18. **Armstrong, M. J., Litvan, I., Lang, A. E., et al.** (2013) Criteria for the diagnosis of corticobasal degeneration. *Neurology*, **80**, 496–503.

19. **Wenning, G. K.**, **Litvan, I.**, **Tolosa, E.** (2011) Milestones in atypical and secondary Parkinsonisms. *Mov Disord*, **26**(6), 1083–95.
20. **CurePSP**. Available at: http://www.psp.org
21. **The MSA Coalition**. Available at: https://www.multiplesystematrophy.org
22. **PSPA**. Available at: http://www.pspassociation.org.uk
23. **PSP Australia**. Available at: https://www.psp-australia.org.au
24. **The German PSP Society**. Available at: https://www.psp-gesellschaft.de
25. **Louis, E. D.** (2014) Essential tremor: from bedside to bench and back to bedside. *Curr Opin Neurol*, **27**(4), 461–7.
26. **International Essential Tremor Foundation**. Available at: http://www.essentialtremor.org
27. **National Tremor Foundation**. Available at: http://www.tremor.org.uk
28. **Tremor Research Group**. Available at: http://www.tremorresearchgroup.org/
29. **Donaldson, I.**, **Marsden, C. D.**, **Schneider, S. A.**, **Bhatia, K. B.** (2012) Clinical approach to movement disorders. In: Donaldson, I., Marsden, C. D., Schneider, S. A., Bhatia, K. B. (eds). *Marsden's Book of Movement Disorders*. Oxford: Oxford University Press.
30. **Hermann, A.**, **Walker, R. H.** (2015) Diagnosis and treatment of chorea syndromes. *Curr Neurol Neurosci Rep*, **15**(2), 514
31. **Gittis, A. H.**, **Kreitzer, A. C.** (2012) Striatal microcircuitry and movement disorders. *Trends Neurosci*, **35**(9), 557–64.
32. **Hermann, A.**, **Walker, R. H.** (2015) Diagnosis and treatment of chorea syndromes. *Curr Neurol Neurosci Rep*, **15**, 514.
33. **Roos, R. A.** (2010) Huntington's disease: a clinical review. *Orphanet J Rare Dis*, **5**, 40.
34. **International Huntington Association**. Available at: http://www.huntington-assoc.com
35. **Cross country for Huntington**. Blog. Available at: https://crosscountry4huntington.wordpress.com/jeroendeschepper/
36. **Huntington's Disease Lighthouse Families.** Available at: http://hdlf.org
37. **Hereditary Disease Foundation**. Available at: http://www.hdfoundation.org/new-index
38. **Albanese, A.**, **Bhatia, K.**, **Bressman, S. B.**, **et al.** (2013) Phenomenology and classification of dystonia: a consensus update. *Mov Disord*, **28**(7), 863–73.
39. **Epidemiological Study of Dystonia in Europe (ESDE) Collaborative Group** (2000) A prevalence study of primary dystonia in eight European countries. *J Neurol*, **247**(10), 787–92.
40. **Tarsy, D. Simon, D. K.** (2006) Dystonia. *N Engl J Med*, **355**(8), 818–29.
41. **Dystonia Advocacy Network**. Available at: http://dystonia-advocacy.org
42. **Dystonia Living** (2016) Dystonia blogs from around the world (7 August 2016). Available at: http://dystonialiving.blogspot.it/2016/08/dystonia-blogs-from-around-world.html
43. **Novotny, D.** (2016) Bionic dystonic: how I advocate for dystonia awareness. Foxfeed Blog. Available at: https://www.michaeljfox.org/foundation/news-detail.php?bionic-dystonic
44. **Down with Dystonia**. Available at: https://www.facebook.com/pg/downwithdystonia/posts/?ref=page_internal
45. **Dystonia Medical Research Foundation**. Available at: https://www.dystonia-foundation.org
46. **Abell, S.**, **Ey, J.** (2009) Tics in childhood. *Clin Pediatr (Phila)*, **48**(7), 790–1.
47. **Hallett, M.** (2015) Tourette syndrome: update. *Brain Dev*, **37**(7), 651–5.

48. **Piedad, J. C.**, **Rickards, H. E.**, **Cavanna, A. E.** (2012) What patients with Gilles de la Tourette syndrome should be treated with deep brain stimulation and what is the best target? *Neurosurgery*, **71**(1), 173–92.
49. **Tourette Associate of America.** Available at: https://www.tourette.org
50. **Tourette's Action**. Available at: https://www.tourettes-action.org.uk
51. **Akbar, U.**, **Ashizawa, T.** (2015) Ataxia. *Neurol Clin*, **33**(1), 225–48.
52. **Mancuso, M.**, **Orsucci, D.**, **Siciliano, G.**, **Bonuccelli, U.** (2014) The genetics of ataxia: through the labyrinth of the Minotaur, looking for Ariadne's thread. *J Neurol*, **261** Suppl 2, S528–41.
53. **Friedreich's Ataxia Research Alliance.** Available at: http://www.curefa.org
54. **UCL Institute of Neurology**. Available at: https://www.ucl.ac.uk/ion/departments/molecular/themes/neurodegeneration/ataxia
55. **Ataxia UK**. Branches and support groups. Available at: https://www.ataxia.org.uk/Pages/FAQs/Category/branches-and-support-groups

Chapter 25
Advocacy for brain tumours

Riccardo Soffietti, Christine Marosi, Roberta Rudà, and Wolfgang Grisold

Introduction

Brain tumours represent an important cause of morbidity and mortality. The incidence of primary intracranial tumours in Western countries is around 10–12 new cases/100,000/year. Meningiomas are the most frequent tumours, followed by gliomas, and the relative frequency of the different histologic types is age dependent. Among elderly patients, glioblastomas and primary central nervous system (CNS) lymphomas are rising in incidence, posing specific challenges to the medical community and health systems. In children the most aggressive tumour types are medulloblastomas and ependymomas. Secondary brain tumours, in particular brain metastases, are so far 7–10-fold more frequent than primary brain tumours, and the increasing incidence over time is due to an improved early diagnosis by MRI and improved survival in many solid tumours by more precise multimodal treatments.

History of neuro-oncology

Neuro-oncology was born as an independent discipline in the 1970s under the leadership of neurosurgeons and neurologists. The field encompassed primary brain tumours, metastatic complications of systemic cancer and non-metastatic complications of malignancy. Jerome Posner, Charles Wilson, William Shapiro, and Victor Levin in the United States and Jerzy Hildebrand in Europe were among the early pioneers. A second generation of neurologists and neurosurgeons who were the students of these leaders entered independent careers in the 1980s. The clinical research efforts led to the development of consortia, the Brain Tumor Cooperative Group in the United States, and the Brain Tumour Group of the European Organisation for Research and Treatment of Cancer (EORTC) in Europe for conducting clinical trials in brain tumours. In the mid-1990s several factors began to change the landscape of neuro-oncology research and patients care. Medical oncologists and radiation oncologists began to turn their attention to the problems of brain tumours, and assumed an increasing role in delivering medical treatments. At this point neuro-oncology was clearly established as a multidisciplinary field, and in 1998 and 1999 two multidisciplinary Scientific Societies (i.e. EANO (European Association for Neuro-Oncology) and SNO (Society for Neuro-Oncology, United States)) were founded, and a new scientific journal, *Neuro-Oncology*, was launched. The last achievement has been the creation of the WFNOS (World Federation of Neuro-Oncology Societies) as an umbrella of the different organizations of neuro-oncology worldwide. To spread the information on neuro-oncological issues, either purely scientific or organizational, a WFNOS magazine (from the previous EANO magazine) has been developed: one of its aims is to stimulate a homogenization of management of brain tumour across the different countries. In parallel, several sections of neuro-oncology have been activated within the medical societies of neurosurgeons, neurologists, medical oncologists, radiologists, radiation oncologists, and pathologists. Last, of utmost importance, nurse and patient organizations are becoming increasingly involved at different levels of daily patient care and clinical trials.

Issues in brain tumours patients

The symptom burden of brain tumour patients reflects the location and extension of the disease. More common symptoms are as follows: cognitive deficits 80%; motor weakness 78%; visual perceptual deficits 53%; sensory loss 38%; bowel/bladder 37%; cranial nerve palsies 29%; dysarthria 27%; dysphagia 26%; aphasia 24%; ataxia 20%; and diplopia 10%. MRI is the gold standard in case of suspicion of a primary brain tumour. The differential diagnosis between neoplastic and non-neoplastic conditions, such as abscesses, encephalitis, tumefactive multiple sclerosis, and vascular lesions can be challenging. In this regard, advanced imaging modalities (MR spectroscopy, perfusion, diffusion, PET with different tracers) are now available in the best developed countries (more or less the Western countries). However, the specificity of these new techniques is not well established and the balance between the need for advanced techniques in uncertain situations and the economical affordability are a matter of debate. Moreover, in several countries with reduced income, CT only is widely available.

Nowadays, surgical resection is performed to an extent as much as possible in order to palliate focal neurological symptoms and intracranial hypertension, and provide tissue for histological diagnosis and molecular characterization. Some recent advances in surgical technology are useful for reducing the morbidity and improving the results in terms of survival. The best example is represented by so called 'awake surgery', which allows intraoperatively a continuous monitoring of the motor, speech and cognitive functions while resecting a tumour (generally a low-grade glioma close to eloquent areas). Overall, awake surgery requires a highly skilled team, including the neurosurgeon, the neuroanaesthetist, the neurophysiologist, the neuropsychologist, and specialized nurses, and significant extra time to exploit the surgical procedure. Thus, it is not surprising that awake surgery is not widely available worldwide, even within the same country.

Similarly, the advances in radiation technology are allowing the delivery of therapeutic radiations (photons, protons, heavy ions) with increased precision due to a better spatial delineation of the target. Stereotactic radiosurgery or radiotherapy permit the treatment of lesions less than 1 cm, and have enlarged the spectrum of diseases that can be successfully treated (brain metastases, recurrent gliomas, residual or recurrent relatively benign tumours, such as meningiomas, neurinomas, sellar tumours). Other technological improvements, such as intensity modulated radiotherapy (IMRT), allow a better sparing of the normal nervous tissue, especially of the brain areas involved in the maintenance of cognitive functions (i.e. hippocampal regions).

Regarding pharmacological antineoplastic therapies, these still rely on conventional cytotoxic agents (i.e. temozolomide and nitrosoureas for gliomas, methotrexate for primary central nervous system lymphoma), but more sophisticated, targeted therapies are being developed, including monoclonal antibodies and small molecules and immunotherapies.

Monitoring of patients over time with neurological and neuropsychological scales and standard MRI is critical for an early detection of tumour progression or neurotoxicity from therapies. However, a correct definition of response or progression can be hampered by the occurrence on MRI of phenomena, such as pseudoprogression and pseudoresponse.

Pseudoprogression consists of an increase or new development of enhancing areas, oedema, and necrosis within a recently irradiated field, mimicking tumour progression. It represents a challenge in the daily clinical practice following chemoradiation for high-grade gliomas[1] or stereotactic radiosurgery for brain metastases.[2] The misinterpretation of pseudoprogression may lead to an erroneous change of strategy (i.e. moving towards an undue second-line treatment instead of waiting for a spontaneous regression).

Thus far, the major clue for a correct diagnosis of pseudoprogression is the persistence of a neurological integrity without steroid need.

Pseudoresponse is typically seen after treatment with anti-vascular endothelial growth factor agents, such as bevacizumab. It is characterized by a reduction of enhancement and oedema, due to a normalization of vessel permeability while the tumour is growing with an infiltrative pattern. The risk is that of continuing an ineffective treatment.

Last, supportive care and palliation in the advanced and end-of-life phases are being increasingly adopted. Hospice care and home care are differently employed in the different countries or even within the same country. In these settings, ethical issues are even more important than medical issues.

In general, the management of brain tumours, that more often are rare tumours, poses to the healthcare system some critical problems in terms of organization. First, the increasing complexity of local treatments, such as surgery and radiotherapy, requires the development of tertiary referral centres, whose definition must be based on precise criteria of expertise, volume of activity, and availability of advanced technologies for molecular markers, neuroimaging, surgery, radiotherapy, and drug delivery. Second, there will be in the near future an increased need of so-called orphan drugs to be supplied to small subgroups of patients with precise molecular alterations to be targeted. Pharmaceutical companies are often reluctant to support clinical trial on potentially active new drugs in rare brain tumours, because of limited economical revenues that can be expected.

For all these reasons, the European Commission has launched a directive in order to develop a network of Centres of Expertise for Rare Solid Cancers, including the CNS tumours that have been called EURACAN. The mission is to create common protocols, predefined pathways for second opinions and complex treatments, and registries to monitor the patterns of care across European countries.

Rehabilitation for brain tumour patients

General concepts

Receiving the diagnosis of a brain tumour means for almost all affected patients and families to be confronted with a still incurable cancer diagnosis and with an individual set of neurological symptoms due to the location and growth pattern of the tumour, with the individual development of tumour surrounding oedema and hence, increased intracranial pressure. The usually short course of the illness, the magnitude of individuality in symptoms and the high variability of their impact on a patient's functional status and quality of life explain the challenge to provide reasonable offers for rehabilitation for those patients. Moreover, most brain tumour patients show (as well as deficits in muscular strength) motor or sensory deficits, disturbance of equilibrium, decreased attention, fatigue, in addition to cognitive deficits that have to be addressed simultaneously in order to assure effectiveness to rehabilitative measures.[3] Nevertheless, there is evidence proving that rehabilitation is able preserving patients' independence and quality of life.[4]

Rehabilitation of neurological symptoms is enabled by the ability of normal brain cells to continuously adapt to the environment. Neuroplasticity is enhanced by providing complex stimuli, favouring the synthesis of neurotrophic factors.[5] Applying the concepts of neuroplasticity allows obtaining measurable benefits in functional recovery in patients with neurological diseases, also in brain tumour patients.[6]

Physical training in brain tumour patients

However, Jones et al. showed that in newly diagnosed brain tumour patients, the muscular strength of thigh muscles as well as cardiorespiratory performance were significantly reduced, reaching only 60% of the values expected for sedentary, age, and sex-matched control persons.[7] The reasons for this deconditioning are yet not fully understood, combining muscular loss due to perioperative inactivity, supraphysiological levels of corticosteroids administered because of brain tumour oedema—and, specific for brain tumours—acidotic muscular damage due to the deregulation of perfusion that is normally regulated by the autonomic nervous system and might be perturbed by the brain tumour itself or its treatment.[8]

These findings underline how important it is to tailor physical training to the individual patient's abilities in order to provide training effectiveness without overstraining the patient's functional capacity. Improvements in muscular strength and mobility were similar in patients undergoing stationary or outpatient rehabilitation programmes suffering from high-grade gliomas as compared to low grade gliomas[4] and for brain tumour patients and stroke patients.[9] A prospective study showed that patients with brain tumours able to maintain a reasonable fitness level (>9 metabolic equivalents of task per week) lived significantly longer than less active patients (with 21.84 (95% CI, 13.32 to ∞) versus 13.03 (95% CI, 11.25–17.37 months).[4] This survival gain is longer than any hitherto observed survival gain obtained by other therapeutic measures.

Cognitive rehabilitation

Attention deficits, fatigue, and focal neurological deficits are amenable to neurologic rehabilitation. Pharmacological interventions, mostly with methylphenidate and other amphetamine derivates have not proven successful in controlled trials,[10,11] but exercise based interventions, as well in stationary rehabilitation or group based training have shown sustained effects lasting for at least six months after end of the training sessions.[11-13] Computer-based training, including virtual reality programs, offer promising opportunities to provide brain tumour patients with challenging, individually tailored, diversified, and around-the-clock available training tools to enhance their cognitive abilities in daily life.[13,14]

Individual assistance for brain tumour patients

Maintaining quality of life for brain tumour patients necessitates lifelong support by a variety of rehabilitation options that can be chosen according to actual patient need. Such integrated rehabilitation programmes combining cognitive, functional and physical training show effectivity and meet the goal of providing feeling of success and prolonged independence for patients with brain tumours[15-17] Still, a lot of research to improve such programmes has to be done.[18]

Systemic cancer and the nervous system

Systemic cancer (either solid or haematologic) detection and treatment is on the agenda of health organizations. Increasingly, the fight against cancer is becoming more successful, and in many patients the transition from an incurable to a treatable condition has occurred. Surgery, which is still the main approach, has received the addition of radiotherapy, chemotherapy, and a number of more targeted and immune mediated approaches. This has dramatically changed the fate for many patients, and cancer cure is feasible for an increasing number of patients.

Obviously, fighting cancer uses strong weapons, which also have a large number of side effects. For several cancers the natural history of treated or untreated patients has changed, which from the perspective of neurology has resulted in a different type of metastatic spread, and a variety of early and late adverse effects.[19]

In addition to treatments, infections and metabolic changes can also leave patients with a severe neurological disability after the cure of a cancer.

Overall, neurological sequelae can be due to either the cancer itself, such as metastasis to the brain, leptomeninges, and vertebral column, or result from cancer treatment as an acute or late effect. In addition, damage to the peripheral nervous system (PNS) and a number of heterogeneous neuropathic pain syndromes can occur.

Radiation therapy is one of the most powerful cancer treatments. Side effects from treatment of the brain are usually classified into acute, delayed, and late complications. Late complications to the CNS can cause cognitive deficits after many years and/or frank radionecrosis. Combination chemotherapy and radiotherapy can cause concerns for brain function[20]: for instance methotrexate can determine severe damage to the white matter in patients pretreated with radiotherapy. CNS damage can be due to chemotherapy alone, as in the case of 'chemobrain' or 'chemofog', especially in patients with breast cancer.[21]

Patients suffering from brain damage can either have focal symptoms, such as paresis, speech disorders, seizures, cognitive disturbances (memory loss, inability to concentrate, and so on) or diffuse encephalopathies. The severity of cognitive disturbances varies, and has an impact on a patient's quality of life.[22]

The PNS is a frequent site of damage from chemotherapy that can cause sensory deficits often resulting in clumsiness, dyscoordination, ataxia, or neuropathic pain. Due to the increased survival it becomes obvious that the sequelae of chemotherapy (CIPN) are not always reversible. Particularly, among young men with seminoma, cancer survivors are 'healed' and continue to suffer neuropathy and neuropathic pain, which affect many activities of daily life.

Cancer pain may have many cancer-related causes, and is often a mixture of different types of pain. Neuropathic pain syndromes following therapy can cause persisting painful neuropathies. Surgical damage of peripheral nerves can also result in neuropathic pain syndromes, and increasingly also phantom pain syndromes, not only after amputation of limbs, but also organs as the breast, rectum, and penis, have been described. As these late sequelae can improve only slightly, efforts have to be made to enhance onco-rehabilitation and also offer permanent support if needed. These late effects are usually in a delayed temporal relation to the cancer treatment. Patients may appear successfully treated for cancer, but suffer from collateral CNS or PNS damage.

Advocacy

There are many aspects in neuro-oncology that require advocacy.

A strong cooperation between general physicians, specialized nurses, and caregivers is essential to build a care team that should integrate the traditional multidisciplinary tumour board (MTB) of the hospital. In this regard, the pathways of cure that are defined by the MTB should be implemented in light of specific needs at home. These include physical barriers, cognitive and psychological problems of patients and relatives, and the relationships between patients and the care team. The efficacy of such interventions is even more critical when the patient is recruited into clinical trials, in which investigations and procedures are more rigid, and there are risks of specific adverse events.

There is a need for better instruments to detect and score cognitive and neurologic deficits. In this regard a neurologic scale (Neurologic Assessment in Neuro-Oncology (NANO) scale) has been recently developed to be validated in future clinical trials.[23] An improved understanding of the effects of cognitive impairment among both the medical community, caregivers, and laypersons is needed to improve social and psychological services.[24] Patients with permanent or persisting disability need advocacy support. Advocacy for proper treatment, permanent, and long-term support and neurorehabilitation are warranted.[25]

The access to proper types of diagnostic and therapeutic measures must be guaranteed, and thus needs advocacy. In particular in the absence of clear-cut guidelines on management patients should be informed of the pros and cons of the different options, the existence of clinical trials, and last but not least must be smoothly discouraged to choose not well defined and uncontrolled modalities that can be found in the web or in the social networks.

Regarding the risk of traditional or novel neurological complications of systemic cancer and treatments it is of utmost importance making oncologists aware of the problem. With the use in some solid tumours (melanoma, NSCLC, and so on) of novel immunotherapies (ipilimumab, nivolumab, pembrolizumab) the risk of immunomediated-reactions to the CNS (hypophysitis, Guillain–Barrè, myositis, myasthenia) has increased. Also general neurologists, when asked for consultation, need to be aware of the specific origin of these 'apparently spontaneous' neurological events.

This can be obtained either at the institutional level or at the level of multidisciplinary Scientific Societies. In this regard ECCO is working to define more precise criteria of management and toxicity evaluation in the different tumour types.[26]

Regarding the issue of survivorship and rehabilitation policy recommendations have been developed by the Cancer Control Joint Action (CanCon) for EU Member States, and consists of five main messages:

1. Cancer survivors' follow-up, late-effect management, and tertiary prevention need to be anticipatory, personalized, and implemented by means of care pathways, with the empowerment of survivors and their relatives.
2. The improvement of early detection of patient's needs and the access to rehabilitation, psychosocial, and palliative care services during the entire course of the disease is required.
3. An integrated and multiprofessional care approach with a coordination of community care providers and services are needed to implement a survivorship care plan.
4. For children, adolescent, and young adult survivors (AYA), health and psychosocial consequences of cancer and its treatments need to be anticipated and addressed through implementation of a survivorship passport, adequate models of healthcare, and coordinated transition to adult medicine.
5. Research in survivorship needs to provide more data on late effects, including genetic predisposition, as well as the added-value and the cost-effectiveness of long-term follow-up, supportive care, rehabilitation, palliative, and psychosocial care interventions.

References

1. **Wen, P. Y.**, **Macdonald, D. R.**, **Reardon, D. A.**, et al. (2010) Updated response assessment criteria for high-grade gliomas: response assessment in neuro-oncology working group. *J Clin Oncol*, **28**, 1963–72.
2. **Lin, N. U.**, **Lee, E. Q.**, **Aoyama, H.**, et al. (2015) Response assessment criteria for brain metastases: proposal from the RANO group. *Lancet Oncol*, **16**, e270–8.
3. **Day, J.**, **Gillespie, D. C.**, **Rooney, A. G.**, et al. (2016) Neurocognitive deficits and neurocognitive rehabilitation in adult brain tumors. *Curr Treat Options Neurol*, **18**, 22–32.

4. **Ruden, E., Reardon, D. A., Coan, A. D.**, et al. (2011) Exercise behavior, functional capacity, and survival in adults with malignant recurrent glioma. *J Clin Oncol*, **29**, 2918–23.
5. **Kolb, B., Teskey, G. C.** (2012) Age, experience, injury, and the changing brain. *Dev Psychobiol*, **54**, 311–25.
6. **Khan, F., Amatya, B., Galea, M. P.**, et al. (2017) Neurorehabilitation: applied neuroplasticity. *J Neurol*, **264**, 603–15.
7. **Jones, L. W., Friedman, A. H., West, M. J.**, et al. (2010) Quantitative assessment of cardiorespiratory fitness, skeletal muscle function, and body composition in adults with primary malignant glioma. *Cancer*, **116**, 695–704.
8. **Schunemann, M., Anker, S. D., Rauchhaus, M.** (2008) Cancer fatigue syndrome reflects clinically non-overt heart failure: an approach towards onco-cardiology. *Nat Clin Pract Oncol*, **5**, 632–3.
9. **Bartolo, M., Zucchella, C., Pace, A.**, et al. (2012) Improving neuro-oncological patients care: basic and practical concepts for nurse specialist in neuro-rehabilitation. *J Exp Clin Cancer Res*, **31**, 82–9.
10. **Gehring, K., Patwardhan, S. Y., Collins, R.**, et al. (2012) A randomized trial on the efficacy of methylphenidate and modafinil for improving cognitive functioning and symptoms in patients with a primary brain tumour. *J Neurooncol*, **107**, 165–74.
11. **Gehring, K., Roukema, J. A., Sitskoorn, M. M.** (2012) Review of recent studies on interventions for cognitive deficits in patients with cancer. *Expert Rev Anticancer Ther*, **12**, 255–69.
12. **Hassler, M. R., Elandt, K., Preusser, M.**, et al. (2010) Neurocognitive training in patients with high-grade glioma: a pilot study. *J Neurooncol*, **97**, 109–15.
13. **Zucchella, C., Bartolo, M., Di Lorenzo, C.**, et al. (2013) Cognitive impairment in primary brain tumours outpatients: a prospective cross-sectional survey. *J Neurooncol*, **112**, 455–60.
14. **Yang, S., Chun, M. H., Son, Y. R.** (2014) Effect of virtual reality on cognitive dysfunction in patients with brain tumour. *Ann Rehabil Med*, **38**, 726–33.
15. **Khan, F., Amatya, B., Drummond, K.**, et al. (2014) Effectiveness of integrated multidisciplinary rehabilitation in primary brain cancer survivors in an Australian community cohort: a controlled clinical trial. *J Rehabil Med*, **46**, 754–60.
16. **Khan, F., Amatya, B., Ng, L.**, et al. (2015) Multidisciplinary rehabilitation after primary brain tumour treatment. *Cochrane Database Syst Rev*, **31**(1), CD009509.
17. **Capozzi, L. C., Boldt, K. R., Easaw, J.**, et al. (2016) Evaluating a 12-week exercise program for brain cancer patients. *Psychooncology*, **25**, 354–8.
18. **Hansen, A., Rosenbek Minet, L. K.**, et al. (2014) The effect of an interdisciplinary rehabilitation intervention comparing HRQoL, symptom burden and physical function among patients with primary glioma: an RCT study protocol. *BMJ Open*, **4**, e005490.
19. **Stone, J. B., DeAngelis, L. M.** (2016) Cancer-treatment-induced neurotoxicity--focus on newer treatments. *Nat Rev Clin Oncol*, **13**, 92–105.
20. **Verduin, M., Zindler, J. D., Martinussen, H. M.**, et al. (2017) Use of systemic therapy concurrent with cranial radiotherapy for cerebral metastases of solid tumors. *Oncologist*, **22**, 222–35.
21. **Argyriou, A. A., Assimakopoulos, K., Iconomou, G.**, et al. (2011) Either called 'chemobrain' or 'chemofog', the long-term chemotherapy-induced cognitive decline in cancer survivors is real. *J Pain Symptom Manage*, **41**, 126–39.
22. **Grober, S. E.** (2002) Resources for treatment of chemotherapy-related cognitive difficulty. *Cancer Pract*, **10**, 216–18.

23. **Nayak, L., DeAngelis, L. M., Brandes, A. A.**, et al. (2017) The Neurologic Assessment in Neuro-Oncology (NANO) scale: a tool to assess neurologic function for integration into the Response Assessment in Neuro-Oncology (RANO) criteria. *Neuro Oncol*, **19**, 625–35.
24. **Boykoff, N., Moieni, M., Subramanian, S. K.** (2009) Confronting chemobrain: an in-depth look at survivors' reports of impact on work, social networks, and health care response. *J Cancer Surviv*, **3**, 223–32.
25. **Hudson, M. M., Ness, K. K., Gurney, J. G.**, et al. (2013) Clinical ascertainment of health outcomes among adults treated for childhood cancer. *JAMA*, **309**, 2371–81.
26. **Beets, G., Sebag-Montefiore, D., Andritsch, E.**, et al. (2017) ECCO essential requirements for quality cancer care: colorectal cancer. A critical review. *Crit Rev Oncol Hematol*, **110**, 81–93.

Chapter 26

Advocacy in dementia

Gorazd B. Stokin

Introduction

Disorders of the mind, which include also dementia with its most disparate behavioural and cognitive features, have notoriously been among the hardest to understand by the patients, families, and the outside world. Logic for this hardship in understanding disorders of the mind ranges from the severe stigmatization spanning across many centuries and most diverse cultures, which traditionally and categorically repelled societies from engaging to understand disorders of the mind, to the relatively late comprehension and translation of the function and dysfunction of the brain to the outside world. Bearing this heritage in mind, dementia has long been defined and interpreted rather differently in different time periods and by different schools of thought and for long ignored as a modern medical entity known today.

Dementia as a modern medical entity can be defined as an acquired and most commonly progressive behavioural and cognitive deficit severe enough to interfere significantly with independency in activities of daily living lasting for more than 6 months and not associated with alterations of consciousness. Today a new case of dementia occurs worldwide every 4.1 seconds.[1] In practical terms, this means that the world faces almost 15 new people needing full support by others in their basic everyday activities every minute. Intriguingly, it was only in the 1970s that Alzheimer's disease has been demonstrated as the major cause of dementia in older people.[2] This finding by Robert Katzman and colleagues not only linked dementia to a specific disease, namely Alzheimer's disease, but it provided credible evidence that refuted the long-standing dogma that dementia in older people corresponds to physiological ageing including age-related vascular changes as the prime aetiopathogenic mechanism leading to dementia. It took almost two decades to translate this finding into common knowledge and this would not have happened if not for successful dementia advocacy!

Dementia progresses through various stages, which all bring different needs to the patients, families, and caregivers and as such ignite different advocacy agendas. In brief, while early stage dementia allows significant independency with a wealth of possible activities and a fairly good quality of life, late-stage dementia brings difficulties with orientation in time and space, erosion of cognitive functions from learning and memory and execution to speech, and difficulties with motor functions eventually leading all to become invariably mute, incontinent, and bedridden. These inherent characteristics of dementia largely prevent dementia patients to act as independent advocates for their diseases. That said, dementia is preceded by a stage where behavioural and cognitive decline does not as of yet interfere significantly with independency in activities of daily living, known as mild cognitive impairment.[3] Mild cognitive impairment offers an excellent window of opportunity for patients on their possible journey to dementia to become proactive and engaged in dementia advocacy. More recent findings suggest that mild cognitive impairment may be preceded on its own by a stage where subjective feeling of behavioural and cognitive decline is not objectivized, known as subjective cognitive impairment.[4]

Although further studies are needed to better understand the relationship between subjective and mild cognitive impairment those afflicted by subjective cognitive impairment represent without any doubt potential 'new breed' of dementia advocates. Although patients with diseases leading to dementia eventually lose their independency in activities of daily living, significant support is available to help them contribute to advocacy efforts. In fact, dementia patients together with their families, caregivers, physicians, scientists, and many others represent a rock-solid body of advocates with an outstanding track record bound to future successes.

Advocacy in dementia

How did advocacy in dementia contribute to dementia care and continues shaping its future? Merit goes to a large extent to the fast pace by which understanding about Alzheimer's disease evolved, which inspired patients, families, physicians, scientists, and many others to develop diverse grassroots movements many of which unified under large advocacy umbrellas. This eventually translated into significant changes in perception and care of dementia globally and into an immediate call for action to assist and serve the ones in need appropriately and with dignity. Importantly, accumulating knowledge about other major diseases leading to dementia, ranging from frontotemporal and Lewy body dementia to vascular diseases and traumatic brain injury, soon followed the path paved by advances in Alzheimer's disease and reinforced dementia advocacy further. More specifically, considering the majority of these diseases present with unique features and difficulties that differ from those observed in Alzheimer's disease, advocacy for these diseases not only strengthened, but also significantly diversified the objectives of advocacy in dementia. In example, hallucinations were only critically addressed in dementia when visual hallucinations were identified as a salient feature of Lewy body dementia.[5]

What motivated and continues motivating patients, families, scientists, physicians, and many others to advocate for dementia? The reasons motivating individuals and organizations to become advocates for dementia are most diverse and originate from personal experiences and frustrations that dementia care is insufficient and needs to improve at local, regional, national, and international levels. At the same time, however, like with any other neurological, medical, or other cause translating into advocacy, it is the inherent characteristics of the cause that carve the objectives of advocacy. In case of dementia these inherent characteristics are, first, that societies have difficulties understanding and accepting behavioural and cognitive deficit such as loss of memory. This contrasts with the relative ease with which they understand

and accept many other diseases such as broken bone or heart attack. Second, the vast majority of diseases underlying dementia remain without a cure. This is a powerful motivation for patients, families, caregivers, physicians, and scientists at large to advocate for more research and its funding with the goal of finding efficient therapies. Third, most diseases that produce dementia have a prolonged course, lasting several years, and this thoroughly wears off families and caregivers. Helping someone with dementia is not a sprint, but a marathon! Exceptions to these diseases leading to dementia, which classically protract over several years, are those causing rapidly progressive dementias (Table 26.1).

These diseases, which still keep being discovered, lead to dementia in less than 2 years from timely diagnosis. Such an example is variant Creutzfeldt–Jakob's disease, also known as the 'mad cow disease', which threatened an epidemic and presented a significant public concern, but managed to become sufficiently contained also thanks to assertive advocacy.[6] Although rapidly progressive dementia carries a notoriously poor prognosis, percentage of diseases leading to rapidly progressive dementia that can be cured turns out to be higher compared with diseases manifesting as classical 'slowly' progressive dementia. This turned out to be a powerful momentum efficiently exploited by advocates raising awareness about autoimmune dementias in particular. Forth, many diseases resulting in dementia manifest with most bizarre constellations of symptoms ranging from hallucinations and delusions to aggression, disinhibition, and nightmares. Many find these symptoms hard to understand, act upon, and solve and this brings this specific symptomatology frequently to the objective of advocacy. Last, but not least, yet perhaps most importantly, dementia care is all around far from optimal, in particular, in low- to mid-income countries, which host the majority of

Table 26.1 Basic characteristics of some of the more common diseases causing dementia

Disease	Causes	Age of onset	Progression*	Treatable
Alzheimer's	sporadic	>65 years old	slow	no
	familial rare		can be rapid	
Frontotemporal	sporadic	<65 years old	slow	no
	familial common			
Lewy body	sporadic	>65 years old	slow	no
	familial rare		can be rapid	
Creutzfeldt–Jakob	sporadic	teens and older	rapid	no
	familial rare			
Autoimmune	sporadic	teens and older	rapid	some
	familial rare			

* Slow progression typically takes 5–15 years, while rapid progression frequently less than 2 years to death. Includes autoimmune dementias such as the anti-NMDA autoimmune encephalitis.

dementia cases. This represents the basis for extensive grassroots movements across the globe with the simple objective of making any change that results in improvement in dementia care a reality.

In contrast to diverse motivations that drive people to advocate dementia care, the advocacy approaches exploited by advocates in their successes are well studied and established. First and foremost, they all rely on impeccable planning in all its steps. Considering advocacy often touches powerful people and organizations, involves public exposure and identifies clearly advocates sticking their neck out, there is simply no space for poor planning in successful dementia advocacy! In other words, successful planning involves defining clearly what problem, shortcoming, or need to develop, update, or otherwise improve will be the objective of the advocacy. And then studying in detail all the facts and the environment, including all the parties involved, to ascertain that select objective can be addressed realistically without major risks in a timely manner. In practice, one should first ask what issue about dementia care is really important, as well as who and why will support and oppose this really important issue? To this end, one needs to clarify how best to convince supporters and as many opponents as possible to accept and support proposed change in dementia care. Moreover, if there are many issues about dementia care one feels strong about, then it might be of benefit to prioritize them based on what are the most important issues, which can be addressed most readily. In this situation all different issues can be economically unified into a single overreaching goal, which can be elegantly structured into short-, mid-, and long-term objectives. Once advocacy objectives are clear each of them requires its own action plan. Action plan consists in specific steps and timeline needed to reach the set objective in addition to identifying needed resources ranging from people and organizations to funding and space. An important role in each action plan is played by its public relations strategy, which consists in developing a clear message, along with a sticky 'soundbite' to be presented repeatedly to the supporting audience, opponents, and public at large by any possible means including various social media. In short, action plans need to be specific, measurable, attainable, realistic, and timely as mnemonically summarized in the acronym SMART (Specific, Measurable, Assignable, Realistic, Time-related). To date, advocacy in neurology, including dementia, advanced to the point that it already proved its impact and significance and as such started being regularly thought to the neurologists. As a result, there are today numerous useful resources available to existing and future advocates in dementia (Box 26.1) with the prime example in advocacy training run by the Palatucci Advocacy Leadership Forum of the American Academy of Neurology.[7]

Past, current, and future endeavours in dementia advocacy can be summarized best by taking into account 5Ws and the H, namely, who, why, when, where, what, and how. Who identifies the advocates, why touches upon their motivation, when describes the Zeitgeist momentum of the advocate, where tells about the environment of the advocate, what explains the objective tackled by the advocate and how reveals the undertaken advocacy strategy. Advocacy in the field of dementia can be divided into the one carried out by patients, families, and caregivers, physicians and scientists, and professional, profit, and non-profit organizations.

Box 26.1 Resources for advocacy in dementia*

Tools for dementia advocates

Community Tool Box—Developing a plan for advocacy

http://ctb.ku.edu/en/table-of-contents/advocacy/advocacy-principles/advocacy-plan/main

South Central Library System Advocacy—Developing ad advocacy plan

http://www.scls.info/pr/advocacy/plan.html

Association for career and technical education—Advocacy Toolkit

https://acteonline.org/advocacy/

American Library Association Advocacy Institute—The Advocacy Action Plan Workbook

http://www.ala.org/advocacy/sites/ala.org.advocacy/files/content/advleg/advocacyinstitute/Advocacy%20Action%20Plan%20-%20revised%2001-09.pdf

Dementia advocacy programmes

Society for Neuroscience

http://www.sfn.org/Advocacy/US-Advocacy-Programs

American Academy of Neurology

https://www.aan.com/go/advocacy/active/palf

Alzheimer Europe

http://www.alzheimer-europe.org

Alzheimer's Association

http://www.alz.org/advocacy/take-action.asp

Alzheimer's Disease International

https://www.alz.co.uk

World Health Organization

http://www.who.int/mediacentre/factsheets/fs362/en/

* The presented materials represent a sample of available tools and programmes in the English-speaking world, while recognizing those available in different languages and different countries.

Patients

Although patients frequently represent the most avid advocates for their neurological diseases, this is not quite the case in dementia advocacy considering its nature precludes most patients from being independently and proactively involved. Accordingly, patients with dementia contribute to advocacy most efficiently when having subjective and mild cognitive impairment, or early stage dementia at most. As dementia advocates they raise awareness about dementia and provide support to dementia care in all aspects of the disease whether physical, emotional, organizational, or financial. A good example of such advocacy is Glen Campbell,[8] an American country icon, who has gone public with his fight against Alzheimer's disease and continued singing on tour while in the early stages of Alzheimer's disease and dementia. In this specific case, Campbell acted as an advocate raising significantly awareness of dementia among his fans and beyond. Another powerful example of patient advocacy in dementia is provided by all those patients with dementia who participate in the patient initiatives organized by Alzheimer Europe, which promotes hearing from and involving patients with Alzheimer's disease and dementia in its agenda. These patients raise awareness of dementia in particular among those directly involved in advancing dementia care such as decision makers and politicians. These patients fuel decision makers and politicians with first-hand description of the problems they are facing while coping with dementia. Last, but not least, is the example of advocacy for a rather recent curable disease-causing rapidly progressive dementia known as anti-NMDA autoimmune encephalitis. Patient Susannah Cahalan describes her experience in battling anti-NMDA autoimmune encephalitis in her book *Brain on Fire—My Month of Madness*.[9] By publicizing her encounter with the anti-NMDA autoimmune encephalitis she explains her experience and success in fighting dementia and thus raises awareness about this new and largely unknown disease. This is of major relevance considering anti-NMDA and many other autoimmune encephalitides, which manifest clinically with dementia, can be successfully treated if recognized in a timely manner.

Families and caregivers

Families experiencing dementia face significant hurdles in their effort to provide the best possible care irrespectively of their status and country of their stay. First, in most cases, when they are initially informed about the diagnosis they learn that there is no cure for the disease-causing dementia. This is always shocking, in particular, if their loved one is younger. Second, they need to learn and accept that their loved one is changed forever and that further changes for the worse will take place. This is particularly difficult for families of patients with rapidly progressive dementia such as sporadic Creutzfeldt–Jakob's disease. The vast majority of families experiences hardship understanding and accepting that their loved one is not quite the same any longer, does not always remember what they recently talked about, and eventually will not recognize their names and faces nor the home as remotely familiar. Particularly difficult to understand and accept for these families is the reality that their loved ones cannot be entrusted many of the everyday duties they have been involved with in the past and that they need increasingly more support in carrying out the very basic daily activities. Importantly, as the time goes by, many families realize that support offered by healthcare and other services does not meet their needs any longer. This is particularly true in advanced dementia where palliative care plays a major role in providing the best possible quality of life and in securing appropriate dignity.

While satisfaction during early medical visits, including diagnostics, may vary depending on the individual healthcare services, location, and country, all families realize sooner or later that they need more dementia care and this one is rarely, if ever, available. They need professional and yet practical advice on how to cope with dementia when their loved one's dementia progresses in its journey. In example, they want to know what to do when dementia precludes their loved ones from understanding why showering or when incontinence becomes incipient and dementia erases subconscious controlled execution of the most obvious in an appropriate action. Third, patients with dementia need regular follow ups to monitor optimal therapeutic measures as well as to identify possible troublesome behavioural changes. Behavioural changes, such as suicidal ideation, depression, apathy, and aggression in Alzheimer's disease and post-traumatic encephalopathy, disinhibition, and various peculiar habits witnessed in frontotemporal dementia and hallucinations, delusions, and nightmares in Lewy body dementia, are all in need of appropriate diagnostics and therapeutic measures. This is often not the case and thus becomes particularly disturbing for the families. And last, but not least, as dementia progresses and families do not manage to provide sufficient and complete care for their loved ones any longer they seek help and realize that transferring their loved one to a dementia care centre is frequently bureaucratically cumbersome and commonly rather costly. All of these reasons, together with many others that are not mentioned here due to space limitation, make families prime advocates for dementia as they experience difficulties with dementia care and this ignites the motivation to advocate for the better.

An excellent example of how family members almost naturally become dementia advocates originates from a recent encounter during a visit by a patient and her family from a less developed country. Discussing the diagnosis of dementia of her mother, the daughter started brainstorming how will she manage? In short, since her father does not know how to cook and clean and does not want to ask for help in town as he does not want people to know what is going on with his wife, she has been travelling every weekend to her home town to cook and clean. At the same time she has a demanding job, plans to get married, and looks forward to having a family of her own. Soon after starting to think aloud she realized that she knows others with parents and other family members suffering from dementia and that possibly the only reasonable way to solve this issue would be to set up a dementia group, which would take care of their loved ones in a newly developed dementia care centre. Although today no one knows whether this idea of a novel grassroots movement will ever start and translate into a dementia care centre the story as such depicts first-hand the difficulties faced by families when confronted with dementia and the momentum that transforms a family member into an 'accidental' advocate. There are several other excellent examples of dementia advocacy by family members. Such an example is Brenda Bouchard of New Hampshire who provides care to her mother and husband and uses her voice to champion the cause at the annual Advocacy Forum of the Alzheimer's Association.[10] Further examples are provided by Nancy Reagan and Maria Shriver, who as public figures contributed immensely to raising awareness about dementia, dementia research, and dementia care in general as a legacy to their beloved husband and father, respectively. Last, but not least, one needs not to forget and acknowledge advocacy by caregivers who are not personally involved in having their family members afflicted by dementia. In fact, empathy, compassion and lengthy experience working with people with dementia makes numerous caregivers strong advocates as on one side they understand complexity of dementia care, while on the other side they witness first-hand lack of efficient chain of care in dementia.

Physicians and scientists

Physicians, most frequently general practitioners, neurologists, psychiatrists, and geriatricians, are directly involved in the diagnostics, therapeutics, follow-up, and care in general for patients with dementia. As such they are on one side regularly exposed to hardship and difficulties faced by their patients and families, while on the other side experience successes and limitations of the healthcare services they are part of in the attempt to provide the best possible care. As a result, the empathy and compassion they sense regularly, together with their determination to do their best for the patients, puts them into a unique position to advocate for better dementia care. The ones taking advantage of this opportunity to become dementia advocates engage in most diverse agendas ranging from securing access and optimizing time spent with physicians, including promotion of telemedicine, improving the quality of, and implementing novel diagnostic methods and providing novel therapeutic approaches. These approaches range from clinical trials, to participating in advocacy forums, such as recently popularized Alzheimer cafes,[11] promoting development and improvement of memory clinics and dementia centres, and providing their expert knowledge to governmental and other organizations involved in dementia care.

Dementia advocacy by a physician is exemplified by Aleš Kogoj, a psychiatrist from Slovenia, who together with a handful of colleagues founded 'Forget me not', Alzheimer Slovenia, in 1997 and soon after developed a gerontopsychiatric unit offering inpatient and outpatient, including day-care, services almost exclusively to patients with dementia in addition to contributing continuously to national guidelines for dementia diagnostics, therapeutics, and dementia care in general.[12] Another excellent example is represented by Daniel Potts, neurologist from Alabama, who became an avid dementia advocate witnessing the transformation of his father from a saw miller to a painter on his journey with Alzheimer's disease. This experience led Potts to become a proactive dementia advocate by co-authoring several books[13] focusing on improving caregiving and serving as the national media spokesman for Alzheimer's and related diseases by the American Academy of Neurology among other activities. One more example is provided by Robert Will, neurologist from Scotland, who founded the Creutzfeldt–Jakob Surveillance Unit in United Kingdom, later extended this effort to a global surveillance network, contributed significantly to the discovery of variant Creutzfeldt–Jakob disease, while advocating continuously for better understanding and care of patients with Creutzfeldt–Jakob's disease and rapidly progressive dementia.[14]

Several other dementia experts ranging from psychologists, dementia nurses, and social workers contribute significantly as dementia advocates. In fact, dementia advocacy would not be the same without them! Motivation for their advocacy stems from empathy, compassion, and encountering roadblocks on their way helping patients with dementia. An excellent example is Beth Johnson, a Red Cross nurse from Stoke-on-Trent, who devoted her life to caregiving. She established the Beth Johnson Foundation, which is proactively involved in advocacy for better dementia care.[15] A more recent example is provided by the initiative of Admiral Nurses of the Dementia UK who devote their work exclusively to help, improve, and advocate on behalf of people afflicted by dementia.[16]

Poor efficacy of current therapeutic approaches, together with the fact that the vast majority of diseases causing dementia remain incurable, puts neuroscientists in the spotlight to advance our understanding of the mechanisms underlying development of diseases causing dementia to the point that will allow designing more efficient therapies—if not cures. As a result, there is a great demand by the patients, families, and the public in general to learn whether and when will the next scientific discoveries bring better diagnostics and above all therapeutics of dementias. Neuroscientists commonly respond promptly to these demands and many of them develop into skilful advocates in dementia. Rationale for neuroscientists to advocate dementia is manifold, but often lies in their altruistic desire to be connected and understand dementia and to share their knowledge and discoveries with people afflicted by dementia as well as with those who invariably contribute to dementia research. Moreover, neuroscientists contribute to advocacy in many other ways such as serving as advisors and spokesmen for diverse research institutions, foundations, industry, and governmental organizations all involved in advancing dementia care. Excellent examples of neuroscientists advocating dementia globally are provided by John Hardy, a geneticist from England, who played a pivotal role in linking faulty genes to Alzheimer's and related disorders and by Ronald Peterson, a neurologist from Minnesota, who furthered our understanding of early stages of Alzheimer's diseases, including major contribution to defining mild cognitive impairment.

Non-governmental organizations

Professional associations provide umbrellas that unify, promote, and propel various dementia related activities into the future. In brief, such associations raise awareness about dementia, provide educational tools for patients, families, caregivers, general public as well as for scientists and healthcare providers, organize a plethora of meetings and conferences, which allow for continued learning and exchange of experiences about dementia, raise funding to support research and advance dementia care initiatives further, serve as dementia experts in regional, national, and international organizations and as such provide excellence in advocacy and advocacy resources about dementia.

Example of a professional association advocating for dementia is the Alzheimer's Association. Founded in 1980, The Alzheimer's Association, which provides patients, families, and public at large with extensive and most practical information about dementia, including behavioural and other features accompanying dementia, recruits patients with dementia and families to get involved in furthering dementia care, supports research to gain new knowledge about dementia with the aim of ultimately finding better therapies, updates patients and their families about new and ongoing clinical trials, offers valuable resources to healthcare professionals involved in dementia care and acts as the major pillar in representing, advocating, and fighting for dementia locally, nationally, and internationally. Furthermore, Alzheimer's Association raises awareness and contributes to dementia care in many other ways, in example, about a decade ago Alzheimer's Association contributed to making the exhibition of William Utermohlen, painter from Philadelphia, exploring his personal experience with Alzheimer's disease through the paintings, a reality.[17] There are several excellent professional organizations involved in dementia advocacy besides Alzheimer's Association, which include among others Alzheimer Europe, which focuses extensively on dementia programmes and policies, Alzheimer's Disease International, which promotes global dementia advocacy and many others such as the Alzheimer Society Canada and the Alzheimer's Australia. Importantly, all other major diseases causing dementia also have their own professional associations, such as the Lewy Body Society, the Association for Frontotemporal Degeneration, and the Brain Injury Society, among others.

In the past decade governments have finally acknowledged the overreaching threat of a dementia epidemic and as a result many governments have recognized dementia as their top healthcare priority. This has automatically transformed governments into dementia advocates, which translates into increased funding for dementia care and, particularly in Europe, to a significant effort to develop national strategies and action plans to fight dementia. Along the same lines, the World Health Organization has recognized dementia as a major health threat to the humanity worldwide and in response drafted the Global Action Plan on the Public Health Response to Dementia 2017–2025. Similarly, the United Nations recently recognized dementia as an important cause of morbidity that contributes to the global non-communicable disease burden and concluded that non-communicable disease prevention programmes and healthcare interventions need to provide equitable access to effective programmes for these illnesses.

Healthcare organizations, including healthcare providers and insurance companies, often provide communities with information about dementia care. Although their primary goal is to a large extent to offer their services to the community, they also play an important role in advocacy of dementia care. Considering majority of people relies on healthcare organizations for their healthcare and therefore consult with them regularly, these organizations represent an often overlooked, but powerful player in dementia advocacy. Similar is true for the pharma industry. Although the pharma industry has been notoriously perceived as driven primarily by profit, its research and development plays a major role in designing, testing, and producing novel therapies. In line with this thought, the industry does contribute significantly to advocacy of dementia care in addition to raising awareness about dementia, being involved in educating about dementia, and in many other dementia-related activities.

Discussions

Current state of the art advocacy in dementia offers to established and aspiring advocates an unprecedented number of tools, programmes, and other resources, which have already been proven to be efficient and successful. Despite all of these each advocacy objective is intimately linked to specific motivation, bold judgement, diverse experiences, and skills unique to every individual advocate. Furthermore, each advocacy objective is specific to the environment where is should be carried out and as such brings along specifics regarding the people, including their set of mind, customs and traditions, and particularities of involved organizations from the economical, legal, and political perspective. Accordingly, despite of all the available tools, programmes, and other resources, each advocacy objective needs to be considered to be exclusive in its own right. This means that each and every advocacy objective needs to be evaluated based on advocates strengths and weaknesses and the knowledge about the specific environment individually. To this end, advocates may benefit greatly by bringing aboard an experienced advocate as a mentor, or by engaging in brainstorming sessions with their close and trustworthy peers. Such an approach will increase the odds that selected objective will be fulfilled realistically and in a timely manner. Importantly, while selecting their objective, each advocate needs to evaluate all the risks involved in carrying out the action plan specific to the objective. One ought to remember that advocacy brings around changes and although these changes are for the better of those afflicted by dementia and/or involved in dementia care, such changes may not be in advantage of everyone and thus not supported and accepted by all.

Moreover, such changes may lead to resistance and opposition, which most commonly targets the advocate and not all advocates are able or ready to take it. To this end, advocates need to reflect whether there is enough strength and commitment to withstand possible 'counter-advocacy', which may involve public scrutiny and confrontation with powerful individuals and organizations. Last, but not least, advocates need to address whether they are in any conflict of interest when entertaining their objective since direct personal benefit driving advocacy objective is most likely bound to failure. Bearing all of these in mind, advocates in dementia are desperately needed considering that, despite all of the successes in dementia advocacy, challenges ranging from the need for earlier diagnostics and more efficient therapeutics to optimizing timely dementia care, in particular, in low- to mid-income countries, remain unsolved. So this is the call for dementia advocates to rise and shine!

Acknowledgement

This work was supported by the European Social Fund and European Regional Development Fund Project Magnet No. CZ 02.1.01 /0.0/0.015_003/0000492.

References

1. **World Health Organization** (2005) The epidemiology and impact of dementia. Current state and future trends. Available at: http://www.who.int/mental_health/neurology/dementia/en
2. **Katzman, R.** (1976) Editorial: The prevalence and malignancy of Alzheimer's disease. A major killer. *Arch Neurol*, **33**(4), 217–8.
3. **Stokin, G. B.**, **Krell-Roesch, J.**, **Petersen, R. C.**, **Geda, Y. E.** (2015) Mild cognitive impairment—an old wine in a new bottle. *Harv Rev Psychiatry*, **23**(5), 367–76.

4. **Reisberg, B., Gauthier, S.** (2008) Current evidence for subjective cognitive impairment (SCI) as a pre-mild cognitive impairment (MCI) stage if subsequently manifest Alzheimer's disease. *Int Psychogeriatr*, **20**(1), 1–16.
5. **Ballard C., McKeith I., Harrison R., et al.** (1997) A detailed phenomenological comparison of complex visual hallucinations in dementia with Lewy bodies and Alzheimer's disease. *Int Psychogeriatr*, **9**(4), 381–8.
6. **Cousens, S., Smith, P. G., Ward, H., et al.** (2001) Geographical distribution of variant Creutzfeldt–Jakob disease in Great Britain 1994–2000. *Lancet*, **357**(9261), 1002–7.
7. **American Academy of Neurology**. Palatucci Advocacy Leadership Forum. Available at: https://www.aan.com/conferences-community/leadership-programs/palatucci-advocacy-leadership/
8. **Peoplecelebrity** (22 June 22 2011) Available at: http://people.com/celebrity/singer-glen-campbells-alzheimers-diagnosis/
9. **Cahalan, S.** (2012) *Brain of Fire—My Month of Madness*. New York: Free Press.
10. **Alzheimer's Association**. Standing strong on shifting sand: An Alzheimer's Advocate's Story. Available at: http://blog.alz.org/standing-strong-on-shifting-sand-an-alzheimers-advocates-story/
11. **Alzheimer's Aid Society of Northern California**. Available at: http://alzaid.org/AlzCafe.html
12. **Talan, J.** (2016) News from the Palatucci Advocacy Forum: bringing a national dementia plan to Slovenia. *Neurology Today*, **16**(10), 7.
13. **Potts, D. C., Woodward Potts, E.** (2011) *A Pocket Guide for the Alzheimer's Caregiver*. Tuscaloosa, AL: Dementia Dynamics, LLC.
14. **Creutzfeldt–Jakob Disease International Support Alliance**. Available at: http://cjdisa.com/friends-and-advisors-group/professor-robert-will-md/
15. **Beth Johnson Foundation**. Who was Beth Johnson? Available at: https://www.bjf.org.uk/about-us/who-was-beth-johnson
16. **DementiaUK**. Helping families face dementia. Admiral nursing. Available at: https://www.dementiauk.org/how-we-help/admiral-nursing/
17. **Harrison, E. M.** (2013) Understanding suffering: Utermohlen's self-portraits and Alzheimer's disease. *Nurse Education*, **38**(1), 20–5.

Chapter 27

Advocating for orphan diseases in neurology

Fritz Zimprich

Introduction

As can be seen throughout this book, advocacy in all its forms is key to improving the situation of patients disadvantaged by a disease. This is particularly true for patients with so-called rare disorders, who face several problems on top of those experienced by patients with more common diseases.[1,2] Rare diseases are defined as life-threatening or chronically debilitating disorders that affect less than 1 in 2,000 individuals in the European Union (EU) or fewer than 2,000 individuals in the United States. Although heterogeneous in a medical sense, from an advocacy and political perspective rare disorders are often summed up under a common group because sufferers of these conditions share a number of similar problems.[1,3-5]

Although the name 'rare' would, at first glance, suggest that the problems associated with these diseases are infrequent ones because of the rarity of the individual disorders themselves, in fact the opposite is true. Due to the large number of different disorders—there are between 5,000 and 8,000 rare diseases on record—a considerable proportion of the population is affected by one or the other rare disease. In Europe, it is estimated that between 6% and 8% of all people suffer from a rare condition.[1,2,5,6]

Despite their high aggregate numbers, rare diseases have been historically neglected in comparison to disorders with a more frequent prevalence, which is why they received the meaningful alternative label as orphan diseases. The historical low priority attached to orphan diseases has led to numerous tangible problems for affected patients and their families.[5]

Problems patients with rare diseases face

The low awareness and comparatively limited knowledge among most health professionals (disregarding a few dedicated experts) for any individual rare disease means the patients and their families usually face a long delay before their disease is diagnosed. It is not unusual for years or even decades to pass from the first symptoms until the condition is correctly identified. In the intervening period, patients not only suffer from the uncertainty of not knowing their diagnosis but also have to bear unnecessary medical interventions.[1-3,5]

A second frequently encountered problem is that, due to the often very limited information on the natural history of rare diseases, sufferers are left with many unanswered questions about their future prognosis or how to lead their lives. The lack of familiarity of medical doctors with the sparse but available literature compounds this problem and forces patients and their families to become experts themselves. Expert patients are, however, often viewed with suspicion by medical professionals.[7-11]

Another problem is the increasingly fragmented nature of medical services along different medical specialties or even subspecialties. Patients with rare (i.e. genetic) diseases often have multisystemic organ manifestations, which means that they have to negotiate with different professionals to get their symptoms treated in an environment where communication between specialists is not automatic.[3,12-14]

Such experiences are indeed reality and common place. This was clearly documented in a survey by EURORDIS, an umbrella organization for patients with rare diseases in Europe. As summarized in their book *The Voice of 12,000 Patients*, 25% of patients had to wait between 5 and 30 years for the correct diagnosis and had to consult 20 physicians on their way to the final diagnosis. Some 18% reported rejection by medical professionals because of their complex problems and, on average, patients needed nine medical services for their treatment, which they experienced as poorly coordinated.[13]

Perhaps most importantly, there is a lack of specific treatments for the overwhelming majority of rare diseases. The development of drugs for rare disorders is challenging due to a number of reasons. Given the small markets for such drugs, the financial incentives for pharmaceutical companies are limited from the outset. Moreover, clinical trials are more difficult to perform in rare diseases due to recruitment problems or getting patients to the trial sites and due to the lack of natural history data or proven outcome parameters among other issues. This results in a lower success rate of clinical trials for orphan drugs in comparison to non-orphan drugs.[8] Not counting specific therapies, the focus of medical care therefore only lies in the improvement of the patients' quality of life by a pure symptomatic treatment of complications.[1-3,15,16]

In the minority of cases where treatments exist, patients often face problems of getting access to these treatments. Orphan drugs are usually very expensive on a per patient basis. Therefore, healthcare providers, if they pay for the drugs at all, may restrict the reimbursement to subgroups, such as they were (maybe very narrowly) defined in clinical trials or tie their approval to other hurdles. In addition, on their way to get approval for orphan drugs patients may experience the general misconception and prejudice that public financing for their expensive therapies will exhaust the limited resources of healthcare systems.[1,2,17,18]

It must be borne in mind that the above-mentioned problems come in addition to those caused by the disorder itself. As most rare diseases are genetic in origin they particularly affect young patients, who are thus doubly disadvantaged as the disease often negatively influences normal development or may be associated with a severe disability. Combined these problems may lead to a substantial financial and social burden for the affected families.[3]

Given all these difficulties, the unmet needs and the high total number of patients, it can be said that rare diseases represent one on the most important and challenging issues facing our health systems today. Advocacy groups for rare diseases have recognized this problem for decades and have been lobbying for an improvement of the situation on behalf of their patients.[2,5,17]

In fact, mainly owing to the pressure of advocates for patients with rare diseases governments and healthcare providers are increasingly acknowledging these deficits and have initiated and promoted various action plans or have even enacted specific legislation to improve the care for patients with orphan diseases.[2,4,5,19,20] In other instances advocacy groups have directly acted to correct disadvantageous situations. The following paragraphs will highlight a few illustrative examples of such successful direct or indirect advocacy activities. But first, the question must be addressed who advocates for patients with rare diseases.

Who advocates for patients with rare diseases?

There are of course many different types of advocacy and advocates that may play a role for rare diseases as for other disorders. With regards to rare diseases, there are however two types of advocates that stand out: patient advocacy groups and advocacy by medical professionals.

Patient advocacy groups

Due to their unmet needs, patients with rare diseases themselves or their relatives started to organize themselves into patient support groups. Apart from a few early exceptions this process began in the second half of the last century and really took off in the 1990s when the numbers of such groups grew rapidly. Initially, patient support groups were usually concerned with patient education and with practical and psychological support for their members. With time, many of these organizations evolved into highly professional 'disease advocacy organizations' also known as patient advocacy groups (PAG) with a much broader scope of aims.[4,10,21-28] Examples of individual patient advocacy groups are the support groups for lysosomal storage diseases or Duchenne muscular dystrophy or pseudoxanthoma elasticum to name just a few.[22,25,28,29] In an attempt to join their efforts and increase their weight umbrella organizations were eventually formed, such as the National Organization for Rare Disorders (NORD) with over 250 individual member patient advocacy groups, the Genetic Alliance, a coalition of over 600 disease advocacy organizations or the European Organisation for Rare Diseases (Eurordis) with over 700 member organizations (Table 27.1).

When patient support groups started to take on a more active advocacy role they faced, as lay organizations, initial resistance from the professional medical community. It was however soon realized that PAG can play an enormously important role in advancing the cause of rare diseases in several ways. They can be crucial in bringing forward research for rare diseases or the development of orphan drugs. They are able to motivate the public and may trigger supporting political changes, and they can connect research groups, pharmaceutical companies, and other stakeholders with each other and get them to focus on the important goals.[4,23,27]

In fact, the emergence of PAG is now commonly seen as one the most significant developments in the field of rare diseases. This has, for example, been acknowledged

Table 27.1 Selected Internet resources in the field of advocacy for rare diseases

Name	Description	References
National Organization for Rare Disorders (NORD)	An umbrella organization for patient advocacy groups	39
European Organisation for Rare Diseases (EURORDIS)	Alliance of patient advocacy organisations	40
Genetic Alliance	Alliance of patient advocacy organisations	41
Orphanet	A portal for rare diseases and orphan drugs	42
EU Rare Diseases	European Commission website on rare diseases	43
RD Action	EU programme that aims to improve knowledge on rare diseases and orphan drugs	44
The International Rare Diseases Research Consortium (IRDiRC)	Consortium that teams up researchers and organizations investing in rare diseases research	45
The Genetic and Rare Diseases Information Center (GARD)	NIH-financed programme to provide the public with access to current, reliable, and easy-to-understand information about rare or genetic diseases	46

by the National Institutes of Health (NIH)-funded Rare Diseases Clinical Research Network programme (RDCRN), which promotes the establishment of consortia for the research into closely related rare diseases.[21] Each consortium is required to include PAG as research partners. Within such networks, PAG are instrumental in reaching out to the patients' communities by disseminating information about the activities of the consortia, they help in recruiting patients for clinical studies or registries, and they may provide partial funding or logistic support for meetings. They are also considered essential for specifying the direction of research by bringing in the patients' perspective.

PAG, as non-profit organizations, are well suited for these tasks. They usually have a slender and flexible organizational structure with low maintenance costs relying on the voluntary work of their members. Most importantly, they are the stakeholders with the strongest incentive to advance research and drug development for their respective diseases and are therefore in a position to remain focused on their long-term aims.[30]

Several surveys have shown that, nowadays, most PAG are indeed engaged in research-related activities. Though many of the smaller volunteer organizations still struggle to reach their goals, there is now a growing body of literature and guidance by bigger advocacy groups or umbrella organizations to help them increase their effectiveness.[23]

Advocacy by medical professionals

Apart from patient advocacy groups, the support and advocacy of medical professionals can be crucial for individual patients but also for issues concerning rare diseases in general.[31,32] Physicians are used to committing themselves in their daily work to patients. Because of their professional experience and central position in the health system, they often have a good understanding what is needed by patients and how best to achieve it. Beyond this personal engagement for individual patients, many professional medical bodies also call for doctors to be engaged in public advocacy activities. The American Medical Association, for example, endorses actions by physicians 'to promote those social, economic, educational, and political changes that ameliorate the suffering and threats to human health and well-being that he or she identifies through his or her professional work and expertise'.[31] Indeed, there are many examples of how physicians have used their unique positions (i.e. the public trust they enjoy and the privileged access to decision makers in the health system, to the benefit of disadvantaged patient groups). The spectrum of possible advocacy actions is broad and ranges from advocating reallocation of resources at a local level to serve specific patient groups, to engagement with the media or advising politicians. However, it is also recognized that there is the need for more formal advocacy training at the postgraduate and even undergraduate level.[31,32]

Regarding rare diseases, the commitment to specialize in a rare disease field, to commit oneself to treat patients with the disease, to engage in clinical or basic research or to provide specific training and mentoring to younger colleagues in the field can be as well regarded as important forms of advocacy.

Examples of advocacy actions in the field of rare diseases

Which kinds of advocacy actions are in most demand? If we want to get an answer to this question we should consider the most urgent, unmet needs of patients with rare diseases.

Listening to patient advocacy groups, pressing problems are the usual delay of the diagnosis, the insufficient knowledge on rare diseases, the lack of effective treatments but also inadequate medical services and financial problems resulting from having to live with a chronic rare disease.

The last two points mainly call for policy or political actions to change the way healthcare systems are organized and often touch on questions of financial solidarity towards underprivileged members of the society.[3,5] The first mentioned needs, however, call for 'research advocacy' (i.e. efforts to promote research and drug development for rare diseases). Additionally, it is in this field where the most successful advocacy actions have been made in the last decades by PAGs and medical professionals. Some of these research-related achievements and open needs will be presented in the next few paragraphs.

Advocacy to empower patients and educational activities

Empowerment of patients (or caregivers) in the context of chronic diseases can be defined as the patient's ability to acquire information that will help her or him to communicate and cooperate with medical professionals to better manage their diseases. The World Health Organization views empowerment of patients as a 'prerequisite for health' and 'a self-care strategy of patient essential to improve health outcomes and quality of life'.[7] Empowerment is particularly necessary for patients with rare diseases, where the diseases-specific knowledge among medical professionals is less readily available. Though some healthcare professionals may still view expert patients with suspicion, it is now largely acknowledged that informed and empowered patients will have better health outcomes.[7]

With respect to educational advocacy, patient support groups have played a leading role. This includes the provision of comprehensible information about the nature of the diseases in question, any potential complications, how to adopt beneficial lifestyles, and how to navigate the respective healthcare system. Information is usually disseminated via the Internet, by printed material, or by direct individual contacts over telephone hotlines or in support group meetings. In general, the presented information is highly relevant and professional. Examples for this can be found on nearly every homepage of PAG, who often view this activity as their core task. Some organizations, such as the Myasthenia Gravis Foundation of America, even produce highly regarded educational material for medical professionals.

Finally, there is also an ever-increasing component of self-advocacy by patients, who use the Internet to collate information regarding their diseases from various sources, though this can also have drawbacks as the information is not curated and can lead to false or even dangerous advice.[33]

Political advocacy to change laws in favour of rare diseases

Well-targeted political advocacy by a patient organization can certainly have a major beneficial impact. Excellent examples for this are provided by the regulations regarding 'orphan drugs' (i.e. drugs for rare diseases) which were first enacted in the United States and later on in many other countries.[1,2,4,9,15,20,28,34,35] Historically, the development of drugs for rare disorders was severely neglected because of missing incentives for pharmaceutical companies which were reluctant to spend huge sums on drugs for a niche markets without a reasonable hope of achieving a return on their investment. In the 1980s the patient advocacy organization NORD campaigned to establish a more functional incentives system. This led in 1983 to the passing of the Orphan Drug Act which provides financial advantages to drug companies developing medicines for rare diseases, such as a prolonged market exclusivity or a waiver for certain fees.[1,15] This act has since been generally acknowledged as a landmark law and has certainly served patients with rare diseases well. More than 350 orphan drugs have been approved in the United States since this law, in comparison to 10 in the decade before the law.[1]

Another example of successful political advocacy can be seen in the recommendations concerning rare diseases issued by the European Council to its member states, which were made as a consequence of the raised awareness of the existing problems due to the incessant action of advocating groups. These recommendations include the specification of national action plans on rare diseases to promote relevant issues such as the identification of qualified centres of expertise for the diagnosis and care of rare diseases. The proposals also include many specific policies regarding the advancement of research and it was further recommended that patient representatives should be involved in all relevant activities such as issues of patient empowerment.[2]

Another form of important political advocacy is the indirect lobbying pursued by PAG on funding agencies to increase spending on research for rare diseases. A study investigating such activities has concluded that such lobbying has helped to increase the funding for rare disease programmes considerably.[36,37] This form of lobbying usually takes place via political channels, which results in the expression of political preferences on research topics and aims without interfering with the peer review process of research proposals.

Advocacy to influence research agendas and drug development

Research and drug development for rare diseases is in many respects more difficult in comparison to common diseases. Above all, it is a bigger challenge to achieve the gold standard of large randomized placebo-controlled trials because of the lower number of patients that can be recruited and because outcome parameters are mostly less well developed.[1,2,15] In addition, it has to be considered that patients with a serious disease and a lack of other options, as is often the case with rare diseases, might be more willing to take risks when testing new drugs. For the same reason, it may be problematic to assign patients with a life-threatening disease on placebo when a drug with a reasonable chance of being effective is tested.[3,29]

Advocates for patients with rare diseases have also argued that clinical trials account too little for quality-of-life parameters or other outcomes valued by patients and their families. Small improvements perhaps not considered worthwhile by trial organizers in the quest for cures may be very important nonetheless for patients. Another frequent complaint is that inclusion criteria are too narrow disregarding patients who might otherwise contribute to the scientific knowledge in different trial designs.[3] Given these issues advocates for rare diseases have long demanded to allow exceptions from the otherwise strict rules regulatory bodies demand of new drugs as these often constitute too big hurdles.

As a result of these shortcomings PAG have become increasingly involved in the design of research agendas over the last decades. The need to do so was also acknowledged by funding bodies, such as the demand of the NIH to have PAG included as research partners in their RDCRN research consortia or by the creation of a Patient Centred Outcomes Research Institute. Similarly, in Europe, patient organizations may be co-funded and integrated in consortia by the European Research Programmes on Rare Diseases (as, for example, in E-rare call).[2,9,21,22]

An example of a very successful involvement of a patient advocacy group in the formulation of a research and drug development agenda is the case of the Parent Project Muscular Dystrophy group.[29] This advocacy group for muscular dystrophy managed, in collaboration with many different stakeholders, to prepare a draft guidance document on behalf of the Food and Drug Administration (FDA) to assist the industry in the development of drugs for Duchenne muscular dystrophy. In this document, many of the above-mentioned patients' views could be considered.

Research advocacy in the shape of various practical measures to support research and drug development

One of the main bottlenecks for research in rare diseases is the difficulty in recruiting sufficient patient numbers, be it for clinical studies or natural history studies. The latter type of study is considered a prerequisite for drug developments and the only way to characterize the phenotypic heterogeneity and the disease course of untreated patients. Many patient advocacy organizations have realized this obstacle and have started to organize disease registries to support and accelerate research by functioning as a resource of patients for studies.[8,10,21,23,27,30,38]

Some of the umbrella organizations even host special tools to facilitate the creation of international disease specific registries or contribute to biorepository databases for rare diseases (http://rarediseases.org/patient-orgs/registries).[38] The role of rare diseases advocates in directly supporting specific research projects can even go beyond that. Many organizations are active in direct fundraising to support favoured research programmes which might otherwise not receive financing or in other instances they might support individual young researchers in the hope of promoting a career in the field of the given rare disease.[21,23,32]

A third and very important practical way that advocacy groups can facilitate research is by acting as catalysts for studies (i.e. by promoting networks of scientists). They could simply achieve this by hosting meetings to bring interested researchers and other stakeholder such as members of the industry and government agencies together. They could also kick-start emerging research programmes by providing early funding. Being at the centre of such networks means that patient advocates also have the opportunity to communicate to researchers the relevant needs of patients and thus influence the direction of healthcare policy.[21,25,30]

Conclusions

Though patients with rare diseases are still exceptionally disadvantaged due to several problems related to the rarity of their disorders, things have started to improve for some disorders. This can be attributed to a large extent to the emergence of professional PAG and their successful engagement on several fronts.

The experience of the last decades has shown that there is a multitude of avenues by which advocacy actions can advance the scientific knowledge on rare diseases, the treatment options, and the care of patients suffering from those disorders. The task ahead will be to further develop this repertoire of possible advocacy measures and to successfully apply them to many more rare disorders.

References

1. **Tambuyzer, E.** (2010) Rare diseases, orphan drugs and their regulation: questions and misconceptions. *Nat Rev Drug Discov*, **9**(12), 921–9.

2. **Taruscio, D., Capozzoli, F., Frank, C.** (2011) Rare diseases and orphan drugs. *Ann Ist Super Sanita*, **47**(1), 83–93.
3. **Kesselheim, A. S., McGraw, S., Thompson, L., O'Keefe, K., Gagne, J. J.** (2014) Development and use of new therapeutics for rare diseases: views from patients, caregivers, and advocates. *Patient*, **8**(1), 75–84.
4. **Dunkle, M., Pines, W., Saltonstall, P. L.** (2010) Advocacy groups and their role in rare diseases research. In: Posada de la Paz, M., Groft, S. C. (eds). *Rare Diseases Epidemiology*. Dordrecht: Springer Netherlands, pp. 515–25. (Advances in Experimental Medicine and Biology; vol. 686).
5. **Forman, J., Taruscio, D., Llera, V. A., et al.** (2012) The need for worldwide policy and action plans for rare diseases. *Acta Paediatrica*, **101**(8), 805–7.
6. **Groft, S. C.** (2014) A past with uncertainty, a future with hope—rare disease day 2014 from a USA perspective. *Orphanet J Rare Dis*, **9**(1), 31.
7. **Aymé, S., Kole, A., Groft, S.** (2008) Empowerment of patients: lessons from the rare diseases community. *Lancet*, **371**(9629), 2048–51.
8. **Woodward, L., Johnson, S., Walle, J. V., et al.** (2016) An innovative and collaborative partnership between patients with rare disease and industry-supported registries: the Global aHUS Registry. *Orphanet J Rare Dis*, **11**(1), 154.
9. **Mechler, K., Mountford, W. K., Hoffmann, G. F., Ries, M.** (2015) Pressure for drug development in lysosomal storage disorders—a quantitative analysis thirty years beyond the US orphan drug act. *Orphanet J Rare Dis*, **10**(1), 249–9.
10. **Walkley, S. U., Davidson, C. D., Jacoby, J., et al.** (2016) Fostering collaborative research for rare genetic disease: the example of niemann-pick type C disease. *Orphanet J Rare Dis*, **11**, 161.
11. **Straub, V., Bertoli, M.** (2016) Where do we stand in trial readiness for autosomal recessive limb girdle muscular dystrophies? *Neuromuscul Disord*, **26**(2), 111–25.
12. **The Lancet, Editorial** (2009) Listening to patients with rare diseases. *Lancet*, **373**(9667), 868.
13. **EURORDIS** (2009) *The Voice of 12,000 Patients. Experiences and Expectations of Rare Disease Patients on Diagnosis and Care in Europe.* Available at: https://www.eurordis.org/IMG/pdf/voice_12000_patients/EURORDISCARE_FULLBOOKr.pdf
14. **Kent, A., Oosterwijk, C.** (2007) A patient and family perspective on gene therapy for rare diseases. *J Gene Med*, **9**(10), 922–3.
15. **Haffner, M. E.** (2006) Adopting orphan drugs—two dozen years of treating rare diseases. *N Engl J Med*, **354**(5), 445–7.
16. **Heemstra, H. E., van Weely, S., Büller, H. A., Leufkens, H. G. M., de Vrueh, R. L. A.** (2009) Translation of rare disease research into orphan drug development: disease matters. *Drug Discovery Today*, **14**(23–24), 1166–73.
17. **Schieppati, A., Henter, J.-I., Daina, E., Aperia, A.** (2008) Why rare diseases are an important medical and social issue. *Lancet*, **371**(9629), 2039–41.
18. **Hogan, M.** (2016) (R)evolution: toward a new paradigm of policy and patient advocacy for expanded access to experimental treatments. *BMC Med*, **14**(1), 17–4.
19. **Yang, J., Manolio, T. A., Pasquale, L. R., et al.** (2011) Genome partitioning of genetic variation for complex traits using common SNPs. *Nat Genet*, **43**(6), 519–25.
20. **Couzin, J.** (2005) Advocating, the clinical way. *Science*, **308**(5724), 940–2.

21. **Merkel, P. A., Manion, M., Gopal-Srivastava, R., et al.** (2016) The partnership of patient advocacy groups and clinical investigators in the rare diseases clinical research network. *Orphanet J Rare Dis*, **11**(1), 66.
22. **Lavery, C.** (2006) Role of patient support groups in lysosomal storage diseases. In: Mehta A, Beck M, Sunder-Plassmann G (eds). *Fabry Disease: Perspectives from 5 Years of FOS*. Oxford: Oxford PharmaGenesis, Chapter 12.
23. **Landy, D. C., Brinich, M. A., Colten, M. E., Horn, E. J., Terry, S. F., Sharp, R. R.** (2012) How disease advocacy organizations participate in clinical research: a survey of genetic organizations. *Genet Med*, **14**(2), 223–8.
24. **Isaacs, D.** (2015) Advocacy. *J Paediatr Child Health*, **51**(8), 747–8.
25. **Boon, W., Broekgaarden, R.** (2010) The role of patient advocacy organisations in neuromuscular disease R&D—the case of the Dutch neuromuscular disease association VSN. *Neuromuscul Disord*, **20**(2), 148–51.
26. **Pinto, D., Martin, D., Chenhall, R.** (2016) The involvement of patient organisations in rare disease research: a mixed methods study in Australia. *Orphanet J Rare Dis*, **11**(1), 261-15.
27. **Terry, S. F.** (2013) Disease advocacy organizations catalyze translational research. *Front Genet*, **4**, 1–5.
28. **Terry, S. F., Terry, P. F., Rauen, K. A., Uitto, J., Bercovitch, L. G.** (2007) Advocacy groups as research organizations: the PXE International example. *Nat Rev Genet*, **8**(2), 157–64.
29. **Furlong, P., Bridges, J. F. P., Charnas, L., et al.** (2015) How a patient advocacy group developed the first proposed draft guidance document for industry for submission to the U.S. Food and Drug Administration. *Orphanet J Rare Dis*, **10**(1), 1535–9.
30. **Gallin, E. K., Bond, E., Califf, R. M., et al.** (2013) Forging stronger partnerships between academic health centres and patient-driven organizations. *Acad Med*, **88**(9), 1220–4.
31. **Earnest, M. A., Wong, S. L., Federico, S. G.** (2010) Perspective: physician advocacy: what is it and how do we do it? *Acad Med*, **85**(1), 63–7.
32. **Griggs, R. C., Batshaw, M., Dunkle, M., et al.** (2009) Clinical research for rare disease: opportunities, challenges, and solutions. *Mol Genet Metab*, **96**(1), 20–6.
33. **Morgan, T., Schmidt, J., Haakonsen, C., et al.** (2014) Using the Internet to seek information about genetic and rare diseases: a case study comparing data from 2006 and 2011. *JMIR Res Protoc*, **3**(1), e10–0.
34. **Hedges, D., Burges, D., Powell, E., et al.** (2009) Exome sequencing of a multigenerational human pedigree. *PLoS One*, **4**(12), e8232.
35. **Scheindlin, S.** (2006) Rare diseases, orphan drugs, and orphaned patients. *Mol Interv*, **6**(4), 186–91.
36. **Reardon, S.** (2014) Lobbying sways NIH grants. *Nature*, **515**(7525), 19–9.
37. **Hegde, D., Sampat, B.** (2015) Can private money buy public science? Disease group lobbying and federal funding for biomedical research. *Management Science*, **61**(10), 2281–98.
38. **Rubinstein, Y. R., Groft, S. C., Bartek, R., et al.** (2010) Creating a global rare disease patient registry linked to a rare diseases biorepository database: Rare Disease-HUB (RD-HUB). *Contemp Clin Trials*, **31**(5), 394–404.
39. **National Organization for Rare Disorders (NORD)**. Available at: https://rarediseases.org
40. **EURODIS: Rare Diseases Europe**. Available at: http://www.eurordis.org
41. **Genetic Alliance**. Available at: http://www.geneticalliance.org

42. **Orphanet**. Available at: http://www.orpha.net/consor/cgi-bin/index.php?lng=EN
43. **European Commission**. Rare diseases. Available at: https://ec.europa.eu/health/rare_diseases/policy_en
44. **RD Action**. Available at: http://www.rd-action.eu
45. **IRDiRC**. Available at: http://www.irdirc.org
46. **Genetic and Rare Diseases Information Center**. Available at: https://rarediseases.info.nih.gov

Chapter 28

Palliative care

David Oliver

What is palliative care?

The World Health Organization (WHO) defines palliative care as:

> 'An approach that improves the quality of life of patients and their families facing problems associated with life-threatening illness, through the prevention and relief of suffering, early identification, and impeccable assessment and treatment of pain and other problems, physical, psychosocial, and spiritual.'[1]

Thus, palliative care primarily aims to encourage the involvement of the person and their family in the management of their disease. They should be involved in the necessary decisions and the professionals should be ensuring that the person's views and aims are upheld (i.e. that they are advocating for the person and their family). The family carers are seen as part of the 'whole patient in the context of their family' and so the support of the carers is very important—in their own right, as well as in their role of supporting the patient.

Palliative care encompasses a wide variety of care services. Specialist palliative care is provided by a specialist team, who have specific training in palliative care and the main area of their work is the provision of palliative care of patients, and their families, who have more complex needs.[2] All professionals in healthcare should be able to provide a palliative care approach for all patients they see using the principles outlined earlier in the WHO definition, but they may have limited training in palliative care and this is only part of their overall workload.[2] Thus neurology services should be able to provide a palliative care approach for the patients they are caring for with an openness to discussion and providing support for patients and families throughout their disease progression, but they may need specialist help for more complex issues, whether physical, psychosocial, or spiritual.[3,4]

However, for neurological patients there may be particular issues that need to be faced, in particular cognitive change, communication difficulties, due to dysarthria or dysphasia, the variability in disease progression, the awareness of palliative care for these conditions and the many different teams that may be involved.

Issues altering advocacy in neurology

Information

Many neurological diseases may be completely unexpected and new to patients. They may find it be very difficult to understand and react to the information given to them, and their family. Moreover, the giving of a diagnosis may not always be a clear and satisfactory process, as neurologists discussing these issues may find it difficult and may not have received training or education in communication.[5] There may be specific fears associated with the disease, particularly when there is a genetic component to the disease. For instance, a person with Huntington's disease (HD) may have particularly difficult memories and experiences from other family members who have died from the disease, and this may in turn alter how they cope with the news that they are also affected.[6]

Careful communication and explanation is necessary. This is a process of the learning about the disease over a period of time, with support from the wider multidisciplinary team. It is also important that the neurologist giving the diagnosis is knowledgeable about the disease and its progression, management, and care so that the patient, and their family, can receive the information they need.[7]

Cognitive change

Many patients with neurological disease face cognitive change, which may progress to dementia, when they may lose capacity to make decisions about themselves and their care. These cognitive changes may be subtle initially and so careful assessment of capacity and cognition may be needed. The changes, especially when associated with behavioural changes, may be noticed first by family members and close carers, who will need to be involved in the wider assessment.[8]

The number of teams

Many patients with progressive neurological disease will develop multiple problems, often including many different teams. These teams may all have their own particular ethos and attitudes and may or may not collaborate effectively with other teams.[9] This can be confusing for all concerned and may certainly affect the involvement of patient and family in decision-making, as conflicting advice may be given which can confuse all involved. This will affect the ability for any advocacy, particular as the patient deteriorates and faces death, when they may be less able to attend hospital or specialist clinics.

Recognition of deterioration/need for palliative care input

The recognition of the need for palliative care may be complex for all involved—patient, family, and professionals. Progressive neurological diseases may deteriorate at differing rates and in a very individual way. The changes may be subtle and not noticed at first, thus not allowing the gradual changes to be recognized. This recognition is important as it can allow patients and families to make appropriate decisions about the future care

The recognition of the later stages of disease progression is also important, to enable preparations to be made for the care of the patients and family. This may be ensuring decisions to have certain management are made, such as to the use of ventilation; the decision that certain interventions would not be appropriate, such as a Do Not Attempt Resuscitation Order; the provision of medication to relieve symptoms and distress at the end of life; and the time of planning and discussion of the wishes of the person—such as their wishes for care, place of care, and place of death, the preparation of a will or funeral plans, and the time for discussion and preparation of family members.[10]

There have been suggestions to help in this recognition:

- The 'surprise question'—'Would you be surprised if this patient died in the coming 6 to 12 months?'[11]
- The use of certain triggers; in particular it has been suggested that the following triggers may be seen more commonly and in combination in the last few months of life:
  - swallowing problems
  - recurring infection
  - marked decline in functional status
  - first episode of aspiration pneumonia
  - cognitive difficulties
  - weight loss
  - significant complex symptoms[12,13]

  There were also suggested triggers for the main neurological conditions.[12,14] Initial studies have shown that the number and frequency of triggers do increase nearer to death, especially aspiration pneumonia.[14]
- There are other systems to help predict the need for palliative care, such as Supportive and Palliative Care Indicators Tool (SPICT)[15] and the Marie Curie Triggers for Palliative Care.[16] These again use suggested triggers but are, as yet, not fully evaluated.

It is very important that the palliative care needs are recognized, so that patients and their families can then discuss and make decisions about their care in accordance with their own wishes. This may need to be discussed in advance of the need, due to the risk of cognitive or communication decline, in which case advance care planning may be necessary—see the next section, 'Chronicity of disease'.

Chronicity of disease

Every person with a progressive neurological disease will deteriorate in an individual way, with great variability. Many patients will deteriorate very slowly, such as for Parkinson's disease (PD) where the time from diagnosis to death may be 20–30 years. The slow progression of the disease may cause all involved—patient, family, and professionals involved in the care—to leave making any decisions or discussing future care until either the final stages of the illness, when an emergency occurs, such as aspiration pneumonia, or until capacity is lost due to cognitive change. The changes are so gradual that the seriousness of the disease progression is difficult to recognize. The awareness of triggers, as described earlier, may allow these changes to be more easily identified and the appropriate action taken.

Patient-related advocacy—on a micro-level

The aim of all patient care should be to enable the person to retain autonomy in their decisions. This may be defined as the informed preference or consent to whatever we do or what is done to us.[17] This would allow the most appropriate and acceptable decision to be made for the person, according to their wishes. This is often complex, because to make a decision the person will need:

- **Information**
  This needs to be accurate and in a form that can be understood by the person. However, the information may be modulated by many different aspects, including fear, anger, delay in obtaining information, and family pressure.
- **Ability to understand and appropriately use this information**
  This may be affected by cognitive change, depression, or anxiety, as well as communication issues, such as deafness, language issues, or autism.
- **Time to decide—with the opportunity to discuss the issues in greater depth.**
  This may be limited on occasions in an emergency situation, when an intervention is necessary urgently or the person's state could be severely compromised or they could die.
- **Ability to communicate the decision made.**
  This may be reduced due to cognitive change but could also be severe speech issues such as dysphasia or dysarthria.

In the United Kingdom, the Mental Capacity Act proposes that all people should be assumed to have capacity to make decisions and there is an assessment process to decide if the person has capacity: assessment of any support they may need to understand, weigh up the decision, make judgements about the information and then make and communicate their decision.[10] The person with capacity should be encouraged to express their autonomous decisions, even in the palliative care phase of disease progression. This should include advocacy that the person makes decisions on the management and treatment they receive, but there is an imperative to ensure that they are given the information and support to make these decisions and express their autonomy. This will include listening and involvement of the wider family and carers—who may be able to provide this support for the patient. They may have their own concerns and prejudices that affect their feelings and attitudes to decision-making. The prime aim should be to allow the person themselves to make any decisions, and the family's role will be to support them during this process.

However, many families feel that they should be making decisions on the person's behalf. They may particularly be against certain decisions being discussed with the patient—for instance, their wishes about place of death or the interventions they wish or refuse at this time. This may be due to their own fears and concerns, and often they do not want to 'upset' the patient. The reality, both ethically and legally, is that the decision should lie with the person, if possible. Careful discussion and explanation may be necessary to show family members that they may have to help the person with this decision and the person cannot be excluded.

The support needed may involve the social and care aspects as well, including the care of family members; how to support and inform children within the family; their understanding of the disease, its progression, and the future; their own particular emotional and psychological needs; along with issues and changes in the roles within a family—perhaps as the patient can no longer work, the family become more dependent on his wife's salary, and she has to undertake roles that he would have taken as his before the illness.[7] Moreover, there are the usual challenges that may occur within families with the changes within the life cycle of a family—births, children leaving home, school issues, marriages, day-to-day stresses—that carers have to face, with the additional stress of providing caring for the patient. Families and carers will have different experiences from the past and have their own vulnerabilities and physical and social resources which they have used before to cope with crises and difficulties that have occurred.[18]

Financial issues may also become more pronounced, particularly as the patient becomes more dependent, unable to work themselves, and maybe only being able to cope at home if the spouse/partner have also given up work. Advice on the possible allowances and pensions may be crucial in allowing the care of the patient to be at home. Advocacy within the complexity of the social relief system may be very important for the whole family.

Carers face increasing demands—in physical care, emotional support for the patient, financial dependency, increasing childcare involvement—and have their own emotional response to the disease progression. Careful assessment of these needs is important.[7] There is a need to support carers, to allow the care of the person with the neurological disease to be maximized. This may take the form of practical care support and these needs to be consistent and flexible to cope with the disease variation and progression. Often this support can be too little, too late. There is also the need to listen to the carers' concerns and support them with the changes they face—fears of deterioration and the possibilities of the dying phase and possible distress.[4,7]

Advance care planning

Anyone may wish to express their views as to the care they would like to receive in the future, so that even if they have lost the ability to express their view due to loss or communication or capacity or consciousness their wishes are known. This is particularly so for a person with a progressive neurological disease, when cognitive loss or altered ability to communicate may be likely scenarios. Thus advance care planning (ACP)—the expression of your views as to future care—is very important.[10]

The way ACP may be undertaken will vary from country to country. In many countries an advance directive (AD) can be used to express treatments a person does not wish to receive or care they would like to receive. In many legislatures such AD are legally binding, if certain statements are made.

A person may often be able to choose a person to act as a proxy/advocate making decisions on their behalf if they are unable to make the decision. This person could be asked by the professional team what the person would have wanted and the proxy/advocate can answer on their behalf. This will again vary in different legislatures but many countries do allow the power of attorney or proxy.[10]

The use of ACP can be difficult as people may be reluctant to discuss future plans. This reluctance may be for the patient, who does not want to face their deterioration and possible death, who could feel that it 'if I talk about it, it will happen', or concerns of upsetting their family. Families and carers may also be reluctant for these discussions as they fear the future for themselves and do not want to 'upset' the patient, or fear that planning ahead is 'giving up hope'. Professionals may also be reluctant to hold these discussions as they do not want to upset patients, fear the reactions of families, fear 'taking away hope', and find the discussion too difficult, especially as they may have little training in this difficult area of communication.

However, with careful discussion and explanation ACP may be possible—from knowing the views of the patient and family to a more legalistic plan which can be mandatory. It is also important for all involved to realize that ACP will only be used if the person has lost the ability to make the decision—from loss of communication or capacity—and if they are able to make a decision themselves this would always take precedence.[10]

Discussion and planning for end of life

Many patients will wish to be involved in the many decisions about their management and their deterioration, including their wishes for their death. This may include their views of where they wish to be cared for and where they wish to die—these do need to be differentiated, may vary, and may not be clearly expressed. Studies have shown that someone may talk of their place of care, where they do not wish to die, but professional teams may misconstrue this as their wish for place of death.[19] There may also be the need to discuss whether the person would wish to have more invasive therapeutic actions taken, such as tracheostomy and ventilation or cardio-pulmonary resuscitation. These discussions are needed before the event because if no decision is made, the 'fall back' position will be for intervention and active treatment.

In these discussions if we are to really advocate for the patient, we need to have clarity as to what they wish to discuss. There may be discussion about dying—the place of death, their fears of what may happen, how their family will cope, their fears of distress and the process of dying-or may be of death itself—of possible judgement/heaven/hell—for which there is no answer.[20,21] However it is essential to answer the correct question, and allow the person the opportunity to express their concerns.

Families and carers may wish to be sure of the person's views, as they wish to be able to express these views on their behalf. However many families fear these discussions, and fear that hope will be lost and distress caused. It is important to clarify the role of ACP and enable families to be clear as to why it may be so important, so that the person's wishes are known and they can still be involved in decision making, even if they have lost capacity.

Professionals also have the same fears of ACP, and find the discussions difficult.[22] There may be a need for training and the opportunity to practise these conversations. The wider multidisciplinary team should be involved, and it may be a specific team member, who has a closer relationship with the person and their family, who can lead on these discussions.

Involvement early in the disease progression

In the past palliative care has been primarily associated with the care of people with cancer, although people with neurological diseases were admitted to St Christopher's Hospice, the first of the modern hospices committed to patient care, education and research, in 1967 very soon after it opened.[22] There has been increasing pressure to include all disease groups and to base the involvement of palliative care services on need rather than diagnosis.[2,23] There has been an increase in the care of people with some neurological diseases, particularly amyotrophic lateral sclerosis (ALS), and recent guidelines and a consensus paper from the European Academy of Neurology (EAN) and the European Association of Palliative Care (EAPC) has recommended increased palliative care for neurological disease.[23]

However, there is often the sense that palliative care may only be appropriate at the end of life, or the later stages of disease progression.[4] This has partly been due to the need to restrict limited services but there has been resistance in people with neurological disease, families, and carers and professionals to involve palliative care, as it was thought that this was related to end-of-life care and was seen negatively.[4] There have been documents suggesting that earlier involvement is important and helpful, as the initial care at the time of diagnosis or initial deterioration can form the relationships with the caring team and patient and family, and reduce the problems later in the disease progression.[24] Moreover, research has shown that palliative care does not increase mortality or shorten life[25] but rather improves quality of life and reduces the symptom burden for patients and family carers.[25]

It has been suggested that the involvement of palliative care could be on an episodic basis, according to need. In the past palliative care was seen to be appropriate only at the end of life (Fig. 28.1(a)) and over the past few years there has been greater awareness of the advantages of increasing palliative care and working collaboratively over the disease's progression (Fig. 28.1(b)). The needs-related involvement suggests that palliative care may have increased input throughout the disease progression, with involvement when there are specific issues—whether physical, psychosocial, or spiritual—see Fig. 28.1(c).[26] There is also evidence in neurological disease that the way the diagnosis is imparted initially may influence the entire disease progression, with fear and distress engendered by the poor communication of the diagnosis and the development of fears of a distressing death—even though with good palliative care this is very rare.[4,24] Carers need to be considered, along with the patient, so that their particular concerns and fears can be addressed.[7]

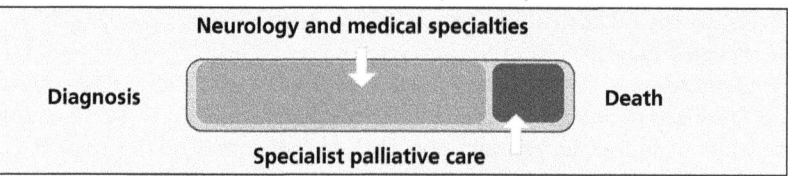
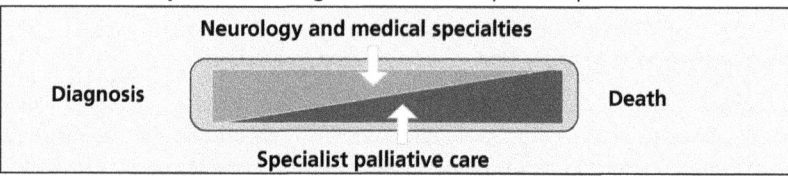
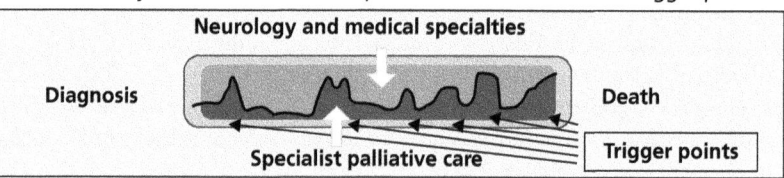

Fig. 28.1 The role of palliative care—differing modes of involvement.
Reproduced from Bede P, Hardiman O, O'Brannagain D, An integrated framework of early intervention palliative care in motor neurone disease as a model to progressive neurodegenerative disease, Poster at European ALS congress, Copyright (2009), with permission from Peter Bede.

Wider issues in advocacy—the meso issues

Many of the issues that arise for individual patients may also affect the wider population. For instance the awareness of palliative care and the attitudes of patients, families, and professionals may develop within the wider community. Often the discussion in the media is of the distress of a neurological disease, with overemphasis on the possibility of distressing symptoms and a distressing death. In some countries this has been accentuated by the discussions of hastened death. In the United Kingdom, the proponents of assisted dying have often involved people with neurological disease, often ALS or HD, and stressed the fears of distress in their arguments for patient choice and autonomy and assisted dying.[27,28] There is a need for the advocacy of patients to receive the appropriate care they require, which may be palliative care.

Within healthcare economies, nationally, regionally, and locally, there may be varying understanding of the issues involved in the care of people with neurological disease. There may be a need for patients, patient support organizations, and professional teams to advocate for people with neurological disease. This may be particularly important in the care of people with rarer diseases, when there may be limited understanding of the needs and experiences of patients and their families. For instance, those commissioning health services may be unaware of the difficulties of care for neurological diseases, which are rare but also genetic, such as Huntington's disease. For other patient groups families may be expected to provide care and support, but for the HD family, who may be facing their own future if they know they have the gene and will develop the disease at a later time, this care may be too difficult.[6]

Even within hospitals there may be a need for advocacy for patient needs. When a patient has a rare disease, and most neurological diseases are individually uncommon, the hospital medical and nursing teams may have little knowledge or experience of caring for the issues involved. The patient, family, and patient organizations may know more than the professionals, which can lead to conflict, unless the professional teams realize that they need to use the expertise that families and carers provide.

International advocacy—the macro level

There is increasing awareness of the role of palliative care in the care of people with neurological disease, with the publication of guidelines[23] and collaboration between both areas of care. The EAPC and EAN consensus document on neurological palliative care has stimulated the establishment of an EAPC Reference Group, which aims to continue to develop this collaboration and look at research into the area.[29] This Group will continue to provide advocacy for palliative care and enable education and training for both areas—with sessions at conferences of both the EAPC and EAN, and looking at increasing collaboration with the World Federation of Neurology.[29] There are also plans to develop a core curriculum on neurological palliative care—so that there is clarity of the educational needs for professionals in training and as part of continuing education. This would encourage increasing knowledge of palliative care for neurology services and increasing awareness and knowledge of the issues faced in neurology for those in palliative care.

There is increasing awareness and pressure for palliative care to be seen as a basic human right.[30] It has been suggested that all people with needs as they deteriorate and face the end of life should be able to receive palliative care. This is not universal across the world, as many areas do not have palliative care services, or others have limited care, often only to cancer care or only at the end of life. This may particularly apply to neurological patients, as there are barriers to care, as just explained, with the need to change attitudes and feelings of patients, families, and carers and professionals.

There are also issues for the availability of medication across the world. It is estimated that 5,500 million people (83% of the world's population) live in countries with low or non-existent access to medication to control pain and only 15% of the people requiring palliative care receive the care they need.[31] This means that there are millions people dying in pain without easy availability of opioid medication. Opioids can be used safely for pain—pain is a problem for 76% ALS patients, 82% in MS, and 62% in PD—and other symptoms such as general discomfort (skin pressure pain), dyspnoea, and distress at the end of life.[32]

There is also a need to advocate for increased education in palliative care and end-of-life care.[33] These areas are not always a high priority with medical, nursing, and paramedical education. However there is increasing pressure for all courses—undergraduate, postgraduate, and continuing education—to focus on palliative care. There is increasing evidence of undergraduate medical education responding to this challenge and in many countries all medical students do receive some training in communication skills and palliative care.[32] The EAN/EAPC consensus document has recommended increased education in palliative care for neurologists in training and as part of ongoing continuing medical education and at the same time increased training in neurology for specialist palliative care professionals.[23] Within neurology there is also pressure for all neurologists to provide palliative care, and receive the education and training they require.[3]

Conclusion

There is increasing evidence of the importance of providing palliative care for neurological patients, particularly those with progressive or degenerative disease. There is the need for all involved in the care of people with neurological disease to advocate for the most appropriate care, so that these people can maintain as good a quality of life as possible and die with dignity and without distress.

References

1. **World Health Organization** (2002) WHO Definition of Palliative Care. Available at: http://www.who.int/cancer/palliative/definition/en/
2. **Higginson, I. J.** (2015) Palliative care delivery models. In: Cheney, N. I., Fallon, M. T., Kaasa, S., Portenoy, R. K., Currow, D. C. (eds). *Oxford Textbook of Palliative Medicine*, 5th edition. Oxford: Oxford University Press, pp. 112–14.
3. **Creutzfelt, C. J., Robinson, M. T., Holloway, R. G.** (2016) Neurologists as primary palliative care providers. Communication and practice approaches. *Neurol Clin Pract*, **6**, 1–9.
4. **Oliver, D.** (2014) Palliative care for people with progressive neurological disease: what is the role? *J Palliat Care*, **30**, 298–301.
5. **Aoun, S. M., Breen, L. J., Howting, D., et al.** (2016) Receiving the news of a diagnosis of motor neuron disease: what does it take to make it better? *Amyotroph Lat Scler Frontotemporal Degener*, **17**, 168–178.
6. **Travers, E., Jones, K., Nichol, J.** (2007) Palliative care provision in Huntington's disease. *Int J Palliat Nurs*, **13**, 125–30.
7. **Campbell, C. W., Chandler, B. J., Smith, S.** (2012) Holistic care: psychosocial and spiritual aspects. In: Oliver, D. (ed.). *End of Life Care in Neurological Disease*. London: Springer, pp. 96–8.
8. **Abrahams, S., Newton, J., Niven, E., Foley, J., Bak, T. H.** (2014) Screening for cognition and behaviour changes in ALS. *Amyotroph Lat Scler Frontotemporal Degener*, **15**, 9–14.
9. **Oliver, D., Watson, S.** (2012) Multidisciplinary care. In: Oliver, D. (ed.). *End of Life Care in Neurological Disease*. London: Springer, pp. 113–27.
10. **Chapman, S.** (2012) Advance care planning. In: Oliver, D. (ed.). *End of Life Care in Neurological Disease*. London: Springer, pp. 133–42.
11. **Thomas, K., Armstrong Wilson, J., GSF Team** (2011) *Prognostic Indicator Guidance (PIG)*, 4th edition. London: The Gold Standards Framework Centre in End of Life Care.

12. **Oliver, D., Silber, E.** (2012) End of life care in neurological disease. In: Oliver, D. (ed.). *End of Life Care in Neurological Disease*. London: Springer, pp. 19–25.
13. **The National Council for Pallitive Care** (2010) End of life care in long term neurological conditions. National End of Life Care Programme 2010. Available at: http://www.nai.ie/assets/98/E29C88A6-9CA5-06B3-E74D285E3C0695A2_document/End_20life_20care_20long_20term_20neuro_20conditions.pdf
14. **Hussain, J., Adams, D., Allgar, V., Campbell, C.** (2014) Triggers in advanced neurological conditions: prediction and management of the terminal phase. *BMJ Supp Pall Care*, **4**, 30–7.
15. **Supportive and Palliative Care Indicators Tool (SPICT)**. Available at: http://www.spict.org.uk/the-spict/
16. **Marie Curie** (2015) Triggers for palliative care. Improving access to care for people with diseases other than cancer. Available at: https://www.mariecurie.org.uk/globalassets/media/documents/policy/policy-publications/june-2015/triggers-for-palliative-care-full-report.pdf
17. **Randall, F., Downie, R. S.** (2010) *End of Life Choices: Consensus and Controversy*. 2010. Oxford. Oxford University Press, pp. 17–19.
18. **Payne, S.** (2007) Resilient carers and caregivers. In: Monroe, B., Oliviere, D. (eds). *Resilience in Palliative Care—Achievement in Adversity*. Oxford: Oxford University Press, pp. 83–97.
19. **Agar, M., Currow, D. C., Shelby-James, T. M., Sanderson, C., Abernethy, A. P.** (2008) Preference for place of care and place of death in palliative care: are these different questions? *Pall Med*, **22**, 787–95.
20. **Lambert, S.** (2014) Spiritual care. In: Oliver, D., Borasio, G. D., Johnston, W. (eds). *Palliative Care in Amyotrophic Lateral Sclerosis: From Diagnosis to Bereavement*, 3rd edition. Oxford: Oxford University Press, Chapter 11.
21. **Oliver, D. J., Turner, M. R.** (2010) Some difficult, decisions in ALS/MND. *Amyotroph Lat Scler*, **11**, 339–43.
22. **Clark, D.** (2002) *Cicely Saunders. Founder of the Hospice Movement. Selected Letters 1959–1999*. Oxford: Oxford University Press.
23. **Oliver, D. J., Borasio, G. D., Caraceni, A., et al.** (2016) A consensus review on the development of palliative care for patients with chronic and progressive neurological disease. *Eur J Neurol*, **23**, 30–8.
24. **Oliver, D.** (2014) Palliative care. In: Oliver, D., Borasio, G. D., Johnston, W. (eds). *Palliative Care in ALS—From Diagnosis to Bereavement*, 3rd edition. Oxford: Oxford University Press, Chapter 2.
25. **Veronese, S., Gallo, G., Valle, A. et al.** (2015) Specialist palliative care improves the quality of life in advanced neurodegenerative disorders: Ne-PAL, a pilot randomized controlled study. *BMJ Supp Pall Care*, **23**(6), 331–42.
26. **Bede, P., Hardiman, O., O'Brannagain, D.** (2009) An integrated framework of early intervention palliative care in motor neurone disease as a model to progressive neurodegenerative disease. Poster at European ALS congress, Turin.
27. **Young, E.** (2016) My mum's decision changed my view of assisted dying. *BMJ*, **352**, 64–5.
28. **Heath, I.** (2012) What's wrong with assisted dying. *BMJ*, **344**, 35.
29. **European Association for Palliative Care** (2016) Palliative Care in Neurology Reference Group. Available at: http://www.eapcnet.eu/Corporate/AbouttheEAPC/ProjectsandTaskforces/EAPCReferencegroups/NeurologyRG.aspx

30. **Gwyther, L., Brennan, F., Harding, R.** (2009) Advancing palliative care as a human right. *J Pain Symptom Manage*, **38**, 767–74.
31. **World Health Organization** (2016) Public health dimension of the world drug problem including in the context of the Special Session of the United Nations General Assembly on the World Drug Problem, to be held in 2016. **WHO Executive Board 138th session. Provisional agenda item.** Available at: http://apps.who.int/gb/ebwha/pdf_files/EB138/B138_11-en.pdf
32. **Oliver, D.** (1998) Opioid medication in the palliative care of motor neurone disease. *Palliat Med*, **12**, 113–15.
33. **Forbes, K., Gibbins, J.** (2015) Teaching and training in palliative medicine. In: Cheney, N. I., Fallon, M. T., Kaasa, S., Portenoy, R. K., Currow, D. C. (eds). *Oxford Textbook of Palliative Medicine*, 5th edition. Oxford: Oxford University Press, pp. 146–53.

Chapter 29

Advocacy for epilepsy: From the shadows to centre stage: Stand up for epilepsy

Jules C. Beal and Solomon L. Moshé

The burden of epilepsy

An estimated 65 million people worldwide have epilepsy, and more than two million new diagnoses are made each year,[1,2] making epilepsy the most common serious chronic neurologic disease.[3] It is a disease that can develop at any age, and can affect people of any ethnicity, gender, or socioeconomic status. In some instances it may be related to a genetic aetiology, or it can occur in association with metabolic disorders, structural abnormalities, infection, brain injury, or numerous other factors that affect people of all walks of life in all parts of the world. These varying aetiologies can affect the types of seizures people have, and a new seizure classification scheme has been developed that emphasizes the importance of the underlying mechanisms.[4]

Beyond the seizures that characterize the disease, comorbid conditions and medical complications are common. Additional neurologic disorders are present in about 40% of people with epilepsy.[5] These include autism, learning and cognitive disabilities, and physical impairments such as paresis, spasticity, and feeding and swallowing difficulties. In some cases, even the electroencephalogram (EEG) abnormalities between seizures (i.e. interictal spikes), are thought to contribute to intellectual disability. Individuals with epilepsy are more likely than those without to sustain injuries related to burns, falls, drowning, and motor vehicle accidents.[6] The mortality rate in individuals with epilepsy is more than twice that of the general population,[7] and there is a more than a 20-fold increase in the risk of sudden death for people with epilepsy compared to those without.[8] The available medical treatments for epilepsy are themselves often associated with medical complications, including organ damage, bone marrow suppression, tremor and ataxia, weight loss or weight gain, hair loss, and birth defects, among other problems.[9]

Even when seizures are controlled, people with epilepsy face numerous challenges. Epilepsy is highly associated with both depression and anxiety. One in three individuals with epilepsy also has depression, and people with depression are more likely to develop epilepsy.[5] People with epilepsy are often subjected to discrimination, misunderstanding, and social stigma in addition to the stress of living with a chronic and unpredictable condition. Their ability to drive is often restricted. They may be prohibited from participating in sports and physical exercise due to misunderstandings about potential risks.[10] They suffer a loss of autonomy, and are frequently faced with limitations in employment options, educational opportunities, and marriage possibilities due to both social stigma and physical limitations.[11] Some people with epilepsy who have seizures that are relatively well-controlled may be able to lead a 'normal' life. However even then the occurrence of breakthrough seizures, which are often completely unpredictable, could derail this at any time.

The disease burden imposed by epilepsy on a global scale, then, is immense. Severe epilepsy was ranked fourth in terms of disability weight out of 220 medical conditions in a recent study evaluating global burden of disease.[12] Among neurological diseases, epilepsy has been ranked second after stroke in terms of years of potential life lost.[13] This degree of morbidity and mortality carries significant economic implications as well, both for individuals and for society at large. An analysis of the healthcare costs of neurologic diseases in Canada found that epilepsy ranked second in terms of total direct healthcare costs, and also ranked second in terms of indirect costs due to premature death and disability.[14]

The incidence of epilepsy is higher in low-income countries,[15] and individuals with epilepsy living in low-income countries are a particularly vulnerable population. They have higher mortality rates, which has been attributed to episodes status epilepticus, seizure related accidents, and sudden unexplained death in epilepsy (SUDEP).[6,16] They also have limited access to appropriate medications, either due to unavailability or prohibitive cost.[17,18] In fact, the treatment gap for epilepsy exceeds 75% in low-income countries and 50% in middle-income countries, as opposed to 10% in high-income countries.[19] This disparity makes it much more difficult for people with epilepsy in low-income countries to live normal, productive lives, and has negative implications for public health and for overall economic and social development.[1,19]

Barriers to care

According to the World Health Organization Atlas of Epilepsy Care, the most significant barriers to the treatment of epilepsy are: insufficient medication supply (reported in 53.2% of countries); insufficient diagnostic facilities (51.9% of countries); ignorance and social stigma (43.6%); lack of skilled personnel (40.4%); and economy (39%).[20] These barriers exist to a certain extent in all societies, and in many cases are closely intertwined with each other. For example, there may be insufficient medications and facilities in a particular region as a result of economic difficulties, or a lack of skilled personnel may be because widespread misunderstanding and stigma deters professionals from learning about epilepsy (Fig. 29.1).

As mentioned earlier, the treatment gap, or the number of people with epilepsy who do not receive timely and appropriate treatment, is greatest in developing countries where essential medicines may not be available or may be too expensive.[17,18] It has been estimated that 80% of the world's anti-epileptic medications are sold in 20% of the world's countries,[21] and that approximately three-quarters of epilepsy patients in developing nations do not receive adequate treatment.[22] This inequity is particularly unfortunate given the fact that epilepsy treatment can be relatively inexpensive: phenobarbital, for

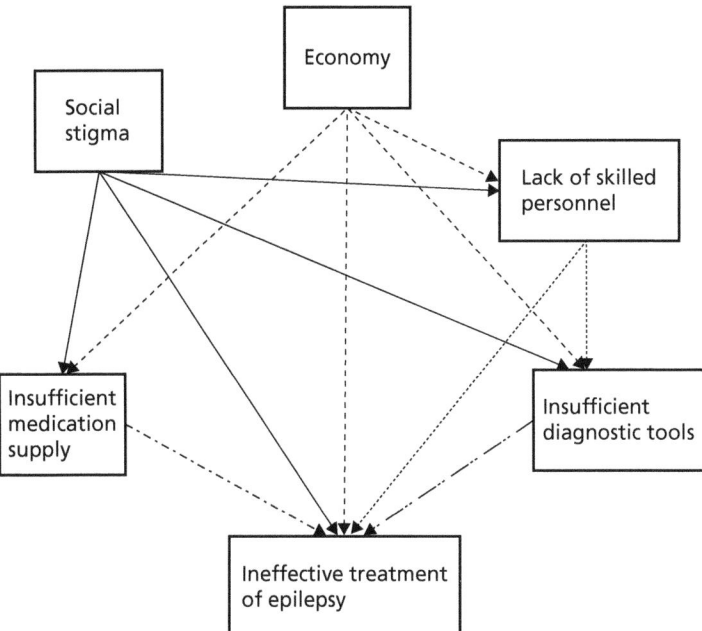

Fig. 29.1 Barriers to epilepsy care. Many of the most significant reported barriers to the treatment of epilepsy are closely interconnected with each other. For example, economic difficulties can cause there to be an insufficient supply of medications and can have a direct impact on the lack of skilled personnel and lack of diagnostic tools and facilities in a region, besides directly impairing individuals' access to medications (i.e. prohibitive cost). Social stigma can lead to fewer people who want to treat epilepsy (lack of skilled personnel), can directly impact access to treatment in the sense that individuals try to hide their condition and don't seek treatment, and may contribute to insufficient diagnostics and insufficient medication supply insofar as it may influence public policy and legislation. Lack of skilled/educated personnel leads to directly to suboptimal treatment and also suboptimal diagnosis and absence of new diagnostic tools.

example, has been estimated to cost approximately three US dollars per person for a yearly supply;[23] however it may be unavailable or significantly more expensive in developing countries.[18] It is important to bear in mind as well that treatment gaps do exist in different forms, even in high-income and resource-rich societies.[6,19] These gaps may become apparent with regard to the use of appropriate treatment protocols, the time from disease onset to treatment, and availability of non-medication treatment modalities such as surgery or diet. The cost of treatment, who actually receives treatment, and the use of treatment guidelines can vary tremendously from place to place.

The treatment gap, then, is closely associated with a knowledge and awareness gap.[6] In other words, there may be a lack of knowledge or an incomplete understanding regarding epilepsy, its implications, and available treatment options and protocols. For example, the conceptualization of epilepsy as a symptom versus a disease, and understanding the difference between primary epilepsy and provoked seizures, may change the way the condition is approached. Physicians may not be equipped to diagnose specific syndromes that have specific treatments, or may not be aware of the comorbidities that may further complicate care. There are also other gaps in general knowledge regarding epilepsy, such as understanding the reasons for the decreased life span, the role of interictal spikes, comorbidities of epileptic lesions, and the processes underlying the development and continuation of epilepsy. Better understanding of these issues will make healthcare providers better able to diagnose and treat people with epilepsy.

Among the general population, lack of knowledge about epilepsy leads to misunderstanding, discrimination, and social stigma. In some societies, epilepsy may not be a priority condition, or may not be viewed as a medical issue at all. People with epilepsy who feel stigmatized often try to hide their condition from their family or community members. This in turn impairs their access to appropriate medical care and treatment options. Education of the general population regarding epilepsy may help reduce stigma and misconceptions, resulting in increased access to appropriate care.[24]

Ongoing advocacy

Overcoming these barriers to epilepsy care requires a coordinated multinational effort, focusing on advocacy for improved epilepsy-related research, legislation, public education, and support networks. In 1997 the World Health Organization (WHO) partnered with the International League Against Epilepsy (ILAE) and the International Bureau for Epilepsy (IBE) to establish the Global Campaign Against Epilepsy and the subsequent 'Out of the Shadows' campaign. The goal of these campaigns was to increase awareness and foster acceptance of epilepsy, and to improve access to treatment and services for individuals with epilepsy. Their stated vision was 'to create a world in which no person's life is limited by epilepsy'.[25] This partnership was able to provide a platform to raise public awareness and understanding regarding epilepsy and reduce social stigma and social impediments to care. They were also able to work with various health departments to develop strategies for addressing and dealing with epilepsy, including education, training, treatment, research, and prevention and identifying regions where treatment gaps existed.

As a result of this collaboration, regional conferences on epilepsy as a public health priority were organized in all the WHO regions, involving a total of 130 countries. Regional reports and regional declarations on epilepsy were produced during these conferences. The purpose of these reports is to provide epidemiological information regarding epilepsy, with the goal to use them as an advocacy tool and to open dialogue with government agencies and healthcare providers. An atlas of epilepsy resources in various countries entitled 'Epilepsy Care in the World' was completed in 2005. This publication provided information on the burden of epilepsy in different regions, and involved 160 participating countries including more than 97% of the world's population.[20]

Under the umbrella of the Global Campaign Against Epilepsy, Demonstration Projects were undertaken in several countries. These are projects designed to provide further information on the burden of epilepsy in these regions, and to develop interventional models, integrate epilepsy into existing healthcare systems, educate medical personnel, and ideally dispel stigma and reduce the treatment gap. The projects have been successful both in raising awareness and in altering policy. After the initiation of the Demonstration Project in Brazil, for example, epilepsy was officially adopted by the Ministry of Education as a theme to be considered in elementary education. In Korea, epilepsy was renamed from Gan-zil, or a 'convulsive disease', to Noi-jeon-jeung, or 'cerebroelectric disorder' in an effort to demystify the condition and more accurately reflect its pathophysiology. One of the most successful Demonstration Projects was in China, where they were able to effectively show that a larger portion of the population than previously estimated was affected by epilepsy, and demonstrate the unmet needs of people with epilepsy in that country. This ultimately led to government funding for epilepsy care and education at the primary care level, particularly in rural areas, which was also demonstrated to be a cost-effective approach to caring for epilepsy patients. The project initially involved 6 provinces and 2.5 million people, and has been extended to involve 18 provinces and 75 million people. As a result of this project, the treatment gap in China has dropped by about 13%.[6,26]

The Global Campaign and the 'Out of the Shadows' movement also resulted in the publication of a document, 'Basic Principles and Guidance Instrument for Developing, Adopting, and Implementing Epilepsy Legislation' published in May of 2012. The purpose of this document is to serve as a guide for advocacy groups, lawyers, policymakers, and governments to 'to develop new legislation on epilepsy or to revise and reform existing legislation and regulations related to epilepsy, thus leading to better care and services and improved living conditions for people with epilepsy throughout the world'.[27]

In a separate movement, the WHO launched the WHO Mental Health Gap Action Programme (mhGAP) in 2008. This programme is geared towards helping to facilitate interventions by non-specialist healthcare workers for a variety of conditions pertaining to neurology and mental health in low- and middle-income countries. Recognizing that there are fewer neurologists and epilepsy specialists in these countries compared to high-income countries, epilepsy was included as a priority disease for intervention in this programme.[28]

The ILAE and IBE also engage in various projects to raise public awareness of epilepsy. The slogan 'Stand up for epilepsy with one voice' has been adopted for the ILAE's global anti-discrimination campaign. As part of this effort they engage in various projects designed to demystify epilepsy and correct common misconceptions. As an example, they partnered with the European Football Association to organize an event in June of 2009 just before the European Championship semi-finals. This consisted of two short matches played by athletes with epilepsy from all over Europe, as well as former professional players who dedicated their time to help raise awareness and make the point that people with epilepsy can and should be able to live a normal life.[25] The idea of using athletics to raise epilepsy awareness eventually led to the publication of a collection of photos entitled 'Stand up for Epilepsy: Sports and Epilepsy Project', showing images of famous athletes from around the world posing with children and young people with epilepsy, many of whom are themselves aspiring athletes. The purpose of the collection is 'to convey the message that these well-known celebrities have no prejudice against epilepsy and that people with epilepsy can achieve their goals'.[29]

In 2011, the ILAE and IBE engaged in a joint campaign to support the Written Declaration of Epilepsy at the European Parliament. To accomplish this, national organizations, local affiliations, and individuals came together to provide members of Parliament with information about the needs and barriers facing those with epilepsy. The Declaration was approved, and the following year more than 50 million euros were allocated towards epilepsy research by the European Commission.[6,30] Similarly the WHO Region of Americas developed and released a Pan American Action Plan on Epilepsy in 2011, working in conjunction with the ILAE, the IBE, and many governments within the region to promote epilepsy awareness.

In May of 2015 the World Health Assembly unanimously approved a resolution on the 'Global Burden of Epilepsy and the Need for Coordinated Action at the Country Level to Address its Health, Social and Public Knowledge Implications'.[1] This resolution was again the result of collaboration with the ILAE and the IBE, as well as other organizations including the World Federation of Neurology (WFN) and Health Action International, and direct involvement from national governments. Official statements in favour of the resolution were made by 42 countries, some of which also spoke on behalf of other nations, and 19 of these countries became co-sponsors of the resolution.[6]

The World Health Assembly resolution encourages WHO members states to strengthen policies surrounding epilepsy and to devote resources towards implementing evidence-based plans and actions with regard to epilepsy and epilepsy management. This includes specific recommendations on promoting epilepsy education, establishing national healthcare plans for epilepsy, and overcoming barriers to care for individuals with epilepsy. Member states are encouraged to implement strategies for improving access to treatment, augmenting epilepsy research and, in some cases, integrating epilepsy care into primary healthcare.[1,6]

The resolution has provided a platform to promote epilepsy awareness and to convince national governments to actively take steps towards improving epilepsy care, education, and research. It has also acted to further strengthen the relationship between the ILAE, IBE, and WHO in addressing the needs of people with epilepsy, and provided additional opportunities for collaboration with other organizations such as the WFN and Health Action International. After the resolution passed, for example, the WFN dedicated World Brain Day 2015 (22 July 2015) to epilepsy and invited the WHO, ILAE, and IBE to participate.[31]

Future directions

Advocacy in epilepsy has made great strides over the past 20 years. However, the worldwide disease burden of epilepsy remains substantial, as do the various barriers to treatment encountered by people with epilepsy. Going forward, the ongoing work to improve the lives of people with epilepsy will continue to focus on enhancing education, collaboration, and research, and on improving medical care for individuals with epilepsy, increasing their access to treatments, fighting discrimination and stigma, and closing the treatment gap.[25] This will require coordinated action and political commitments at the national level, and also the continued direct involvement of national societies, local associations, and community leaders. In many regions this may also require the involvement of traditional healers and sensitivity to cultural beliefs and practices.[24] Individuals with epilepsy and their families and friends can and should play an increasingly important role in supplementing or even driving advocacy work, particularly in the age of social media.[6]

One of the concrete ways in which these groups and individuals can advocate for improved epilepsy care is by pushing for epilepsy-friendly legislation. This can include legislation supporting access to care for individuals with epilepsy, legislation protecting these individuals themselves from discrimination, and legislation to make epilepsy and epilepsy education a priority condition for healthcare organizations and systems.

In response to the World Health Association Resolution, the ILAE, IBE, WFN, and WHO are planning to continue to work together to develop specific recommendations to guide in the implementation of national and regional epilepsy action plans and legislation. These recommendations will again focus on low- and middle-income countries and will cover diagnosis, access to medications, and medical care, access to social services, counteracting stigma and discrimination, and promoting epilepsy research. They also plan to conduct a review of past activities to determine the best models that have been used to address the burden of epilepsy. They will make this review and documentation widely available.[6] The 'Basic Principles and Guidance Instrument for Developing, Adopting, and Implementing Epilepsy Legislation', published as part of the Global Campaign Against Epilepsy in 2012, provides similar practical recommendations for organizations and individuals working to advocate for the implementation of epilepsy-friendly legislation.[27]

Access to anti-seizure medications remains a specific major concern that can be addressed by appropriate legislation: in many low-income countries these medications are either not available at all or are significantly more expensive than in higher income countries.[18] The WHO publishes a list of essential medications every two years, which includes medications that should be available at affordable prices at all times within functioning health systems. It is important to ensure that essential seizure medications remain on this list.[24] Well-crafted legislation should be able to improve availability and affordability of seizure medications, and continue to emphasize their critical importance.

Ongoing epilepsy education will continue to be an important tool in the future of epilepsy advocacy. Education decreases stigma as well as leading directly to improved availability of diagnostic modalities, treatments, and skilled medical personnel. Essential to improving epilepsy education will be the widespread sharing of information and tools, such as diagnostic algorithms and treatment guidelines that can be accessed all over the world.[25] Epilepsy educational tools will need to be made widely available at appropriate levels for neurologists and epilepsy specialists, as well as primary care providers. To this end, organizations such as the ILAE or IBE can continue to develop and update standardized educational materials that can be widely dispersed. The education of medical providers should also extend to specific training for nurses and social workers, who both provide crucial primary care services and build essential healthcare networks for individuals with epilepsy.[25]

In terms of education of the public, the continuation of the Demonstration Projects and similar community-based projects will provide continued education regarding the burden of epilepsy and the unmet needs of those faced with epilepsy. Other initiatives similar to the 'Stand up For Epilepsy Sports and Epilepsy Project'[29] can be undertaken to raise awareness of epilepsy and fight the stigma and discrimination with which it is often associated. These initiatives may be spearheaded by national and international organizations, local affiliates, and importantly individuals with epilepsy and their families and supporters.

Ongoing research support and creative approaches to advancing epilepsy research continue to be essential in the work to improve the lives of those with epilepsy. In particular translational research, bridging the gap between the laboratory and clinical applications, will continue to be extremely important. Promoting this type of work will involve demonstrating the importance of epilepsy research to both clinicians and basic scientists. Clinicians will need to be educated in basic science, and bench researchers educated in clinical epilepsy.[25] Research in the developing world will necessitate reinforcement of infrastructure and augmentation of local resources. Again, epilepsy-related education will be paramount. 'Twinning', in which research groups in industrialized countries and emerging countries are paired together, may help to foster epilepsy research in these areas.[24] Training programmes for researchers and opportunities for them to conduct research in their countries are also essential. The goals may be facilitated by assistance from national and international advocacy organizations.[25]

New areas of research already being explored include the identification of biomarkers that can predict epileptogenesis, and the search for medications that can prevent the development of epilepsy as opposed to treating its symptoms (i.e. anti-epileptogenic medications as opposed to anti-seizure medications). A large, international, multicentre study called the Epilepsy Bioinformatics Study for Antiepileptogenic Therapy, or EpiBioS4Rx, has begun to look at exactly these questions with regard to patients with traumatic brain injury. Their aim is to involve a mixture of research scientists, clinicians, health organizations, professional societies, and patients and patient organizations in this project, and to make the results of their studies widely available to the entire epilepsy community.[32]

Ideally, future epilepsy research will involve both small and large research groups, and will continue to involve partnerships between researchers and special interest groups. The focus of epilepsy research may vary by region, depending on common causes of epilepsy within a given area (e.g. infection, trauma, perinatal causes, and others).[25] New animal models may need to be developed and new treatments must be cultivated. Complementary and alternative medicines should be investigated, as should botanicals that may be able to be grown in remote regions.[24]

Conclusion

Epilepsy is a disease that disrupts the lives of many people of all ages and all ethnicities, all over the world. It is an unpredictable and often debilitating disorder that is often stigmatized and poorly understood. Over the past 20 years, advocacy efforts have made great strides towards improving epilepsy education, fighting stigma, and beginning to close the treatment gap for those who suffer from this disease. As research progresses and better treatments, and possibly cures, are discovered, it is important to continue to advocate that government agencies make epilepsy a priority. We must emphasize that essential medications need to be readily available, and that an infrastructure must be in place to support people with epilepsy. We must work to improve public education, to improve access to treatments, and to establish clear therapeutic and research guidelines. Medical professionals need to be educated on how to manage epilepsy, and appropriate diagnostic tools must be made widely available. Old treatment models that may not adequately address the real needs of people with epilepsy need to be modified, and country-specific standards for epilepsy care must be developed. It is only through collaboration between advocacy groups, governments, and individuals that real progress can be made towards a world in which no one's life is limited by epilepsy.

Acknowledgements and disclosures

Solomon L. Moshé is the Charles Frost Chair in Neurosurgery and Neurology and has received funding by grants from NIH NS43209 and 1U54NS100064, CURE Infantile Spasms Initiative, US Department of Defense (W81XWH-13-1-0180), the Heffer Family and the Segal Family Foundations, and the Abbe Goldstein/Joshua Lurie and Laurie Marsh/Dan Levitz families. He serves as Associate Editor of *Neurobiology of Disease*, and is on the editorial board of *Brain and Development*, *Pediatric Neurology*, and *Physiological Research*. He receives from Elsevier an annual compensation for his work as Associate Editor in *Neurobiology of Disease* and royalties from two books he co-edited. He received a consultant's fee from Eisai and UCB.

References

1. **World Health Organization** (2015) *Global Burden of Epilepsy and the Need for Coordinated Action at the Country Level to Address Its Health, Social, and Public Knowledge Implications.* Resolution WHA68.20, 26 May 2015. Available at: http://www.ilae.org/visitors/News/documents/WHO-Epilepsy-2015.pdf
2. **Leonardi, M.**, **Ustun, T. B.** (2002) The global burden of epilepsy. *Epilepsia*, **43**(Suppl. 6), 21–5.
3. **Moshé, S. L.**, **Perucca, E.**, **Ryvlin, P.**, et al. (2015) Epilepsy: new advances. *Lancet*, **385**, 884–98.
4. **Scheffer, I. E.**, **Berkovic, S.**, **Capovilla, G.**, et al. (2017) ILAE Classification of the epilepsies position paper of the ILAE Commission for Classification and Terminology. *Epilepsia*, **58**(4), 512–21.
5. **de Boer, H. M.**, **Mula, M.**, **Sander, J. W.** (2008) The global burden and stigma of epilepsy. *Epilepsy & Behavior*, **12**, 540–6.
6. **Covanis, A.**, **Guekht, A.**, **Li, S.**, et al. (2015) From global campaign to global commitment: the World Health Assembly's resolution on epilepsy. *Epilepsia*, **56**(11), 1651–7.

7. **Lhatoo, S. D., Johnson, A. L., Goodridge, D. M., et al.** (2001) Mortality in epilepsy in the first 11 to 14 years after diagnosis: multivariate analysis of a long-term, prospective, population-based cohort. *Ann Neurol*, **49**, 336–44
8. **Ficker, D. M.** (2000) Sudden unexplained death and injury in epilepsy. *Epilepsia*, **41**(suppl 2), S7–12.
9. **Luoni, C., Bisulli, F., Canevini, M. P., et al.** (2011) Determinants of health-related quality of life in pharmacoresistant epilepsy: results from a large multi-center study of consecutively enrolled patients using validated quantitative assessments. *Epilepsia*, **52**, 2181–91.
10. **Capovilla, G., Kaufman, K. R., Perucca, E., Moshé, S. L., Arida, R. M.** (2016) Epilepsy, seizures, physical exercise, and sports: a report from the ILAE task force on sports and epilepsy. *Epilepsia*, **57**(1), 6–12.
11. **Fiest, K. M., Birbeck, G. L., Jacoby, A., et al.** (2014) Stigma in epilepsy. *Curr Neurol Neurosci Rep*, **14**, 444.
12. **Salomon, J. A., Vos, T., Hogan, D. R., et al.** (2012) Common values in assessing health outcomes from disease and injury: disability weights measurement study for the Global Burden of Disease Study 2010. *Lancet*, **380**(9859), 2129–43.
13. **Thurman, D. J., Hesdorffer, D. C., French, J. A.** (2014) Sudden unexpected death in epilepsy: assessing the public health burden. *Epilepsia*, **55**, 1479–85.
14. **Government of Canada and Neurological Health Charities Canada** (2014) *Mapping Connections—An Understanding of Neurological Conditions in Canada*. Ottawa, Canada: Public Health Agency of Canada.
15. **Newton, C. R., Garcia, H. H.** (2012) Epilepsy in poor regions of the world. *Lancet*, **380**, 1193–201.
16. **Ding, D., Wang, W., Wu, J., et al.** (2013) Premature mortality risk in people with convulsive epilepsy: long follow-up of a cohort in rural China. *Epilepsia*, **54**, 512–17.
17. **Meyer, A. C., Dua, T., Boscardin, W. J., et al.** (2012) Critical determinants of the epilepsy treatment gap: a cross-national analysis in resource-limited settings. *Epilepsia*, **53**, 2178–85.
18. **Cameron, A., Bansal, A., Dua, T., et al.** (2012) Mapping the availability, price, and affordability of antiepileptic drugs in 46 countries. *Epilepsia*, **53**(6), 962–9.
19. **Meyer, A. C., Dua, T., Ma, J., et al.** (2010) Global disparities in the epilepsy treatment gap: a systematic review. *Bull World Health Organ*, **88**, 260–6.
20. **World Health Organization** (2005) International Bureau for Epilepsy and International League Against Epilepsy. *Atlas: Epilepsy Care in the World*. Available at: http://www.who.int/mental_health/neurology/Epilepsy_atlas_r1.pdf
21. **Jallon, P.** (1997) Epilepsy in developing countries. *Epilepsia*, **38**, 1143–51.
22. **Meinardi, H., Scott, R. A., Reis, R., Sander, J. W.** (2001) The treatment gap in epilepsy: the current situation and ways forward. *Epilepsia*, **42**, 136–49.
23. **Brodie, M. J., Kwan, P.** (2012) Current position of phenobarbital in epilepsy and its future. *Epilepsia*, 53 Suppl 8, 40–6.
24. **Beal, J. C., Moshé, S. L.** (2013) Stand up for epilepsy: the global campaign. In: Gusev, E. I., Guekht, A. B. (eds). *Epilepsy: Translational, Clinical, and Social Aspects*. Moscow: Ankinron, pp. 17–23
25. **Moshé, S. L.** (2009) The International League Against Epilepsy at the threshold of its second century: challenges and opportunities. *Epilepsia*, **50**(12), 2508–13.

26. **World Health Organization. Regional Office for the Western Pacific** (2009) *Epilepsy Management at Primary Health Level in Rural China: WHO/ILAE/IBE Global Campaign Against Epilepsy Demonstration Project.* Manila: WHO Regional Office for the Western Pacific. Available at: http://www.who.int/iris/handle/10665/254615
27. **Global Campaign Against Epilepsy** (2012) *Basic Principles and Guidance Instrument for Developing, Adopting and Implementing Epilepsy Legislation.* May, 2012. Available at: http://www.globalcampaignagainstepilepsy.org/wp-content/uploads/2010/02/Basic-Principles-final.pdf
28. **World Health Organization** (2008) *MhGAP Intervention Guide for Mental, Neurological and Substance Use Disorders in Non-Specialized Health Settings.* 2008. Available at: http://www.who.int/mental_health/publications/mhGAP_intervention_guide/en/
29. **International League Against Epilepsy** (2013) Stand up for Epilepsy: Sports and Epilepsy Project. Available at: https://www.ilae.org/about-ilae/public-policy-and-advocacy/epilepsy-and-sport-project-stand-up-for-epilepsy
30. **Perucca, E.** (2014) The European declaration on epilepsy: past, present and future. *Epilepsy & Seizure,* **7,** 14–22.
31. **World Federation of Neurology** (2015) World Brain Day 2015. Available at: https://www.wfneurology.org/world-brain-day-2015
32. **Epilepsy Bioinformatics Study for Antiepileptogenic Therapy (EpiBioS4Rx).** Available at: http://epibios.loni.usc.edu/

Chapter 30

Advocacy for patients with headache

Timothy J. Steiner and Jes Olesen

Introduction

Headache disorders have always been at the bottom of the heap of neurological disorders. This is evidence not only of the pressing need for advocacy on behalf of patients with headache but also, sadly, of the enduring failure of advocacy in the past.

Why headache commands so little respect may never be fully explained, and it is very difficult to explain when, in 2016, headache disorders were shown by the Global Burden of Disease (GBD) Study to be the second highest cause of disability among all diseases worldwide.[1] Several contributory reasons can nonetheless be identified, none of which suggest that this is an irredeemable situation.

To begin with, headache disorders receive little attention in undergraduate medical curricula throughout the world—4 hours' teaching on average, in 4–6 years, according to the World Health Organization (WHO).[2] Doctors accordingly qualify with little understanding of headache disorders, and consequently little interest in them. Later, in postgraduate training, the primary headaches are rarely seen among hospital inpatients because they are virtually never a cause for hospital admission. Headache is frequently encountered as a symptom of other diseases, but the focus then is on the underlying disorders, and the headache often ignored. Migraine, tension-type headache, and cluster headache may be common in neurological outpatients, where they present no neurological, imaging, or laboratory abnormalities or other biomarkers to interest trainees in this specialty. They are even more common in primary care, where doctors untrained to treat headache achieve poor outcomes in dissatisfied patients who eventually give up the quest for effective care. Among the general public there is at best insouciance towards and at worst a joking disdain for headaches,[3] which are often trivialized as 'normal', a minor annoyance, or an excuse to avoid responsibility. This is coupled with a general disbelief that headache disorders have a biological basis, or that they can genuinely be disabling or life-impairing. Rather, they are attributed to psychological factors and 'stress', a notion reinforced in the public's mind by the fact that migraine is predominantly a female disorder and, at worst in this style of thinking, clearly associated with menstruation.

The low esteem granted to headache disorders is self-perpetuating. Few doctors are motivated to push for improvements in headache care, let alone for the structured headache services that WHO recommends.[2] Policymakers responsible for healthcare, and granting authorities who effectively control research, are inevitably influenced by these factors, particularly the lack of public clamour for change[3]; their decisions, made critically, invariably reflect them.

The case for advocacy in headache

Headache disorders, responsible for more disability than all other neurological disorders combined,[1] are arguably more in need of advocacy than any other group among these disorders.

The scientific argument

Despite minuscule funding, scientific progress in headache disorders over the last 30 years has been amazing. An international headache classification hierarchically ordering the many different headache disorders and setting out explicit diagnostic criteria for each of them has, through several revisions,[4-6] been accepted and taken into general use all over the world. This has provided a bedrock for sound epidemiological studies, which have not only demonstrated their high prevalence in every world region and among rich and poor countries alike[1,7] but also transformed awareness of the global burden attributable to them. Over 16 years, in increasingly better informed GBD studies, migraine has ascended the ranks of top causes of disability worldwide, from nineteenth in GBD 2000[8] to seventh in GBD 2010,[9,10] sixth in GBD 2013,[11] third in GBD 2015,[7,12] and second in GBD 2016.[1] Meanwhile, tension-type headache was introduced in GBD 2010,[9,10] while medication-overuse headache was first included in GBD 2013—and ranked eighteenth highest cause of disability.[11] With its precise definitions, the classification has underpinned excellent genetic studies, so that 38 genetic variants are currently known to be significantly associated with migraine.[13] Brain blood flow studies have demonstrated the likely link between migraine aura and cortical spreading depression.[14] Migraine can now be treated with effective drugs that are both selective and highly specific.[15]

Migraine at least, therefore, has been solidly demonstrated as a neurobiological disorder, while several similar advances are taking place for cluster headache.

The public health argument

The prevalence of primary headache disorders in the general population is now very well documented in most world regions.[1,9,11,12,16] Tension-type headache and migraine are, respectively, the second and third most common diseases in the world.[9] The global one-year prevalence of migraine among adults is currently estimated at almost 15%, although recent studies with better methodology generally find higher values, and this estimate will rise.[17] Migraine preferentially affects young adults, and is the *top* cause of disability among those aged less than 50 years.[17] Tension-type headache affects more people, but in many cases only mildly or infrequently, so that it contributes less to global disability.[1,9,11,12,16,17]

These two disorders are mostly episodic. At least 2% of adults worldwide have headache on 15 days a month or more (that is, on more days than not). Among the manifest disorders is medication-overuse headache, with a prevalence ranging between 0.5% and 7%.[18] This condition is a secondary headache,[5,6] but it occurs mostly as a consequence of mismanagement of migraine and is itself eighteenth among the worldwide causes of disability.[11] Cluster headache may affect only one in 1,000 adults, but it is among the most severe pains known to mankind,[5,6] and highly disabling to those affected.

The totality of pain engendered by these disorders is enormous. Pain is disabling, as are some of the other symptoms common especially in migraine, such as nausea. It is not surprising that, collectively, headache disorders are among the top causes of disability in the world.[1-3,7-12,16,17]

Furthermore, there are over 200 other types of headache.[6] These include chronic post-traumatic headache, a major cause of disability among soldiers and athletes, and in countries where accident rates are high.

The financial argument

It is equally not surprising that headache disorders are responsible for much lost productivity. The annual economic costs of headache disorders in Europe have been estimated in one study at over EUR 40 billion[19] and in another, taking into account both absenteeism and reduced productivity among those at work with headache, at well over EUR 100 billion.[20] Over 90% of costs are indirect, consequential upon lost productivity. In China, where headache prevalence is below the global mean, it nonetheless depletes gross domestic product (GDP) by an estimated 2.24%.[21] In India, with a high one-year migraine prevalence of 25.2%,[22] productivity loss attributable to headache at population level, every single day, is 3.0%, a loss likely also to be reflected in diminished GDP.[23] These numbers place headache disorders among the most costly of neurological disorders (only dementia and perhaps stroke are more so), the consequence of their being, by a wide margin, the most disabling.[1]

As the economic studies show, the direct costs of headache (the resources sunk in treating it) are less than one-tenth of the total costs.[20,24] Since the primary headache disorders are to a very large extent treatable, greater advertent investment in headache care will predictably not only bring substantial improvements in public health but also be cost-saving at societal level.[2]

The failure of advocacy so far

These are compelling messages, but they have not yet reached the consciousness of health policymakers.[3,17] In Europe, where the funding of brain disorders has been estimated in relation to their costs, headache disorders were found to be the least funded of all neurological disorders.[25] In the United States (US), funding for headache by the National Institutes of Health has been equally poor—far below that of other, less costly neurological disorders. Paradoxically, the funding of headache disorders is dwarfed by marketing budgets for painkillers to treat headache.

Yet, as we have described, sound data create a solid basis for advocacy for headache. The public health messages are clear enough. First, good healthcare can alleviate much of the symptom burden of most headache disorders, thereby mitigating both the humanitarian and the financial costs that arise from them. Second, none of the five essential components of effective healthcare for headache is beyond the capabilities of primary care: awareness of the problem; correct recognition and diagnosis; avoidance of mismanagement; appropriate lifestyle modifications; and informed use of cost-effective pharmaceutical remedies. For the vast majority of those who need it, effective treatment requires no expensive equipment, tests, or specialists. Third, therefore, structured headache services can be based in primary care, and low-cost for this majority. Such services are WHO's recommended solution, and would have most patients effectively and cost-effectively treated in primary care by general practitioners (GPs) educated with basic knowledge, and only the small proportion who truly need them managed in specialist services.[2]

Advocates have used these data and argued these messages throughout the world. In the Americas and Europe, and to a lesser extent in other world regions, both lay and professional headache organizations include advocacy among their purposes. Next are some examples. In the United Kingdom, a group of charities including the Migraine Trust, the Organization for Understanding Cluster Headache (OUCH), and the British Association for the Study of Headache (BASH) lobby Parliament through the All-Party Parliamentary Group on Primary Headache Disorders.[26] The most important output of this group, a publication pithily summarizing the problem ('Headache disorders—not respected, not resourced'),[27] has no more led to policy change than did the publication by BASH of 2,000 detailed and evidence-backed proposals for headache service organization. The Migraine Association of Ireland does much to raise awareness, and, with the country's president as their patron,[28] has had some influence on policy. In Norway, Norsk Hodepineselskap among others lobbied for a National Headache Competence Centre, which duly opened at the Norwegian University of Science and Technology (NTNU) in Trondheim.[29] The Danish Headache Centre in Copenhagen was this year (2018) accommodated in a new specially designed building,[30] made possible by a very large donation from a private foundation that was itself the fruit of concerted advocacy. These are important but nonetheless limited successes: in none of these countries are there structured headache services in the form recommended by WHO.[2] In the Lombardy Region of Italy, legislative support for such services has been gained, but this appears to be a unique triumph for advocacy in Europe. In the US, Headache on the Hill (HOH) is an annual congressional advocacy event co-sponsored by the American Headache Society, each year lobbying approximately 130 members of Congress on behalf of those with disabling headache disorders. A direct outcome of HOH in 2016 was the Safe Treatments and Opportunities to Prevent Pain Act ('STOP Pain Act'),[31] signed into law in July. Congress now directs National Institutes of Health (NIH) to fund *pain* research to an extent commensurate with pain's societal burden. How this law will increase funding for research on headache disorders is yet to be seen. What is clear is that, if full benefit is to be had, *headache's* societal burden needs to be firmly quantified.

Thus it is difficult to discern any substantial gains from all this advocacy effort. Perhaps the advocates have been too few in number, have failed to speak in unison, or are regarded in a world of limited resources merely as spokesmen for vested interests.

Whatever the reasons, not only does headache research remain pitifully underfunded, but also care for headache patients is miserable in most countries.[2] Headache disorders may be largely treatable, but *still* they are among the highest causes of disability worldwide.[1,17] The principal reason why this and the other burdens of headache persist is failure of health policy. It is not sufficient that efficacious therapies exist: healthcare resources must be allocated, and healthcare systems put in place, so that these therapies are delivered to all who need them—everyone whose quality of life is affected by headache. This is not happening. Structured headache services are yet to be found in most countries of the world. There is nowhere near enough teaching of GPs to equip them for their role,[2] and throughout the world there are very few dedicated headache centres to support them.

Advocacy for headache has, so far, equally failed. But, with ever-growing evidential support, this failure is surely remediable.

WHO and the Global Campaign against Headache

More than any other health authority, WHO has acknowledged the public health importance of headache disorders, and acted as advocate for headache on a macro level.[2,32-35] Together with the UK-registered non-governmental organization *Lifting The Burden* (LTB), WHO launched the Global Campaign against Headache in 2004.[36] LTB was admitted into official relations with WHO in 2011.[37] cementing this collaboration. This milestone event was itself achieved through prolonged and persistent advocacy.

LTB's priority since the campaign launch has been to gather the data upon which successful advocacy must be mounted. This was much needed. Even up to 2007, very little was known of the prevalence or burden of any headache disorder for more than half the people of the world: those living in most of the Western Pacific Region, including China, all of Southeast Asia including India, all of Eastern Europe including Russia, most of the Eastern Mediterranean Region, and most of Africa.[16] Filling these knowledge gaps was consequently the campaign's first objective.[38]

Collaborating with many local investigators and, crucially, with successive GBD studies,[1,9,11,12] the Global Campaign informed the latter by conducting new population-based surveys—so far in Georgia, Russia, China, Mongolia, Nepal, India, Saudi Arabia, Pakistan, Morocco, Zambia, and Ethiopia, with others planned in South America and West Africa. This concerted data-collection effort replaced many of the assumptions of earlier GBD studies with empirical data, so supporting increasingly accurate estimates.[17] It was by this means that migraine became recognized as a top cause of disability worldwide,[1,17] medication-overuse headache was ranked eighteenth,[11] and GBD 2016 established headache disorders collectively as second.[1] For the US Congress, and all other agencies that influence resource allocation to headache research or care, there is no longer any doubt regarding headache's societal burden.

LTB itself is not primarily an advocacy organization, but it recognizes advocacy as a key means of achieving its stated purpose, which is to reduce the burden of headache worldwide.[36-38] Therefore the Campaign's second objective (using knowledge from the first) is to persuade governments and other health-service policymakers, healthcare providers, people directly affected by headache and the general population of this simple fact: that headache must, on the clearest evidence, have higher healthcare priority.[36-38] In 2011, in a joint publication with LTB, WHO sent this message to all the Ministries of Health of the world:

> 'The facts and figures ... illuminate the worldwide neglect of a major cause of public ill-health and reveal the inadequacies of responses to it in countries throughout the world.'[2]

Nothing more starkly apt can be said.

Conclusions

Advocacy for more headache research and better headache care has been largely in vain so far. Despite irrefutable evidence of the prevalence, burden, and cost of headache disorders, it may be that results will come only after a very long haul. But it is crucially important that advocacy continues, because the huge need for headache care is largely unmet throughout the world.[2] The arguments for change are now unanswerable—but they have to be put to those who can make change happen. In addition, it appears they will have to be repeated, again and again.

There are glimpses of light and small successes here and there, and these may help advocacy in other parts of the world. Actions at national levels must combine in collaboration with the Global Campaign against Headache. The International Headache Society is now bringing together all advocacy groups, along with representatives of regulatory agencies and of pharmaceutical and biotechnology companies, aiming to determine advocacy priorities and identify opportunities for advocacy everywhere. If they work together, the many national and supranational professional and lay groups will find previously closed doors are, at last, slowly opening.

References

1. **Vos, T., Abajobir, A. A., Abbafati, C., et al.** (2017) Global, regional, and national incidence, prevalence, and years lived with disability for 328 diseases and injuries for 195 countries, 1990–2016: a systematic analysis for the Global Burden of Disease Study 2016. *Lancet*, **390**, 1211–59.
2. **World Health Organization and *Lifting the Burden*** (2011) *Atlas of Headache Disorders and Resources in the World 2011*. Geneva: WHO.
3. **Katsarava, Z., Steiner, T. J.** (2012) Neglected headache: ignorance, arrogance or insouciance? *Cephalalgia*, **32**, 1019–20.
4. **International Headache Society Classification Subcommittee** (2004) *The International Classification of Headache Disorders*, 2nd edition. *Cephalalgia*, **24** (Suppl 1), 1–160.
5. **International Headache Society Classification Subcommittee** (2018) *The International Classification of Headache Disorders*, 3rd edition. *Cephalalgia*, **38**, 1–211
6. **Steiner, T. J., Stovner, L. J., Vos, T.** (2016) GBD 2015: migraine is the third cause of disability in under 50s. *J Headache Pain*, **17**, 104.
7. **World Health Organization** (2001) *The World Health Report 2001*. Geneva: WHO, pp. 19–45.

8. **Vos, T., Flaxman, A. D., Naghavi, M.**, et al. (2012) Years lived with disability (YLDs) for 1160 sequelae of 289 diseases and injuries 1990–2010: a systematic analysis for the Global Burden of Disease Study 2010. *Lancet*, **380**, 2163–96.
9. **Steiner, T. J., Stovner, L. J., Birbeck, G. L.** (2013) Migraine: the seventh disabler. *J Headache Pain*, **14**, 1.
10. **Vos, T., Barber, R. M., Bell, B.** (2015) Global, regional, and national incidence, prevalence, and years lived with disability for 301 acute and chronic diseases and injuries in 188 countries, 1990–2013: a systematic analysis for the Global Burden of Disease Study 2013. *Lancet*, **386**, 743–800.
11. **GBD 2015 Disease and Injury Incidence and Prevalence Collaborators** (2016) Global, regional, and national incidence, prevalence, and years lived with disability for 310 diseases and injuries, 1990–2015: a systematic analysis for the Global Burden of Disease Study 2015. *Lancet*, **388**, 1545–602.
12. **Gormley, P., Anttila, V., Winsvold, B. S.**, et al. (2016) Meta-analysis of 375,000 individuals identifies 38 susceptibility loci for migraine. *Nat Genet*, **48**, 856–66.
13. **Olesen, J., Friberg, L., Olsen, T. S.**, et al. (1990) Timing and topography of cerebral blood flow, aura, and headache during migraine attacks. *Ann Neurol*, **28**, 791–8.
14. **Olesen, J., Diener, H.-C., Husstedt, I. W.**, et al. (2004) Calcitonin gene-related peptide receptor antagonist BIBN 4096 BS for the acute treatment of migraine. *NEJM*, **350**, 1104–10.
15. **Stovner, L. J., Hagen, K., Jensen, R.**, et al. (2007) The global burden of headache: a documentation of headache prevalence and disability worldwide. *Cephalalgia*, **27**, 193–210.
16. **Steiner, T. J., Stovner, L. J., Vos, T., Jensen, R., Katsarava, Z.** (2018) Migraine is *first* cause of disability in under 50s: will health politicians now take notice? *J Headache Pain*, **19**, 17.
17. **Westergaard, M. L., Holme Hansen, E., Glümer, C.**, et al. (2014) Definitions of medication-overuse headache in population-based studies and their implications on prevalence estimates: a systematic review. *Cephalalgia*, **34**, 409–25.
18. **Gustavsson, A., Svensson, M., Jacobi, F.**, et al. (2011) Cost of disorders of the brain in Europe 2010. *Eur Neuropsychopharmacol*, **21**, 718–79.
19. **Linde, M., Gustavsson, A., Stovner, L. J.**, et al. (2012) The cost of headache disorders in Europe: the Eurolight project. *Eur J Neurol*, **19**, 703–11.
20. **Yu, S., Liu, R., Zhao, G.**, et al. (2012) The prevalence and burden of primary headaches in China: a population-based door-to-door survey. *Headache*, **52**, 582–91.
21. **Kulkarni, G. B., Rao, G. N., Gururaj, G., Stovner, L. J., Steiner, T. J.** (2015) Headache disorders and public ill-health in India: prevalence estimates in Karnataka State. *J Headache Pain*, **16**, 67.
22. **Steiner, T. J., Rao, G. N., Kulkarni, G. B., Gururaj, G., Stovner, L. J.** (2016) Headache yesterday in Karnataka state, India: prevalence, impact and cost. *J Headache Pain*, **17**, 74.
23. **Hu, X. H., Markson, L. E., Lipton, R. B., Stewart, W. F., Berger, M. L.** (1999) Burden of migraine in the United States: disability and economic costs. *Arch Intern Med*, **159**, 813–18.
24. **Sobocki, P., Lekander, I., Berwick, S., Olesen, J., Jönsson, B.** (2006) Resource allocation to brain research in Europe—a full report. *Eur J Neurosci*, **24**(10), 2691–93.
25. **All-Party Parliamentary Group on Primary Headache Disorders** (2015) Available at: http://www.publications.parliament.uk/pa/cm/cmallparty/register/headache-disorders.htm

26. **The Migraine Association of Ireland**. Available at: https://www.migraine.ie/about-the-mai/
27. **St. Olavs Hospital**. Nasjonal kompetansetjeneste for hodepine (National Competence Service for Headaches). Available at: https://stolav.no/Sider/Nasjonal-kompetansetjeneste-for-hodepine-NKH.aspx
28. **Danish Headache Center**. Available at: https://www.rigshospitalet.dk/english/departments/neuroscience-centre/danish-headache-center/Pages/default.aspx
29. **United States Congress**. Available at: https://www.congress.gov/bill/114th-congress/house-bill/5249/text
30. **World Health Organization** (2000) *Headache Disorders and Public Health*. Geneva: WHO.
31. **World Health Organization** (2003) *Headache Disorders. Fact sheet no. 277*. Geneva: WHO.
32. **World Health Organization** (2007) *Neurological Disorders: Public Health Challenges*. Geneva: WHO.
33. **Thakur, K. T., Albanese, E., Giannakopoulos, P., et al. (eds).** (2015) *Mental, Neurological, and Substance Use Disorders*. **Disease control priorities**, 3rd edition, Vol. **4**. Washington DC: World Bank.
34. **Steiner, T. J.** (2004) Lifting the burden: the Global Campaign against Headache. *Lancet Neurol*, **3**, 204–5.
35. **Steiner, T. J., Birbeck, G. L., Jensen, R., Katsarava, Z., Martelletti, P., Stovner, L. J.** (2011) The Global Campaign, World Health Organization and *Lifting the Burden*: collaboration in action. *J Headache Pain*, **12**, 273–4.
36. **Steiner, T. J., Birbeck, G. L., Jensen, R., Katsarava, Z., Martelletti, P., Stovner, L. J.** (2010) *Lifting the Burden*: the first 7 years. *J Headache Pain*, **11**, 451–5.
37. *Lifting the Burden*: **the Global Campaign against Headache**. Available at: http://www.l-t-b.org
38. **International Headache Society**. IHS Newsletter Issue 15—December 2016. Available at: http://www.ihs-headache.org

Chapter 31

Advocacy for patients with neuropathic pain

Ligia Onofrei and A. Gordon Smith

Introduction

Pain is nearly universal, yet each person's experience is highly variable. Many different factors contribute to an individual's unique pain experience: genetic factors, mechanism of injury, medical comorbidities, social aspects, variations in coping styles, belief systems, and innate personality traits. Despite this variability, clinicians are faced with using a limited complement of medications and clinical approaches and are often left unsure of how to offer individualized care.

Approximately 100 million Americans suffer from chronic pain, roughly one-third of the population.[1,2] The cost of chronic pain in the United States is staggering, at an estimated $560–635 billion each year.[1] This estimate includes $261–300 billion in medical costs and $300 billion in lost productivity.[1]

Neuropathic pain is defined as 'pain caused by a lesion or disease of the somatosensory system'.[3] Currently, diabetic neuropathy (DPN) and chronic low back pain are the two most common causes of neuropathic pain.[4] Approximately 20 million Americans suffer from neuropathic pain, with older patients more affected than younger patients.[4,5]

Pain has received more attention in recent years at a national level. In 2011, the Institute of Medicine published a report titled 'Relieving pain in America'. This report was a direct result of provisions made by the 2010 Patient Protection and Affordable Care Act that required the Department of Health and Human Services to develop activities that recognized the importance of pain as a public health problem.[6] This report is a blueprint for transforming the approach to pain care in the United States and covers broad topics ranging from the biological basis of pain to the social implications of pain, while touching on the current therapies of pain and current state of research.[6] Advocacy can be approached at multiple levels and from different perspectives: patient, physician, health system, and governmental. Each will be reviewed.

Patient-level advocacy

From a patient's viewpoint, care for pain should be simple: if one suffers from pain, one should be able to have easy, affordable, rapid access to comprehensive treatments and interventions that offer pain relief. Care should be personalized, taking into account one's unique circumstances, and access to the full spectrum of appropriate therapies should be readily available. The reality, however, is that care for pain is complicated by a large number of factors including mode and timing of care delivery, availability of effective interventions, and cost. Current treatment modalities for neuropathic pain include medications, operative procedures, physical modalities, regional anaesthesia, neuro-augmentation modalities such as spinal cord stimulators (SCS), implantable drug delivery systems, comprehensive pain rehabilitation programmes (PRP) such as interdisciplinary pain centres, and complementary and alternative medicine modalities.[7]

Despite the theoretically abundant choices available, the efficacy of each individual intervention is limited. In clinical trials, only 10–25% more of the patients in the intervention group achieved greater than 50% pain intensity reduction when compared to the placebo group.[3] The number needed to treat (NNT) to achieve greater than 50% reduction in pain intensity over 12 weeks for neuropathic pain agents is 4 to 6 for duloxetine (at a dose of 60–120 mg/day), gabapentin (at a dose of 1,200 mg/day), and pregabalin (at a dose of 600 mg/day for DPN and 300–600 mg per day for postherpetic neuralgia).[8] This implies that only 15–25% of patients achieve benefit. Opioid medications have been used for a large number of disorders including neuropathic pain, but studies point to modest benefits. One Cochrane Collaboration systematic review of the evidence supporting use of oxycodone in the treatment of painful DPN found that oxycodone had only 'moderate benefit' (defined as at least 30% relief or patients who felt they were much or very much improved) in 44% of patients; the same 'moderate benefit' was found in 27% of patients treated with placebo, for an NNT of 5.7.[3] Additionally, opioids are expensive and have potential for significant side effects, addiction, and dependencies.[3] The high side effect profile is reflected in dropout rates as high as 60% over 12 weeks in several clinical trials.[3]

These data highlight the critical importance of developing more effective and better tolerated therapies. Effective advocacy must therefore start with a renewed interest in research. Patients can become their own advocates in this matter by participating in research themselves and encouraging others to do so. Additionally, patient groups can exert influence on government agencies and the government itself to direct funds towards pain research and to change the regulatory environment to favour research and a more efficient drug approval process. Accomplishing this task requires significant mobilization of patient organizations, who would need to engage in lobbying for the interests of their group in addition to meeting regularly with their elected officials.

Beyond the issue of finding appropriate pain relief, patients with chronic pain are faced with many additional concerns: decreased quality of life, difficulty maintaining interpersonal relationships, decreased productivity, at the same time they face higher medical costs.[9] Chronic pain therefore is not a disease that affects only the individual, but also a disease that affects family, friends, and the community at large. The patient's unique circumstances, which includes family and work environment, stress levels, learned behaviours, and cultural views are all important determinants of how pain assessment and management can be approached.[6]

Therefore, effective pain management should extend beyond medications to include a myriad of other approaches including physical therapy, activity modifications, behaviour modifications, cognitive behaviour therapy, and complementary and alternative modalities such as massage, acupuncture, biofeedback, and meditation. Unfortunately, access to alternative therapies and interdisciplinary pain management programmes is frequently restricted or not covered by insurance companies, or co-pays are cost prohibitive.[10]

Access to mental health treatment is of paramount importance when addressing chronic pain, as 40–50% of patients with chronic pain have comorbid mood disorders.[6] While it is not known whether chronic pain is the cause of mood disorders or the other way around, or whether patients with propensity for developing mood disorders also have a higher propensity for developing chronic pain, most studies suggest that depressive disorders tend to occur after the development of chronic pain.[6] Alarmingly, the risk of death by suicide is twice as high in patients with chronic pain compared to patients without pain.[11]

Variable insurance coverage and availability of mental health services, physical therapy, and complementary and alternative treatments are barriers to high-quality pain care. Patients can advocate for improved access to needed care by leveraging their role as consumers of medical services and insurance products. Physicians must advocate, on behalf of their patients, to make vital services available and can work within institutions to create comprehensive clinics in which multispecialty care can be delivered. Development of treatment guidelines that support appropriate use of these therapies will facilitate insurance coverage. Advocates should emphasize that insurance companies will ultimately benefit from access to those services that promise to prevent chronic pain and minimize risk of treatment complications or utilization of high-cost emergency services. If the US healthcare delivery system shifts towards a bundled value-based payment model, healthcare organizations will become incentivized to build delivery systems that optimize earlier access to care.

Physician-level advocacy

Physicians who treat patients with pain often find themselves navigating similar issues to their patients such as availability and coverage of medical treatments and interventions or access to subspecialty care. Physicians also face many unique challenges.

Since primary care physicians treat 52% of chronic pain patients in the United States, the continued education of primary care physicians is of particular importance.[12] While some guidelines for continuing medical education (CME) addressing pain management exist, this has not translated into effective educational programmes, with most physicians and nurses feeling their pain management training to be inadequate.[6,13] In one study of primary care residents, only half felt 'somewhat prepared' to counsel patients about pain management, while 27% felt 'somewhat unprepared' or 'very unprepared', with only 21–26% feeling 'very prepared'.[14] In a survey of 500 primary care physicians at 12 academic centres, only 34% felt comfortable treating people with chronic non-cancer pain.[15]

CME programmes

Even when physicians want to acquire additional training, pain-related CME programmes are frequently limited in scope and applicability and often include only basic or very general information without a discussion of difficult cases. Others focus solely on legal regulations. Physicians and other members of the care team must advocate for their needs as learners, including requesting professional organizations to create CME programmes that encompass a wide spectrum of pain disorders including guidance for management of medically complex or difficult problems, and that impart skills and knowledge that can be easily applied in the daily practice of medicine. Creation of easily accessible, evidence-based guidelines for the treatment of pain such as the guidelines created by the American Academy of Neurology for the Treatment of Painful DPN will help providers improve care.[16]

While access to evidence-based management guidelines is very important for effective pain management, it is also important for physicians to have an intimate understanding of how pain permeates patients' lives and how it affects their function and enjoyment of life. Unfortunately, many patients with chronic pain feel marginalized by, and develop uneasy relationships with, the medical establishment.[6,13] Patients frequently feel that when pain can be ascribed to an underlying disease such as a cancer, their pain is viewed as 'legitimate' or 'real' and they are treated with concern, but that when the cause of their pain is not well defined, they are marginalized, and their pain is dismissed and undertreated.[6] Pain becomes a disease in its own right for those who develop chronic pain, even if no specific aetiology is found.[6] As a community, we must change the culture of how chronic pain is perceived and managed. This type of change can be instituted by teaching medical students the social and psychological aspects of pain, not just about the biological and medical complexities. Currently, while some guidelines exist for continuing medical education, there are no formal core competencies at a medical school level for the evaluation and treatment of pain.[13]

Promoting awareness of healthcare disparities

It is also important to continue educating physicians about healthcare disparities. Race, gender, and socioeconomic status affect health outcomes and it appears these same factors also affect pain care.[17] Minority patients and those who are poor have more severe pain and pain related disability.[9] Unfortunately, minority patients have less access to primary care and patients of lower socioeconomic status are more likely to have insurance plans that limit access to subspecialty pain care or interdisciplinary pain management.[9] African-American patients are at higher risk of not having their pain assessed or treated.[9,17,18] In one study of patients with long bone fractures performed in an Atlanta emergency department, African-American patients were 1.7 times more likely than whites to receive no pain medication despite controlling for multiple confounders.[19] Similar findings were described in Hispanic and elderly patients regardless of race.[18,20] It is important to be aware of these disparities in order to implement corrective strategies.

Advocacy in medical education

Medical education should also prioritize acquisition of the skills needed to become an effective advocate beginning in medical school and continuing through postgraduate and continuing medical education. Most care providers are comfortable with advocating for their patients at an individual level, including lobbying insurance companies for access to needed treatments. Students, residents, and other medical professionals also need to be taught how to advocate for their patients and their communities and ultimately how to advocate for the benefit of society. Unfortunately, while many medical students are involved in advocacy during their undergraduate and medical school years and identify advocacy as an important part of their medical duties, one survey of Canadian residents showed that most are not involved in any advocacy activities due to issues such as insufficient time and rest, as well as stress.[21]

Advocacy in medical residency curricula

Advocacy is not included in most residency curricula and is not addressed in the US residency milestones. Most physicians do not have the skills and knowledge required to initiate an advocacy project, even if they are interested in becoming engaged. It is therefore important to create curricula that support development of advocacy competency. While some have started looking into the potential framework for a curriculum, discussing the challenges associated with implementing, evaluating, and ensuring progression of skills during formative years, no such curriculum has been formally adopted at this time in North American Medical Schools.[22] Advocacy curricula should not become just another checkmark in a logbook, or an artificial benchmark.

Most physicians (and students) are passionate advocates for their patients. Providing them with the tools, platforms, and support required to initiate advocacy efforts focused on their patient communities will enhance the health of patients with neuropathic pain and will serve to further engage providers in their careers and reduce the very high rate of burnout observed in most medical specialties.[23,24] For example, the American Academy of Neurology (AAN) has found new and creative ways of engaging its members with programmes such as the Palatucci Advocacy Leadership Forum (PALF), which offers intensive training for up to 30 AAN members each year, with a broad curriculum covering basic topics pertaining to the legislative process as well as advanced topics such as how to develop relationships with legislators and how to address the media.[25] The AAN also stages a yearly event which brings together neurologists from across the country to Washington DC to advocate to government representatives regarding key issues affecting neurologists and their patients in addition to offering an online course which teaches neurologists the fundamentals of advocacy.[24,25]

Health system and government-level advocacy

The priorities of a health system and society include ensuring that the greatest number of people participate in the workforce, system-level expenditures are kept to a minimum, population health and safety are maximized, and discovery and regulation of new drugs and interventions are supported. The costs associated with pain care are estimated at 560–635 billion dollars in both direct and indirect costs.[1,9] A substantial burden of these costs is borne by commercial insurances including workman's compensation, but Medicare paid approximately $65 billion in 2008 for pain alone, amounting to approximately 14% of all Medicare costs for the year.[6] Since the prevalence of neuropathic pain has been increasing, expenditures can be expected to climb as well. It is therefore of crucial importance to both patients and the healthcare system that pain therapies have demonstrated value, that is maximizing the ratio of benefits/cost. When treatments are ineffective or not as effective as would be desired, the costs to the system rise as patients often attempt to find relief by sequentially trying many different interventions. Development and distribution of rigorous evidence-based treatment guidelines will enhance value by avoiding utilization of therapies for which there is evidence of lack of efficacy.

Research

The importance of research cannot be understated. Enhanced funding of basic and translational research addressing underlying mechanisms of neuropathic pain including *in vitro* studies of potential therapeutic approaches will be necessary to identify new treatments and how best to implement them in populations. The time and resources required to translate exciting preclinical discoveries is daunting, which has made pharmaceutical companies cautious. The average time for taking a drug from preclinical research to clinical approval is 10–15 years, with an average cost of $2.5 billion.[26,27] Critical rate limiting steps in drug development include the failure of phase 2 trials to translate to phase 3 successes. Approaches to improve drug development include advocacy for continued governmental funding of basic and translation research focused on neuropathic pain, increase of incentives for development of new therapies in high priority areas, and support of systemic approaches to maximize efficiency in the drug development pipeline including investing in standing clinical trial networks, such as the National Institutes of Health (NIH)-funded Network for Excellence in Neuroscience Clinical Trials (NeuroNEXT) that leverage shared resources including master trial agreements and central institutional review boards.[28]

Funding

Researchers interested in neuropathic pain face a particularly challenging funding environment. The NIH provides about one-third of all funding for biomedical research in the United States, but funding for pain research accounts for less than 1% of the NIH budget. The overall NIH budget has remaining stagnant.[6,9] There is a striking discrepancy between funding for research and the direct cost for pain care. In 2007 $181 million was spent on pain research, less than 0.1% of the $635 billion annual cost of pain care.[6] There are many stakeholders that could have a larger role in addressing the need for increased research funding and patients and physicians must lobby aggressively for increased funding.

Public–private partnerships

Fostering public–private partnerships is another important strategy for which patients and providers can advocate. The Analgesic, Anesthetic, and Addiction Clinical Trial Translations Innovations Opportunities and Networks (ACTTION) is a public–private partnership including the US Food and Drug Administration (FDA) with the mission to identify, sponsor, and coordinate innovative approaches to neuropathic pain drug development with a focus on clinical trials.[29,30]

ACTTION has resulted in a significant number of publications focused on improved trial design and analysis of psychosocial determinants of pain.[29] The Clinical Trials Transformation Initiative, is a public–private partnership between the FDA's Office of critical path programmes and Duke University, focusing on improving the quality and efficiency of clinical trials.[31]

Another critical initiative with the potential to significantly enhance the quality of care is the Patient-Centered Outcomes Research Institute (PCORI), which was established by the Patient Protection and Affordable Care Act of 2010 as an independent, non-profit organization whose aim is to support projects that will help patients and clinicians make better health decisions by answering important clinical questions that drive practice.[32] PCORI's scope is broad, with studies across many subspecialties. So far, PCORI has funded one large multicentre prospective trial titled Patient-Assisted Intervention for Neuropathy: Comparison of Treatment in Real Life Situations (PAIN-CONTRoLS) to examine which medication is most effective and has fewest side effects for patients with cryptogenic sensory polyneuropathy.[33] There are also opportunities to better integrate clinical trials and comparative effectiveness research into clinical practice.

Integration of research into the clinical setting

There are several tactics to better integrate research into clinical settings. Development of a standardized diagnostic taxonomy for neuropathic pain disorders (such as the one ACTTION is developing) will facilitate development of precision-based therapies that can be more easily translated into clinic.[34] Another tactic is the development and implementation of standardized questionnaires and clinical assessment tools that can be used in clinical practice and research.[35] Currently, research studies do not use consistent scales and measures across studies, limiting comparison of different clinical trials and effectiveness in clinical practice.

Several groups have successfully developed standardized evaluation tools including the Outcome Measures in Rheumatoid Arthritis Clinical Trials (OMERACT), and the Western Ontario and McMaster Universities Arthritis Index (WOMAC) pain and function scale.[6] The Initiative on Methods, Measurement, and Pain Assessment in Clinical Trials (IMMPACT), a programme related to ACTTION, has created databases that support research for osteoarthritis, neuropathic pain, fibromyalgia, back pain, and postsurgical pain.[29,30,35] Creation of national databases that could capture a large volume of information may be of most benefit. The NIH has developed common data elements (CDEs) for a variety of disorders including chronic low back pain.[36] A standardized, integrated system would allow for improved tracking of healthcare utilization along with long-term outcomes, employment, and disability cases. In essence, it would simplify research as clinical data could more easily be used for research, with long-term tracking of desired outcomes integrated as a matter of routine. Also, this would improve clinical care as the tools used in research could then easily transition from trials to clinical practice. This would improve clinical care by giving physicians better ways to track and understand significant changes in their own patients. There needs to be a focus on translating discoveries from clinical trials (efficacy) to general medical practice (effectiveness). Comparative effectiveness research is a focus of PCORI. There needs to be a focus at the national level, with collaboration between care providers, researches, and healthcare systems in order to support T3 (translation to practice—effectiveness) and T4 (translation to communities—population health and outcomes research) translational science. Furthermore, assessing pain at one point in time is not sufficient. The impact of pain on function at work and at home and on the ability of patients to enjoy their life and ability to maintain relationships must be assessed. Mobile technology and 'bio-wearables' promise to facilitate real time data collection from patients in both clinical and research settings.

Patient safety

Patient safety is another national healthcare priority. One example is the recent practice changes mandated as a result of the opioid epidemic. Opioids have been used extensively for pain relief with prescriptions increasing 48% between 2000 and 2009. Abuse of pain medications has led to thousands of accidental deaths.[9] In 2015, more than 15,000 Americans died from prescription opioid overdoses, with twice as many deaths attributed to opioids compared to heroin.[37] Even more alarmingly, there were approximately 2.2 million recreational users of opioids in 2009, of which approximately 18% obtained the medication from their own physicians.[6] In this case, it is the role of the government to advocate for changes that protect the public.

The increased number of deaths coupled with the high rates of abuse and prescription diversion were the catalyst for new laws in the United States aimed at regulating the prescription and use of opioids.[38] The stricter regulations are aimed at reducing the number of patients who are prescribed opioids chronically and the total daily doses used.[39] Unfortunately, the crackdown on opioid prescriptions has left patients feeling deeply frustrated and in some cases desperate.[38] The medical community is divided, with some physicians significantly reducing prescriptions of opioids while others advocate for judicious use of opioids as a continued viable alternative for the management of chronic pain when other options have been exhausted.[39] One unintended consequence has been an increase in the number of heroin overdoses.[40] Another interesting shift is that when patients do not have access to opioid medications, they tend to seek medical care that is more costly than their previous levels of care and that patients tend to report higher levels of pain.[40] While it is estimated that $7.3 billion are saved each year in the United States by preventing opioid overdoses, it is estimated that $12.1 billion are spent on associated outpatient and inpatient costs for additional treatment for pain and for covering lost wages for the patients who survive overdoses.[40]

Education of the public

From a societal viewpoint, it is just as important to focus on prevention of chronic pain as on treatment. It is important to educate the public about prevention of injuries in the home or at work, and promotion of activities which are known to reduce the burden of chronic pain such as regular exercise and controlling weight.[6] Targeted campaigns to reduce tobacco use have been successful, and a similar approach should be taken to alter behaviours that could result in chronic pain. While some conditions may not be preventable, the two top reasons for neuropathic pain-DPN and low back pain, are both conditions in which patient behaviour play significant roles.

Many diabetic patients are unaware of the risk and impact of DPN. DPN affects up to 50% of patients with diabetes and is a major cause for reduced quality of life and healthcare expenditures. The annual direct costs for diabetes care in the United States are $245 billion (DPN accounts for approximately 27% of all direct medical costs of diabetes).[41,42] On average, patients with DPN take 3.8 ± 3.9 prescription pain medications, with 79.2% taking at least one medication and 52.2% taking at least two medications.[41] Medications used included NSAIDs (46.7%), opioids (43.1%), anticonvulsants (27.1%), SSRIs/SNRIs (18%), and tricyclic antidepressants (11.4%).[41] Medication side effects limit the rate of titration and the maximum tolerated dose, with many patients using relatively low doses with suboptimal effects. Despite use of multiple medications, patient-perceived effectiveness was low, with only 23.1% of patients reporting medications to be effective or very effective, and only 22.4% of patients were satisfied with control of their pain.[41] Among those employed, 64.4% reported missing work or described decreased work productivity in the three months preceding the study, with 59% of patients reporting decreased home productivity as well.[41] For most people, high levels of pain with poor quality of life is unacceptable and as such public campaigns showing an accurate description of diabetes and its complications may increase the numbers of patients who are willing to take early steps to treat or reverse it.

Public education can result in lasting benefits as patients may become less likely to engage in negative coping mechanisms that lead to exacerbation of pain and to inappropriately escalate care or request inappropriate treatments or tests, and may be more likely to seek support from family and friends and to observe proven strategies to prevent injuries that may lead to neuropathic pain. Patients seeking information on the causes and treatments of pain often have difficulty finding objective and accurate information. They may be inappropriately offered services that are expensive, time-consuming, and unproven and that may result in inappropriate delay in seeking conventional medical treatment or that may result in harm. Instructional materials for patients must be comprehensive but also written in an accessible manner. Education can take many forms: online modules, fact sheets and pamphlets, radio and TV announcements. It is therefore important for physicians to be involved in the creation of educational materials and to support national efforts for the creation and dissemination of educational materials and campaigns.

Regulation of drugs: Help or hindrance?

While some regulations can be beneficial, others have been perceived as potentially detrimental to scientific exploration. For example, patients have been increasingly advocating for the use and research of medical marijuana, with a significant proportion of patients who feel that the medicinal use of marijuana is useful and that curtailing access to it is an infringement on a person's ability to obtain adequate relief.[43] Many states in the United States and several countries around the world such as Canada, the Netherlands, and Israel have legalized medical marijuana, although physicians continue to have mixed feelings on whether it is an appropriate therapy for a range of conditions, including pain.[43,44] The studies examining medical use of cannabis have considerable variability in the formulation of the cannabis and mode of administration as well as study duration and dose, however several studies suggest potential efficacy.[45,46] Research to determine whether cannabis is an effective therapy for neuropathic pain faces considerable barriers. In the United States, the principal barrier stems from very strict federal regulations, which have limited larger multicentre clinical trials.[47]

Conclusion

The most consistent theme that permeates pain care is that the treatment of pain must be personalized in order to address the individual's experience of pain. It is equally important to develop tools that empower patients to actively participate in the management of their pain.[6] While pain specialists can be very helpful in the management of severe pain, pain specialists and dedicated pain clinics are limited in number and are difficult to access in a timely manner for many patients.

Primary care physicians treat the majority of patients with neuropathic pain; therefore empowerment of primary care is essential. Advocating for access to experienced primary care level pain management in a timely fashion and availability of consultative pain specialists including integrated multidisciplinary and complementary and alternative pain care is a priority. Such a system cannot be created without the involvement of multiple stakeholders, including insurance companies, healthcare systems, patient advocates, governmental payers and regulatory agencies, among many others (refer to Table 31.1 for a summary of current and potential advocacy efforts). The only effective and sustainable path to change is to combine our efforts—at a patient level, physician level, and a national policy level to align our priorities and interests.

Table 31.1 There are numerous challenges to providing excellent patient centred pain care, and in developing new treatments. Examples of some of these challenges and advocacy approaches to addressing them are provided

Challenge	Advocacy solution
Current interventions and medications for pain have limited efficacy	Advocate for more research, fast-track drug approval processes—patients and physicians
Limited availability/coverage of services such as physical therapy, psychological therapies, and complementary and alternative interventions	Lobby insurance companies or mandate at a regulatory level that comprehensive services be made available—patients, physicians, national systems
Physicians have a limited understanding of the psychosocial challenges patients experience due to pain	Change medical school curricula to emphasize the psychosocial dimensions of pain—physicians, patients, national systems
Physicians receive limited and often fragmented education about pain management	Advocate for improved continued medical education programmes that help physicians become effective in the management of pain—physicians, physician organizations, national systems
Physicians have limited knowledge of how to become advocates	Institute curricula at a medical school level or continuing medical education level that teach physicians how to become effective advocates—physicians, physician organizations
Research is needed but is expensive, with limited funding available	Continue to lobby for funding at a national level but encourage other stakeholders such as insurance companies or large healthcare organizations to participate in research—physicians, patient groups
Lack of consistency between clinical and research measures and across studies	Standardize research—physicians, national systems
Increased opioid use has led to safety concerns, with significant limitations in opioid use and increased patient frustration	Continue educating the public about the importance of containing opioid use while continuing to look for alternatives patients, physicians, physician organizations, national systems
Limited educational materials for patients	Create educational materials that address prevention, educate about different medical conditions and best options for treatment—patients, physicians, national systems

References

1. **Gaskin, D. J., Richard, P.** (2012) The economic costs of pain in the United States. *J Pain*, **13**(8), 715–24.
2. **U.S. and World Population Clock.** Available at: http://www.census.gov/popclock/
3. **Gaskell, H., Derry, S., Stannard, C., Moore, R. A.** (2016) Oxycodone for neuropathic pain in adults. *Cochrane Database Syst Rev*, **7**, CD010692.
4. **Nickel, F. T., Seifert, F., Lanz, S., Maihofner, C.** (2012) Mechanisms of neuropathic pain. *Eur Neuropsychopharmacol*, **22**(2), 81–91.
5. **Stroke NIoNDa.** Peripheral Neuropathy Fact Sheet December 2014. Available at: https://www.ninds.nih.gov/Disorders/Patient-Caregiver-Education/Fact-Sheets/Peripheral-Neuropathy-Fact-Sheet
6. **Institute of Medicine (US) Committee on Advancing Pain Research, Care, and Education** (2011) *Relieving Pain in America: A Blueprint for Transforming Prevention, Care, Education, and Research.* The National Academies Collection: Reports funded by National Institutes of Health. Washington, DC.
7. **Turk, D. C.** (2002) Clinical effectiveness and cost-effectiveness of treatments for patients with chronic pain. *Clin J Pain*, **18**(6), 355–65.
8. **Kalso, E., Aldington, D. J., Moore, R. A.** (2013) Drugs for neuropathic pain. *BMJ*, **347**, f7339.
9. **Meghani, S. H., Polomano, R. C., Tait, R. C., Vallerand, A. H., Anderson, K. O., Gallagher, R. M.** (2012) Advancing a national agenda to eliminate disparities in pain care: directions for health policy, education, practice, and research. *Pain Med*, **13**(1), 5–28.
10. **Institute of Medicine (US) Committee on the Use of Complementary and Alternative Medicine by the American Public** (2005) *Complementary and Alternative Medicine in the United States.* Washington, DC: National Academies Press.
11. **Tang, N. K., Crane, C.** (2006) Suicidality in chronic pain: a review of the prevalence, risk factors and psychological links. *Psychol Med*, **36**(5), 575–86.
12. **Breuer, B., Cruciani, R., Portenoy, R. K.** (2010) Pain management by primary care physicians, pain physicians, chiropractors, and acupuncturists: a national survey. *South Med J*, **103**(8), 738–47.
13. **Fishman, S. M., Young, H. M., Lucas Arwood, E., et al.** (2013) Core competencies for pain management: results of an interprofessional consensus summit. *Pain Med*, **14**(7), 971–81.
14. **Blumenthal, D., Gokhale, M., Campbell, E. G., Weissman, J. S.** (2001) Preparedness for clinical practice: reports of graduating residents at academic health centers. *JAMA*, **286**(9), 1027–34.
15. **O'Rorke, J. E., Chen, I., Genao, I., Panda, M., Cykert, S.** (2007) Physicians' comfort in caring for patients with chronic nonmalignant pain. *Am J Med Sci*, **333**(2), 93–100.
16. **American Academy of Neurology (AAN)** (2011) *Treatment of Painful Diabetic Neuropathy. AAN Summary of Evidence-based Guideline for Clinicians.* Available at: https://www.aan.com/Guidelines/Home/GetGuidelineContent/480
17. **Smedley, B. D., Stith, A. Y., Nelson, A. R., Institute of Medicine (US) Committee on Understanding and Eliminating Racial and Ethnic Disparities in Health Care** (2003) *Unequal Treatment: Confronting Racial and Ethnic Disparities in Health Care.* Washington, DC: National Academy Press.

18. **Bernabei, R., Gambassi, G., Lapane, K., et al.** (1998) Management of pain in elderly patients with cancer. SAGE Study Group. Systematic Assessment of Geriatric Drug Use via Epidemiology. *JAMA*, **279**(23), 1877–82.
19. **Todd, K. H., Deaton, C., D'Adamo, A. P., Goe, L.** (2000) Ethnicity and analgesic practice. *Ann Emerg Med*, **35**(1), 11–6.
20. **Tamayo-Sarver, J. H., Hinze, S. W., Cydulka, R. K., Baker, D. W.** (2003) Racial and ethnic disparities in emergency department analgesic prescription. *Am J Public Health*, **93**(12), 2067–73.
21. **Stafford, S., Sedlak, T., Fok, M. C., Wong, R. Y.** (2010) Evaluation of resident attitudes and self-reported competencies in health advocacy. *BMC Med Educ*, **10**, 82.
22. **Flynn, L., Verma, S.** (2008) Fundamental components of a curriculum for residents in health advocacy. *Med Teach*, **30**(7), e178–83.
23. **Hixson, J. D., Johnson, N.** (2015) *Become an Effective Advocate for Your Patients and Specialty*. Minneapolis, MN: American Academy of Neurology.
24. **American Academy of Neurology**. About Neurology on the Hill: American Academy of Neurology. Available at: https://www.aan.com/public-policy/neurology-on-the-hill/about-neurology-on-the-hill/
25. **Henson, L. J., May, E. F.** (2013) A personal journey in advocacy. *Neurol Clin Pract*, **3**(1), 39–43.
26. **Ward, N., Raja, S. N.** (2015) The global burden of neuropathic pain: IASP's educational and advocacy efforts to enhance the management of neuropathic pain sufferers. *Pain Manag*, **5**(2), 69–73.
27. **DiMasi, J. A., Grabowski, H. G., Hansen, R. W.** (2016) Innovation in the pharmaceutical industry: New estimates of R&D costs. *J Health Econ*, **47**, 20–33.
28. ***The Lancet Neurology*** (2012) NeuroNEXT: accelerating drug development in neurology. *Lancet Neurol*, **11**(2), 119.
29. **Analgesic, Anesthetic, and Addiction Clinical Trial Translations, Innovations, Opportunities, and Networks**. Available at: http://www.acttion.org/
30. **Dworkin, R. H., Turk, D. C.** (2011) Accelerating the development of improved analgesic treatments: the ACTION public–private partnership. *Pain Med*, **12** Suppl 3, S109–17.
31. **Clinical Trials Transformation Initiative**. Available at: https://www.ctti-clinicaltrials.org/
32. **Patient-Centered Outcomes Research Institute**. Available at: http://www.pcori.org/
33. **Patient-Centered Outcomes Research Institute**. *Patient-Assisted Intervention for Neuropathy: Comparison of Treatment in Real Life Situations (PAIN-CONTRoLS)*. Available at: http://www.pcori.org/research-results/2013/patient-assisted-intervention-neuropathy-comparison-treatment-real-life
34. **Dworkin, R. H., Bruehl, S., Fillingim, R. B., Loeser, J. D., Terman, G. W., Turk, D. C.** (2016) Multidimensional diagnostic criteria for chronic pain: introduction to the ACTTION-American Pain Society Pain Taxonomy (AAPT). *J Pain*, **17**(9 Suppl), T1–9.
35. **Dworkin, R. H., Turk, D. C., Wyrwich, K. W., et al.** (2008) Interpreting the clinical importance of treatment outcomes in chronic pain clinical trials: IMMPACT recommendations. *J Pain*, **9**(2), 105–21.
36. **NIH U.S. National Library of Medicine**. Common Data Element (CDE) Resource Portal. Available at: https://www.nlm.nih.gov/cde

37. **Rudd, R. A., Puja, S., David, F., Scholl, L.** (2016) Increases in drug and opioid-involved overdose deaths—United States, 2010–2015. *Morbidity and Mortality Weekly Report (MMWR)*, **65**, 1445–52. Available at: https://www.cdc.gov/mmwr/volumes/65/wr/mm655051e1.htm
38. **Freyer, F. J.** (2016) Strict opioid laws hit chronic pain sufferers hard. *The Boston Globe*, June 18. Available at: https://www.bostonglobe.com/metro/2016/06/18/the-other-side-america-war-opioids/i9YYLR0bGWFdP9z1T1pwjI/story.html
39. **American Academy of Pain Medicine** (2013) Use of opioids in the treatment of chronic pain [press release]. 4 February 2013. Available at: http://www.painmed.org/files/use-of-opioids-for-the-treatment-of-chronic-pain.pdf
40. **Kilby, A. (ed.)** (2016) Opioids for the masses: Welfare tradeoffs in the regulation of narcotic pain medications. Thirty-eighth Annual Fall Research Conference, The Role of Research in Making Government More effective. 3–5 November 2016, Washington DC.
41. **Gore, M., Brandenburg, N. A., Hoffman, D. L., Tai, K. S., Stacey, B.** (2006) Burden of illness in painful diabetic peripheral neuropathy: the patients' perspectives. *J Pain*, **7**(12), 892–900.
42. **American Diabetes Association** (2013) Economic costs of diabetes in the U.S. in 2012. *Diabetes Care*, **36**(4), 1033–46.
43. **Sznitman, S. R., Bretteville-Jensen, A. L.** (2015) Public opinion and medical cannabis policies: examining the role of underlying beliefs and national medical cannabis policies. *Harm Reduct J*, **12**, 46.
44. **Kondrad, E., Reid, A.** (2013) Colorado family physicians' attitudes toward medical marijuana. *J Am Board Fam Med*, **26**(1), 52–60.
45. **Deshpande, A., Mailis-Gagnon, A., Zoheiry, N., Lakha, S. F.** (2015) Efficacy and adverse effects of medical marijuana for chronic noncancer pain: Systematic review of randomized controlled trials. *Can Fam Physician*, **61**(8), e372–81.
46. **Lynch, M. E., Campbell, F.** (2011) Cannabinoids for treatment of chronic non-cancer pain; a systematic review of randomized trials. *Br J Clin Pharmacol*, **72**(5), 735–44.
47. **Stith, S. S., Vigil, J. M.** (2016) Federal barriers to Cannabis research. *Science*, **352**(6290), 1182.

Section 5

Outlook, follow-up, results, ending, conclusion, and debriefing

Chapter 32

Continuation or ending and 'debriefing'

Wolfgang Grisold and Thomas Grisold

Introduction

It was originally planned to write two separate chapters: one on 'continuation and ending', and one on 'debriefing'. In the course of writing it became clear that the process of ending and closing a project is closely linked to debriefing.

As compared to the many efforts to create, start, and successfully run advocacy projects, less energy and attention is given to closing or 'ending' them. There are many reasons for this, including loss of interest by participants during lengthy projects, shifts in participant priorities or, more practically speaking, the appearance of cooperation difficulties, or the drying up of funds.

Ending and closing procedures are an essential part of business management and economics.[1] Ending and closing entails debriefing participants, summarizing the whole project, 'harvesting' and exploiting knowledge and experience, and making the experience and knowledge available for future projects.

Any advocacy project can be seen as a project cycle. In optimal circumstances, project accomplishments will persist either in the form of an established procedure, or a valuable achievement, or will bring about changes for the better.

Advocacy projects can end unexpectedly, or prove to be a failure at any time for many reasons (e.g. a change of ownership or leadership, or major changes in project direction).

In any project, persons have various roles, with varying degrees of responsibility. On closing the project, people need to be debriefed, thereby relieving them of their responsibilities and enabling them to comment on and judge achievements, in addition to reflecting on their role in the project. As advocacy projects have a high level of personal engagement and input, often on a voluntary or altruistic basis, closing, ending, and debriefing procedures should be standard in all of them.

Results of an advocacy project

Project ending and closure need to define the results and final achievements noted in Box 32.1.

An advocacy project can be defined as successful if the goals are achieved. Judgement is usually based on the blue print and project definition.

> **Box 32.1 Results of an advocacy project**
>
> 1. Success
>   Complete
>   Partial
> 2. Failure
>   At various time points
> 3. Continuation

If only some of the goals are accomplished, the project is considered a partial success. Indeed in complex advocacy projects this is, by definition, often the case.

Any advocacy project can fail at any stage and for many reasons. It is recommended to thoroughly analyse the project to gain input and knowledge for future projects.

Continuous advocacy projects in which there is a smooth transition from project status to routine practice constitutes a special case (Chapter 16).

Ending and closing

Ending and closing a project has positive aspects, such as the achievement and termination of an effort, but it can also have negative connotations for the persons involved. Project ending can induce a sense of grief, difficulty in letting go, and a persistent desire for continuation. Ending advocacy also means relinquishing the role of advocate, which is a very important, well-described aspect of social advocacy.[2] In the social context, clients must be empowered to act on their own and advocates need to retract and disengage from their role and their particular relationship with the patient.

Two quotes illustrate the aforementioned paragraph:

1. Advocacy is about helping people help themselves. It's about making people stronger—able to speak up for themselves.[2]
2. The main thing is that letting go should always be seen as a good thing—something to be happy and proud about.[2]

Projects have goals, milestones, and marks of achievement. The final goal must always be specified. In analogy to medical studies, it is useful to divide objectives into primary and secondary endpoints. This simple structure is useful for practical purposes during the project and for its finalization, as primary and secondary endpoints are often merged and sometimes confused.

A strategy is needed to achieve the final endpoints, while the action plans and methods must be adhered to and followed during the project. The project will need to follow a structured closing procedure, which ought to be implemented right from the beginning.

Any project leader needs to be aware that interest and engagement, manpower, and resources can potentially become scarce towards the end of a project. This implies that resources and preparations for closure need to be thoroughly planned in advance.

Closing plan

The *closing plan* becomes important as the project progresses, and must incorporate several items (Box 32.2).

Business relations should receive a proper ending and closure in this setting too, and can be used as a template for ending advocacy.[3]

The closing procedure consists of a closure phase, needed to terminate all contracts with participants and to identify and resolve any unfinished items, followed by the close of the project, which formally ends the project phase.

The results need to be stated and formalized, and a post-implementation review should be in place. Learning, harvesting, and post-mortem analysis must be transparent and should be made available for the next project.

Continuation: (example: Chapter 16). Most advocacy projects follow a defined aim and purpose. Their mission, time cycle, the parties involved and 'ownership' of the project should be clearly stated.

Let's take the example of an advocacy project aimed at distributing an expensive treatment to elderly people, who are currently prevented from receiving said treatment due to age restrictions. The aim of the advocacy project is to make the treatment available for this age group. The campaign is conducted, negotiations finally achieve their goal, and the drug becomes available.

This is the template of a successful project: the project is effectively closed, its aim has been fulfilled and the content is implemented.

Projects are often more complex. Even during their lifetime, the scope of advocacy projects can widen, expected limits and boundaries can be exceeded, and the advocacy projects have to be reviewed (content, leadership, ownership).

Debriefing is a term once associated with airline, military, and combat organizations. It serves to relieve a person on duty of his/her responsibilities, but at the same time provides feedback on how a mission has been carried out. The debriefing process has also been used in psychological reviews and in particular crisis and disaster settings.[4]

Debriefing is a process whereby the facilitators[5] and learners re-examine the clinical encounter. This process fosters the development of clinical reasoning and judgement skills through reflective learning processes.[6]

Box 32.2 Content of the closing plan

- Content of the project
- Results
- Financial plan
- Reporting, including to advocates
- Human resources. Ending, closing
- Debriefing of advocacy project participants

Debriefing needs to be well structured and should be implemented in all advocacy projects. Reflection is very important, first for the whole project, involving all members, and second for the individual who is debriefed.

A good example of briefing and debriefing is the case of air pilots, who routinely take part in structured briefing and debriefing procedures. Once the flight is over, debriefing is part of the routine procedure. Debriefing processes have also been described in medicine, as the debriefing of medical personnel and carers in palliative care.[7]

Learning and harvesting

It is important to establish what can be learnt from an advocacy project. Lessons can be learnt from any project at any stage, not necessarily from a completed or a successful project, and should result in guided reflection.

> 'Harvesting' sounds very technical but is a widely adopted scientific term, also used in the context of projects.[8]

Any advocacy project should have defined milestones and needs to be minuted to allow retrospective analysis and to review content, operations, and financial aspects. It is valuable to compare goals with results and to determine why some goals may not have been accomplished, while others have been added, and why some goals may even have exceeded expectations.

This analysis is very useful, not only for the participants, but for everyone concerned; where relevant, the public should be informed. The final results should be discussed, analysed, and knowledge harvested.

Micro, meso, and macro projects

Ending and closing differs according to the type of project, and involvement in the ending and closing procedures increases proportionally with the size of the project.

In particular, it is important to closely follow-up meso and macro advocacy projects from the beginning and to be stringent as regards not only the different endpoints but also project complexity, which can develop during the life of a project.

More stakeholders are involved in larger projects. It is important for all steps of any project to be explained transparently and understandably, to report any possible conflicts of interest, and finally to make a clear, understandable summary. This will enable auditors and stakeholders to see exactly how the project was implemented and concluded.

Post-mortem analysis

One method for post-hoc analysis of projects is referred to as post-mortem analysis (PM), which utilizes several techniques to achieve the best retrospective result. PM is a useful approach to analyse projects in detail after termination (project review/audit/retrospective, post-partum, post-iteration review, report improvement).[9-12]

The PM process focuses on the analysis of the project, taking into account all available aspects. It is used for quantitative analysis (detailing the timeline, hours used, resources deployed) and qualitative analysis, focusing on project content, the quality of the achievements, and the level of satisfaction of all concerned (users, team, stakeholders). The final analysis identifies important elements which can be used for new projects.[13-19]

The use of PM software[11] has been proposed for some applications.

Conclusion

The last chapter of the book is concerned with ending, closing, debriefing, post-mortem analysis, gaining experience, and harvesting knowledge from all advocacy projects.

Much less energy is usually spent on ending projects, compared to the enthusiasm and energy invested to develop and implement projects. This disparity of efforts is well known and is not specific to advocacy projects. Advocacy projects in the field of neurology do, however, have a specific aim: their content is always directly or indirectly patient-related and they are often conducted by altruistic, highly motivated persons. Besides altruistic motives, most projects advocate direct or indirect improvements for patients which carry ethical value.

Optimum, efficient, successful project handling is not simply the personal aim of the participants; it is also an implicit duty inherent in all advocacy projects and participants.

A project can be symbolically likened to books on a shelf, supported on each side by 'bookends'. One side represents the start of the project, which has been amply discussed in previous chapters; the other side can be compared to its ending, which is the topic of the final chapter. The books need both bookends to keep them in place.

The procedures for closure need to be as accurate and substantive as they are for project instalment and interim monitoring. The closing procedure should provide a structured process for debriefing the participants, while the knowledge gained and harvested will depend on the size of the project.

Learning and harvesting is important and will need energy and time; participants' willingness to take part should be clarified from the outset. The debriefing process serves not only to leave the project and responsibility behind but also to offer insight and knowledge.

In summary it can be helpful to implement closing strategies and procedures in all new and planned advocacy projects.

A post-hoc analysis of projects technique is called PM, and has several techniques described to achieve the best retrospective result.

In summary it can be helpful to implement closing strategies and in the procedures in all new and planned advocacy projects.

References

1. **Yonge, O. P., Lee, H., Luhanga, F.** (2006) Closing and not just ending a course. *Nurse Educator*, **31**(4), 151–2.

2. **Tufail, J.** (2007) *Advocacy in Action. The Fourth Book of Speaking Up: A Plain Text Guide to Advocacy*. London and Philadelphia: Jessica Kingsley Publishers.
3. **Jackson, C.** 15 Tips for ending client relationships in a positive way. http://www.trackur.com/15-tips-for-ending-client-relationships-in-a-positive-way
4. **Raphael, B., Wilson, J. P.** (2000) *Psychological Debriefing: Theory, Practice and Evidence*. Cambridge: Cambridge University Press.
5. **Jamalpuri, V., Kline, A., Shepherd, M.** (2016) Debriefing—what, why and how? *Journal of Pediatric Critical Care*, **3**(3), 54–8.
6. **Dreifuerst, K. T.** (2009) The essentials of debriefing in simulation learning: a concept analysis. *Nurs Educ Perspect*, **30**, 109–14.
7. **Aoun, S., Slatyer, S., Deas, K., Nekolaichuk, C.** (2017) Family caregiver participation in palliative care research: challenging the myth. *J Pain Symptom Manage*, **53**(5), 851–61.
8. **Schindler, M., Epplerb, M. J.** (2003) Harvesting project knowledge: a review of project learning methods and success factors. *International Journal of Project Management*, **21**(3), 219–28.
9. **Heyer, F.** (2006) Post-mortem-analysen und erfahrungs-erhebung. Available at: http://www.se.uni-hannover.de/pub/File/kurz-und-gut/ws2005-seminar-exp2/5-PostMortems-Heyer.pdf
10. **Birk, A., Dingsayr, T., Stalhane, T.** (2002) Postmortem: never leave a project without it. Available at: https://pdfs.semanticscholar.org/294d/bed0763f4cd90ff7d6d4f2615350aa120d39.pdf
11. **Collier, B., DeMarco, T., Fearey, P.** (1996) A defined process for project post-mortem review. Available at: https://www.semanticscholar.org/paper/A-defined-process-for-project-post-mortem-review-Collier-DeMarco/b34aded7ed583f447d0fce08204bd16a4ec38152
12. **Kerth, N. L.** (2001) *Project Retrospectives: A Handbook for Team Reviews*. New York: Dorset House Publishing.
13. **Levine, C., Albert, S. M., Hokenstad, A., Halper, D. E., Hart, A. Y., Gould, D. A.** (2006) 'This case is closed': family caregivers and the termination of home health care services for stroke patients. *Milbank Q*, **84**(2), 305–31.
14. **Carter, P. A., Mikan, S. Q., Simpson, C.** (2009) A feasibility study of a two-session home-based cognitive behavioral therapy-insomnia intervention for bereaved family caregivers. *Palliat Support Care*, **7**(2), 197–206.
15. **Di Blasi, Z., Crawford, F., Bradley, C., Kleijnen, J.** (2005) Reactions to treatment debriefing among the participants of a placebo-controlled trial. *BMC Health Serv Res*, **5**(1), 30.
16. **Keene, E. A., Hutton, N., Hall, B., Rushton, C.** (2010) Bereavement debriefing sessions: an intervention to support health care professionals in managing their grief after the death of a patient. *Pediatr Nurs*, **36**(4), 185–9; quiz 90.
17. **Pickett, M., Brennan, A. M., Greenberg, H. S., Licht, L., Worrell, J. D.** (1994) Use of debriefing techniques to prevent compassion fatigue in research teams. *Nurs Res*, **43**(4), 250–2.
18. **Walker, G.** (1990) Crisis-care in critical incident debriefing. *Death Studies*, **14**(2), 121–33.
19. **van den Bergh, N.** (1993) Using critical incident stress debriefing to mediate organizational crisis, change and loss. *Employee Assistance Quarterly*, **8**(2), 35–55.

Chapter 33

Results, outlook, and goals of this book

Wolfgang Grisold, Walter Struhal, and Thomas Grisold

Introduction

The book has been divided into five parts: 'What is advocacy?', 'Why is it needed?', 'What tools can be used?', 'How it is done in different neurological diseases?', and finally, 'What can we learn from this book?' Looking at the multitude of views, targets, and practical approaches, the main goal of this book is to create awareness of advocacy as an important tool, to recognize and use available resources, and implement the concept of advocacy into practice.

We placed strong emphasis on how advocacy looks like in practice, with a strong focus on the context of neurology. The authors provided excellent insights into how advocacy projects can be achieved and they reflected on interesting cases from their own experiences. For example, patient care by a relative, communication at an oncological ward (Chapter 7), the self-advocacy of a patient (Chapter 1), and finally an example of change in the meso-level, where an old institutional concept needed to be changed (Chapter 1).

We also encouraged authors from other fields and with different perspectives to share their insights and experiences. For example, Chapter 3 presented the historical foundations of advocacy; Chapter 16 reported on the organization of the 'SOS Kinderdorf'; and Chapter 11 reviewed activities related to cancer, where advocacy has already been successfully introduced for several diseases.

In the preparation of this book, we were often confronted with the question of what 'advocacy' means. It was often conceived as a rather abstract definition, for an activity which was neither defined consistently, nor was the precise purpose clear. Many discussions circled around the difficult distinction of lobbying and advocacy. Even critical terms, such as 'adverse' or 'counter-advocacy' appeared, and strong emphasis was put on the 'what if', or negative aspects.

One key message that we would like to bring across is that advocacy is a valuable and universally applicable activity. We also hope that the views of the authors have clarified that by and large 'to speak up for a patient', either directly or indirectly, is the core of advocacy. It is not only driven by altruism and the need for positive change, but in the context of this book needs to be seen as an element which is necessary for our professional services, and is often already an implicit or tacit element.

Following Chapter 6, we are aware that 'good' or 'bad' advocacy are not as easy to distinguish for several reasons, such as recurrent issues, present and timely changing concepts, and also aspects of contemporary developments. Furthermore, this chapter also points to a variety of ethical aspects, legal issues, administration, and jurisdiction which have an influence on the judgement of what is good or bad.

As advocacy projects can include many health groups, patients, and carers, transparency of the structures, the envisioned endpoints, and 'ownership' of advocacy projects is important. It is essential to discuss and design advocacy projects in regard to goals, endpoints, and timelines. As any project, advocacy projects can end according to a schedule, reach only some of the defined goals, or they can fail. In reference to Chapter 18 and others, we stress that even accounts where project fail provide valuable material and inspirations for what can be improved or implemented in subsequent projects.

Being an advocate not only means to serve a purpose and be altruistic, but also expose one's own work and position or personal status. This personal exposure of an advocate is part of the commitment, and advocates need to be aware of this.

Messages, resources, content, and tools

Summarizing the chapters and key insights, we propose that there are a few key messages that we want to highlight (Table 33.1).

Advocacy projects

Advocacy projects aim to help, support, and 'balance' and correct inequities. This may sound cynical, considering the large global imbalances in healthcare (Chapters 1 and 14), but one of the major efforts of all advocacy issues has the goal to improve for the better. The treatment gap is a major issue in healthcare, and as described in Chapter 29, worldwide large variations exist.

Even within the construct of advocacy we have to be aware of persons needing even more support as defined by their age, the underprivileged at any age, persons who are unable to participate in a decision process, and the growing number of migrants and refugees (Chapter 12).

Resources

Advocacy projects need resources, and many authors made it clear that the most important is the human resource, which drives development and progress in advocacy. Finances, sponsorship, and funding are important; at the same time advocacy projects should remain independent from the influence of other interests. Examples of the hazard of losing independence are numerous, and sometimes a 'slippery slope' needs to be avoided. The search and identification of possible conflict of interest is of paramount importance.

Table 33.1 Key messages of advocacy, explanations, and relevant chapters

	Explanation	Chapter
Advocacy is universally applicable		1
Resources are often available and need to be identified		1 (Goals)
Anyone can be an advocate, or need advocacy (be an advocate)		1 and 2
Advocacy needs a powerful insight	Advocacy activities should be built on the genuine needs of a patient of patient groups	1 (Epistemology)
Advocacy can be powerful		1
Advocacy can meet resistance		2 (International comparisons)
Advocates are often driven by altruistic motives		1 and 2
Advocacy concerns all health groups, patients, carers, and laypersons alike		1 and 2
Technical details as project management, tools, and end points are essential	Advocates can use various tools to plan and carry out their projects. There are strategies for unexpected barriers, such as procrastination	3
Advocacy can be directed at several levels (micro, meso, macro)		1 and 2
Different advocacy tasks and content need different strategies		1

The resources are not limited to neurologists and professionals but involve other health groups, patients, and laypersons. The chapters indicate that patients, carers, and the public are increasingly conscious of their ability to advocate. It will be important to see and implement these developments in future projects. It is important to not only use the synergy, but also to meet the needs and demands from the level of the persons concerned as advocates. An example of the Patient-Centered Outcomes Research Institute (PCORI) is given in Chapter 7 and the grant applications for MS studies; Chapter 21 illustrates this important development.

Content and tools

Advocacy generally lacks explicit guidelines and a paradigm in which it is embedded. Advocacy aims to improve matters for patients and carers at several levels. As such, it often develops spontaneously, needs time to make the case and content and decision to go ahead. Advocacy often challenges existing structures and naturally will meet obstacles and resistance, which needs to be met and overcome. Advocates need to be aware of these obstacles, and meet them with concern, anticipation, and resilience. In that regard, it might be useful to think of advocacy as a process where one learns new practices and unlearns old ways of doing and seeing (Chapter 1).

There are several tools available. They can be useful instruments but they often need individual adaptation. Examples in this book include conferences, websites, events, and many more. Much can be learnt from professionals such as public relations and media experts on how and by which instruments advocacy projects can be developed.

The examples given in this book on various diseases and medical conditions illustrate that advocacy is not homogenous but needs to adapt to the distinct setting of each subspecialty. It has already been introduced in the context of stroke, MS, ALS, neuromuscular diseases, movement disorders, cancer and neuro-oncology, dementia, epilepsy, and also overarching aspects as palliative care, pain, headache, and the important aspect of orphan diseases.

Level: Micro, meso, and macro

It is important to define the level of advocacy, and to choose the tools for a successful advocacy project. The terminology of micro, meso, and macro level does neither refer to quality nor to importance. A micro advocacy project can be equally important as a meso and a macro project. Thus, size is not a marker of importance, but the size and targets will need respective instruments and strategies.

Relation of physicians, health groups, and patient/carers

The relation of physicians and other health groups and patient are in a constant evolution. At present, paternalistic concepts are increasingly replaced by patient autonomy and shared decision-making. The relations are also influenced by an increasing influence from consumerism.

In addition, there are also major changes in the practice of medicine and institutions (Chapter 7) and many ideas from industrial processes and production are used and implemented in medicine. This may be a benefit for some highly specialized procedures, but may influence the holistic approach to patients negatively.

Advocate-advocatee and self-advocate

To advocate for someone needs an advocate and an advocatee, and increasingly patients and carers are aware of their abilities as self-advocates. This focuses on many levels as obtaining information, access services, be aware of rights and choices, interact with health and social care professionals and services and most importantly communicate and being able to speak up for themselves. A very useful and comprehensive summary can be found on 'take action in many ways'.[1]

Using media

Advocacy projects often need media to raise awareness, communicate, and make their voice heard. Electronic media are used more and more and online resources play an increasing role.

Remaining content and not surface driven will be an important mission of future advocates. Helping to identify useful and science-based content from online resources, and identifying ineffective, unjustified, and often expensive therapies will be one of their mandates.

Major administrative bodies like the FDA[2] do recognize this development. Also patients increasingly share their experiences via social media.[3]

Implementing advocacy into teaching curricula

Chapters 1, 7, and 17 tried to define advocacy, and also selected some of the most important attributes of advocates. In particular, with respect to training, the importance of advocacy has to be implemented into training curricula. One example is provided in Chapter 18 ('International advocacy'), where International Federation of Medical Students Associations (IFMSA) provide students with opportunities to train and improve their advocacy skills. To move advocacy to awareness and from an implicit to a prominent and permanent role is important.

Summary and outlook

Summary and conclusion

Advocacy is a powerful tool, and needs to be used and implemented for the patient directly but also for patient-related issues such as rules, jurisdiction, support, and care.

Any person can be an advocate, or can be in need for an advocate at any time. Advocacy is not a privilege of neurologists and health groups, but also persons, carers, and laypeople can be successfully practising advocacy.

Limitations and further research

This book focuses on advocacy in neurology and neglects advocacy in other medical fields, and in many other contexts as law, social work, issues of politics, and many others.

In medicine the use of the term has increasingly been used in the past, several different concepts, ideas, and strategies are summarized under this term, which as we pointed out has a core of definition and meaning and but finally depends on interpretation and context. Most importantly, intention, value, and goals are subject to contemporary aspects and Zeitgeist. As advocacy is an ever-changing process and subject to timely changes, the content and opinions of this book will have a short half-life.

Acknowledgements

We thank all authors for their cooperation and their various excellent contributions. Throughout this book, we remained open-minded for how advocates approach this topic from various aspects, and we deeply enjoyed the variety of perspectives and solutions that emerged. We also want to thank Oxford University Press for providing a platform for a topic that is considered in countless fields but has received limited attention in neurology. We are confident that this book will decrease this gap. We hope it will inspire advocates and offer useful insights and tools that can be used in their daily work.

References

1. **Brain & Life** (2016) Take action. Available at: https://www.brainandlife.org/the-magazine/article/app/12/1/19/take-action-for-many-patients-and-their-families-advocacy-is
2. **FDA Voice** (2016) A 'roadmap' for navigating patient advocacy. Available at: http://blogs.fda.gov/fdavoice/index.php/2016/03/a-roadmap-for-navigating-patient-advocacy/
3. **Patientslikeme.com**. Social media statistics via Easy Counter. Available at: https://www.easycounter.com/report/patientslikeme.com

Index

Notes *vs.* indicates a differential diagnosis or comparison.
Tables, figures and boxes are indicated by an italic *t, f* and *b* following the page number.
As this book is concerned with advocacy, entries under this term have been kept to a minimum.
Users are advised to look for more specific phrases.

A

AAN *see* American Academy of Neurology (AAN)
ABPI (Association of the British Pharmaceutical Industry), Code of Practice, 238
ACP (advance care planning), 319–20, 320–1
action planning
 case study, 259, 260–1*t*
 neuromuscular disorders, 259
activity modifications, neuropathic pain treatment, 349
ACTTION (Analgesic, Anesthetic and Addiction Clinical Trial Translations Innovations Opportunities Network), 353
AD *see* Alzheimer's disease (AD)
ADA (Americans with Disabilities Act) (US), 258
Adler, Victor, 36
Admiral Nurses of the Dementia UK, 299
Adorno, Theodor, 38–9
advance care planning (ACP), 319–20, 320–1
advance directives
 amyotrophic lateral sclerosis, 246
 cognitive impairment and, 47–8
 family objections to, 320
 handling of, 48
 lack of, 41
 palliative care, 319–20
 research participation, 50
Advocacy Action Plan Workbook, dementia, 295*b*
Advocacy Forum of Alzheimer's Association, 297–8
advocacy, need for, 4–7, 97–9
advocacy types, 105–7
 advocate-centred advocacy, 63–4
 bottom-up advocacy, 8
 caregiver advocacy *see* caregivers
 coalition advocacy, 8
 collective advocacy, 36–9
 community advocacy, 106–7, 107*f*
 counter advocacy, 65–6
 family advocacy *see* family advocacy

grassroot advocacy, 8
grasstop advocacy, 8
guerilla advocacy, 8
healthcare advocacy, 86
health system advocacy *see* health system advocacy
industrial advocacy, 59
international advocacy *see* international advocacy
issue-centred advocacy, 63
legislative advocacy, 8
management advocacy, 74
mediation advocacy, 105
negative self-advocacy, 6
parTisan advocacy, 8
patient advocacy *see* patient advocacy
public relations advocacy, 106
referral resource advocacy, 106
science politics advocacy, 249–50
scientist advocacy, 298–9
self-advocacy *see* self-advocacy
spokesperson advocacy, 105
top-down advocacy, 8
virtual advocacy, 271
advocates
 advocatee self advocate, 372
 centred advocacy, 63–4
 centred projects, 63
AEP (Association of European Psychiatrists), 161
AFET (Allgemeiner Fürsorgeerziehungstag), 167
African-American patients, neuropathic pain, 350
African Union (AU), 153
ageing population, 6
 cognitive disorders in migrants/refugees, 128
 neuropathic pain, 350
Ahari, S, 56
Ali, Muhammad, 146
AI (appreciative inquiry), 27–8
AL (Arab League), international advocacy, 153
All-Party Parliamentary Group on Primary Headache Disorders, 342
ALS *see* amyotrophic lateral sclerosis (ALS)

alternative medicine *see* complementary and alternative medicine (CAM)
Alzheimer Europe, 300
  advocacy dementia, 295b
Alzheimer's Association, 299–300
  advocacy dementia, 295b
  Advocacy Forum, 297–8
Alzheimer's Australia, 300
Alzheimer's disease (AD), 293t
  dementia, 291
  personality impairment, 47
Alzheimer's Disease Interaction, 295b
Alzheimer's Disease International, 300
Alzheimer Slovenia, 298
Alzheimer's Society Canada, 300
AMA (American Medical Association), 307
Amalienbad (Workers Palace), 38
American Academy of Neurology (AAN)
  advocacy dementia, 295b
  Alzheimer's disease, 298
  Neurology on the Hill, 143
  Palatucci Advocacy Leadership Forum, 351
  Palatucci programme, 78, 86, 87, 197–8, 294
  Treatment of Painful DPN guidelines, 350
American Headache Society, 342
American Heart Association, 224
American Library Association Advocacy Institute, 295b
American Medical Association (AMA), 307
American Stroke Association, 224
amyotrophic lateral sclerosis (ALS), 243–52
  advance directives, 246
  advocacy dangers, 245–6
  advocates for, 244–50
  assisted dying, 322
  Austrian response to, 196
  characteristics, 243
  depression, 246
  deterioration, 244
  disease cause, 244
  family advocacy, 246–7
  health policy advocacy, 249
  ice-bucket challenge, 195–6
  incidence/prevalence, 243, 253
  laypeople advocacy, 248–9
  palliative care, 321
  pathological crying and laughing, 246, 248
  pharmaceutical treatment, 249
  physician-assisted suicide & euthanasia, 247
  professional advocates, 247–8
  psychology, 244–5
  quality of life, 245
  reactive depression, 244, 248
  science politics advocacy, 249–50
  social aspects, 246–50
analgesia, head injury, 45
Analgesic, Anesthetic and Addiction Clinical Trial Translations Innovations Opportunities Network (ACTTION), 353
anticonvulsants, diabetic neuropathy, 355

antineoplastic therapies, brain tumours, 283
anti-NMDA antibodies, 296
anti-Parkinsonian drugs, 254
anti-seizure medication access, 333
anti-Semitism, 33–4, 38–9
anti-tobacco alliance, 64–5
anxiety, epilepsy, 327–8
apnoea test, 46–7
application of advocacy, 103–5
  communications, 103–4
  community support, 104
  empowerment, 103
  information, 105
  navigation, 104
appreciative inquiry (AI), 27–8
Arab League (AL), international advocacy, 153
articulation
  failure of, 23–4
  patient needs, 22
  see also communication
ASEAN (Association of South East Asian Nations), 153
ASN (Association of Sri Lankan Neurologists), 226
Aspen Neurobehavioral Conference Workgroup, 42
assisted dying, United Kingdom, 322
Association for Frontotemporal Degeneration, 300
Association of European Psychiatrists (AEP), 161
Association of South East Asian Nations (ASEAN), 153
Association of Sri Lankan Neurologists (ASN), 226
Association of the British Pharmaceutical Industry (ABPI), Code of Practice, 238
ataxia, 274–5
  definition, 274
  diagnosis, 274
Ataxia UK, 275
Atlas: Country Resources for Neurological Disorders (WFN), 156–7
Atlas of Epilepsy Care (WHO), 328, 330
attributes of advocates, 72–4
atypical parkinsonism, 268–9
  see also Multiple System Atrophy (MSA) Coalition
Austad, K E, 56
Australia
  care coordination, 93
  Medical Board of Australia, 58
  PSP Australia, 269
  Royal Australasian College of Physicians (RACP), 58, 59
  Western Health, stroke case study, 220–2
Austria
  ice-bucket challenge, 196–7
  SOS children's villages *see* SOS Children's Villages

Austromarxists, 36
authenticity, advocacy, 73
autoimmune disease, dementia, 293t
autonomy, advocacy, 73
awareness
 epilepsy care barriers, 329–30
 raising in multiple sclerosis, 235

B

back-casting, project management, 182
Baker, Mary, 160
BASH (British Association for the Study of Headache), 342
Basic Principles and Guidance Instrument for Developing, Adopting and Implementing Epilepsy Legislation (2012), 331, 333
Bateman, N, 8, 41
BEBRF (Benign Essential Blepharospasm Research Foundation), 272t
behaviour modifications, neuropathic pain treatment, 349
Behçet's disease, 126–7
Believe & Achieve (B&A), European Multiple Sclerosis Platform, 233
Bender, A, 43
benefits, disabled people, 255
Benign Essential Blepharospasm Research Foundation (BEBRF), 272t
Bernat, J L, 46
Bibile, Senaka, 57
biomarkers, epilepsy, 334
Black, B S, 49
blogging, public relations, 212–13
Blue Latitude Health, 100
bodily knowledge, 24, 26
bottom-up advocacy, 8
Bouchard, Brenda, 297–8
Brain Bee, 141
brain cancer/tumours, 97–111, 281–9
 cognitive impairment, 47
 cognitive rehabilitation, 285
 empowerment models, 99–100, 102
 individual assistance, 285
 issues in, 282–3
 knowledge, help & advice, 100
 patient information journey, 100, 101f
 personality impairment, 47
 physical training, 284
 progression, 282
 rehabilitation, 284–5
 self-management, 100
brain death, 46–7
brain diseases, chosen terminology, 160
brain injury, 43–4
 decision-making process, 50–1
 resuscitation after, 44
 stroke, 45–6
 traumatic brain injury, 292
Brain Injury Society, 300

Brain on Fire - My Month of Madness (Cahalan), 296
brain research, chosen terminology, 160
brains trust, 106–7
Brain Tumor Cooperative Group, 281
Brain Tumour Group, European Organisation for Research and Treatment of Cancer, 281
Brazil, Epilepsy Demonstration Projects, 331
Breuer, Josef, 35
British Association for the Study of Headache (BASH), 342
Brody, H, 57–8
budget, healthcare for, 83–4
businesses, managed healthcare, 84
Busquin, Philippe, 161t

C

Cahalan, Susannah, 296
Call to Action (2015), European Brain Council, 164
CAM *see* complementary and alternative medicine (CAM)
campaigns, 63
Campbell, Glen, 296
Canada
 Heart and Stroke Foundation stroke case study, 223
 Ontario Stroke Study, 223
 Western Ontario and McMaster Universities Arthritis Index (WOMAC), 353
cancer, 114b
 brain cancer *see* brain cancer/tumours
 central nervous system lymphomas, 281
 European Cancer Patient Coalition, 118–19
 European Guide on Quality Improvement in Comprehensive Cancer Control, 115
 European Organisation for Research and Treatment of Cancer, 281
 glioblastomas, 281
 glioma *see* glioma
 Global Colon Cancer Alliance, 117
 International Brain Tumour Alliance, 116–17
 International Kidney Cancer Coalition, 117
 Lung Cancer Europe, 119
 lymphomas, 281
 medulloblastomas, 281
 mortality, 114b
 multidisciplinary tumour board, 286
 patient-centred care, 114–15
 patient empowerment, 113–15
 Recognising European Cancer Nursing project, 116
 sarcoma, 120
 systemic cancer, 285–7
 tumour-directed treatment, 50
 see also ECCO (European CanCer Organization); European Cancer Congress (ECCs)
Cancer Control Joint Action (CanCon), 287

CanMED, 73
cardiovascular disease, ICD-10 vs. ICD-11, 156
care
　barriers in epilepsy, 328–34, 329f
　brain cancer planning, 99
　coordination, 93–4
　palliative care services, 315
　plans, 106
　see also healthcare
caregivers, 97–111
　coaching, 100
　confidence levels, 100, 102
　dementia, 296–8
　education of, 136–8
　neuro-oncology, 286
　relations to other groups, 372–3
Carta de Santiago, 224
case studies
　action planning, 259, 260t
　genetic variability, 257–8
　incurable disease, 90–2
　International Federation of Medical Students' Association, 198–200
　leadership failure, 197–8
　neurofibromatosis, 256–7
　Nigeria stroke support, 225
　nursing, 90–2
　oncology wards, 76–7
　patient needs, 22
　peripheral neuropathy, 256
　resistance to advocacy, 15–16
　self-advocacy, 5–6
　spinal cord injury, 256–7
　stroke, 220–7
catechol-*O*-methyltransferase (COMT) inhibitors, 267
cause-effect cycle, societal issues, 174
CBD (corticobasal degeneration), 268–9
CBT (cognitive behavioural therapy), neuropathic pain treatment, 349
CCI (Childhood Cancer International), 117–18
CDEs (common data elements), neuropathic pain research, 353–4
CEE (Central and Eastern Europe), European Multiple Sclerosis Platform, 231
celebrities, 146–7
Central African Republic, health expenditure, 153
Central and Eastern Europe (CEE), European Multiple Sclerosis Platform, 231
central nervous system (CNS), lymphomas, 281
Centres of Expertise for Rare Solid Cancers, European Commission, 283
Charcot, Jean-Marie, 69
charities, 146–7
　reversal of beliefs, 37–8
chemotherapy, systemic cancer, 286
Childhood Cancer International (CCI), 117–18
children, 6
　migrants/refugees health, 129

neurology education, 140–1
China, epilepsy Demonstration Projects, 331
Chinese Stroke Association (CSA), 225–6
Chiong, W, 48
choice, empowerment skill as, 99
chorea, 270–1
chorea gravidarum, 270
Churchill, Winston, 187, 189
civil wars, migrants/refugees, 124
climate change, migrants/refugees, 124
clinical decision-making, patient activation, 102
clinical trials, 53–4, 55
　burden to patient as, 121
　rare disorder drugs development, 310
closing plans, 365–6, 365b
　advocacy projects, 17
cluster headache, 339, 340
CME (continuing medical education), neuropathic pain, 349–50
CNS (central nervous system), lymphomas, 281
coalition advocacy, 8
cognitive ability, 25
　advocacy in neurology, 316
　driving, 49
cognitive behavioural therapy (CBT), neuropathic pain treatment, 349
cognitive impairment, decision-making and consent giving, 47–8
cognitive rehabilitation, brain tumours, 285
Cohn, Robin, 208
collaboration
　advocacy, 73
　patient needs, 27–8
collective advocacy, 36–9
colonies, migrants/refugees, 123–4
coma, 42
common data elements (CDEs), neuropathic pain research, 353–4
communication
　advocacy, 76–8, 103–4
　mindful communicating, 25–6
　movement disorders, 276t, 277
　palliative care advocacy, 318
　project failure, 188
　proxies, with, 43–5, 73
　see also articulation
community, 104, 106–7, 107f
Community Tool Box, advocacy dementia, 295b
co-morbidities, epilepsy, 327
competencies, nurse advocacy, 92
complementary and alternative medicine (CAM)
　media, 140
　movement disorders, 276t
　neuropathic pain treatment, 349
computed tomography (CT), brain tumours, 282
COMT (catechol-*O*-methyltransferase) inhibitors, 267
confidence levels, caregiver advocacy, 100, 102

conflicts of interest
  advocacy, 62
  Sri Lankan essential drug policy, 58
connections, international advocacy, 202
consanguinity, migrants/refugees, 127
consciousness disorders
  decision-making process, 42
  grades of, 42–3
consent, cognitive impairment, 47–8
consumerism, science *vs.*, 70
content, projects of, 371–2
continuation, 363–8
  definition, 365
continuing medical education (CME), neuropathic pain, 349–50
conventional politics, advocate-centred advocacy, 63–4
Convention on the Rights of the Child, 171, 172
core competencies, physicians, 69
cornerstones of advocacy, 22
corticobasal degeneration (CBD), 268–9
  see also movement disorders
Council for European Union, migrants/refugees health, 128
counter advocacy, 65–6
creative tools
  advocacy, 73
  public relations, 211
Creutzfeldt–Jakob disease, 293t
  sporadic, 296
Creutzfeldt–Jakob Surveillance Unit (UK), 298
cross-border projects, European Multiple Sclerosis Platform, 230
Cross-Committee Working Party on Patient Registries, 236
Cruz-Flores, Salvador, 224
CSA (Chinese Stroke Association), 225–6
CT (computed tomography), brain tumours, 282
culture, 14
  failure of, 193
CURE PSP, 268–9

D

DALYs *see* disability adjusted life years (DALYs)
Danish Headache Centre (Copenhagen), 342
data
  migrants/refugees health, 129
  SOS Children's Villages, 169
debriefing, 363–8
  definition, 365–6
decision-making
  brain injury, 50–1
  cognitive impairment, 47–8
  communication with proxies, 43–5
  consciousness disorders, 42
  end-of-life phase, 51
  patient *vs.* family, 318–19, 320
  shared, 48
  surrogate decision-makers, 44
deconditioning, 284

definition of advocacy, 7–8, 61, 219
deinstitutionalization, SOS Children's Villages, 171–2
dementia, 291–302
  advocacy in, 292–4
  Alzheimer's disease, 291
  care, 292–3, 297
  caregiver advocacy, 296–8
  cognitive impairment, 47
  definition, 291
  diseases causing, 293–4, 293t
  driving ability, 48–9
  family advocacy, 296–8
  non-governmental organizations, 299–300
  patients, 295–6
  physician advocates, 298–9
  public health response recommendations, 157
  research participation, 50
  scientist advocacy, 298–9
  stages of, 291–2
  treatment restriction, 50
Demonstration Projects, Global Campaign Against Epilepsy, 330–1, 334
dependency avoidance, 59
depression, epilepsy, 327–8
de Schepper, Joel, 271
deterioration recognition, advocacy in neurology, 316–17
Deuticke, Franz, 35
developing countries
  epilepsy care barriers, 328–9
  healthcare provision, 83–4
diabetic neuropathy (DPN), 347
  education, 355
Diagnostic and Statistical Manual IV (DSM-IV), tics, 273
Dialectics of Enlightenment (Adorno), 38–9
Die große Mutter, 38
Dirksen, Everett M, 229
disability adjusted life years (DALYs)
  Europe, 154
  migrants/refugees, 125
  non-communicable diseases, 156
disabled people, recognition of needs, 255
discrimination, migrants/refugees, 130
DMRF (Dystonia Medical Research Foundation), 272t, 273
doctors *see* physicians (doctors)
Do Not Attempt Resuscitation Orders, 317
dopamine agonists, Parkinson's disease treatment, 267
DPN *see* diabetic neuropathy (DPN)
driving ability, 48–9
drug development
  neuropathic pain, 348
  rare disorders, 308
DSM-IV (*Diagnostic and Statistical Manual IV*), tics, 273
Duchenne muscular dystrophy, drug development, 310

duloxetine, neuropathic pain treatment, 348
dystonia, 271–3
Dystonia Advocacy Network (DAN), 272
DySTonia Inc, 272*t*
Dystonia Medical Research Foundation (DMRF), 272*t*, 273

E

EAN *see* European Academy of Neurology (EAN)
EANO (European Association for Neuro-Oncology), 281
EANS (European Association of Neurosurgical Societies), 161
EAPC *see* European Association of Palliative Care (EAPC)
Eastern Europe, SOS Children's Villages, 171–2
ECCO (European CanCer Organization), 113–22
  Patient Advisory Committee, 113, 115–16, 116–20
  patient perspective, 120–1
  structure, 115–16
ECCs *see* European Cancer Congress (ECCs)
ECNP (European College of Neuro-Psychopharmacology), 161
economics
  cancer, 114*b*
  headaches, 341
  patient activation, 102
  public relations, 207
  see also finances
ECPC (European Cancer Patient Coalition), 118–19
ECTRIMS (European Committee for Treatment and Research in Multiple Sclerosis), 237
education, 135–41
  advocacy in, 373
  doctors' responsibilities, 69
  epilepsy, 333–4
  importance of, 36
  learning from projects, 366
  palliative care and, 323–4
  public neurology education, 135–6, 136*b*
  rare disorders, 307–8
  targeted groups, 136–41
EFNA *see* European Federation of Neurological Advocacy (EFNA)
EFNS (European Federation of Neurological Societies), 159
EFPIA (European Federation of Pharmaceutical Industries and Associations), 161, 238
Ego, 35
EHA (European Huntington Association), 266
Eisenhower, Dwight, 187–8
elderly care home, Vienna, 15–16
electronic press kits (EPKs), 210
elevator pitches, 181
EMAS (European Medicines Agency), 236
embodying, The Theory U, 29–30, 29*f*
emergency care, neuromuscular disorder, 254

empathy, 73
employment
  multiple sclerosis, 233
  neurological disorders, 144
empowerment
  application of advocacy, 103
  models in brain cancer, 99–100, 102
  morality, 102–3
  patients, 7
  rare disorders, 307–8
EMSP *see* European Multiple Sclerosis Platform (EMSP)
enacting, The Theory U, 29, 29*f*
ENCALS (European Network for the Cure of ALS), 248
encephalopathy, 47
ending, 363–8
  advocacy projects, 17
end-of-life phase, 320–1
  decision-making process, 51
  movement disorders, 276*t*
  palliative care, 321
entitlements, empowerment skill as, 99
EONS (European Oncology Nursing Society), 116
EORTC (European Organisation for Research and Treatment of Cancer), 281
EPA (European Psychiatric Association), 161
EPDA (European Parkinson's Disease Association), 267
ependymomas, 281
EpiBioS4Rx (Epilepsy Bioinformatics Study for Antiepileptogenic Therapy), 334
epilepsy, 327–37
  anxiety, 327–8
  care barriers, 328–34, 329*f*
  children/teacher education, 140–1
  co-morbidities, 327
  depression, 327–8
  education, 333–4
  future work, 332–3
  general knowledge lack, 330
  healthcare costs, 328
  low-income countries, 328
  migrants/refugees, 126
  mortality, 327
  prevalence, 327–8
  symptoms, 327
  treatment access, 333
Epilepsy Bioinformatics Study for Antiepileptogenic Therapy (EpiBioS4Rx), 334
epistemology, 21–32
  definition, 23
EPKs (electronic press kits), 210
equity, 16
essential drug policy, Sri Lanka, 57–9
essential tremor (ET), 269
ET (essential tremor), 269
ethics, 41–52

research, 49–50
treatment restrictions, 50–1
EUnetHTA (European Network of Health Technology Assessment), 237
EuNetMuS, 233
EURACAN, 283
EU Rare Diseases, 306*t*
EUReMS (European Registry for MS), 235
EuropaColon, 117
Europa Donna, 118
Europa Uomo, 118
Europe
  Alzheimer Europe *see* Alzheimer Europe
  Association of European Psychiatrists (AEP), 161
  care coordination, 93
  Central and Eastern Europe, 231
  Council for European Union, 128
  ECCO (European CanCer Organization) *see* ECCO (European CanCer Organization)
  Federation of European Neuroscience Societies (FENS), 161
  Global Alliance of Mental Illness Advocacy Networks - Europe (GAMIAN-Europe), 160
  headache advocacy, 341
  healthcare provision figures, 154, 155*f*
  health information for migrants/refugees, 124
  Lung Cancer Europe (LuCE), 119
  Lymphoma Coalition Europe (LCE), 118
  Melanoma Patient Network Europe (MPNE), 119
  Myeloma Patient Europe (MPE), 117
  rare disorders prevalence, 303
  Recognising European Cancer Nursing (RECaN) project, 116
  social healthcare system, 85
  Stroke Alliance for Europe (SAFE), 224
  VOT (value of treatment) for brain disorders in Europe, 163
European Academy of Neurology (EAN), 160
  European Federation of Neurological Advocacy and, 266
  palliative care, 323, 324
European Association for Neuro-Oncology (EANO), 281
European Association of Neurosurgical Societies (EANS), 161
European Association of Palliative Care (EAPC), 321
  palliative care, 323, 324
European Brain Council, 159–66
  Call to Action (2015), 164
  creation, 160–1
  FP6 advocacy, 161, 161*t*
  FP7 advocacy, 162
  FP8-Horizon 2020, 163
  FP9, 163–5
  funding for FP5/FP6/FP7, 161*t*, 162–3
  Year of the Brain (YOTB 2014), 164–5

European Cancer Congress (ECCs)
  2015, 121
  patient care, 120
European CanCer Organization *see* ECCO (European CanCer Organization)
European Cancer Patient Coalition (ECPC), 118–19
European Code of Good Practice in MS, 232, 235
European College of Neuro-Psychopharmacology (ECNP), 161
European Commission
  Centres of Expertise for Rare Solid Cancers, 283
  PARENT Joint Action (cross-border PAtient REgistries iNiTiative), 236
European Committee for Treatment and Research in Multiple Sclerosis (ECTRIMS), 237
European Council, rare disorders, 308–9
European Federation of Neurological Advocacy (EFNA), 160
  European Academy of Neurology and, 266
  movement disorders, 265–6
  Neurology Advocacy Awards, 266
  Patient Advocate Workshops, 266
European Federation of Neurological Societies (EFNS), 159
European Federation of Pharmaceutical Industries and Associations (EFPIA), 161, 238
European Football Association, epilepsy advocacy, 331–2
European Guide on Quality Improvement in Comprehensive Cancer Control (CanCon), 115
European Huntington Association (EHA), 266
European Medicines Agency (EMAS), 236
European Men's Health Forum, 118
European Month of the Brain (2013), 164
European MS Nurse Survey (MS-NEED), 232
European Multiple Sclerosis Platform (EMSP), 229–41, 239*f*
  annual conferences, 232
  Believe & Achieve, 233
  challenges, 238
  Code of Good Practice, 233*t*
  cross-border projects, 230
  data collection, 233
  European Code of Good Practice in MS, 232
  foundation, 230
  future work, 238–40
  major projects, 231–3
  MS Barometer, 232
  Nurse PRO training programme, 232
  Path to Participation, 233
  Patient and Consumer Working Party membership, 233
  project website, 233
European Network for the Cure of ALS (ENCALS), 248

European Network of Health Technology
    Assessment (EUnetHTA), 237
European Network of National Patient Registries
    in Multiple Sclerosis, 233
European Oncology Nursing Society
    (EONS), 116
European Organisation for Rare Diseases
    (Eurordis), 305, 306t
European Organisation for Research and
    Treatment of Cancer (EORTC), 281
European Parkinson's Disease Association
    (EPDA), 267
European Parliament, Written Declaration of
    Epilepsy, 332
European Psychiatric Association (EPA), 161
European Registry for MS (EUReMS), 235
European Research Programmes on Rare
    Diseases, 309
European Task Force on Disorders of
    Consciousness, 42–3
European Union (EU), white paper
    drafting, 142
EURORDIS, 304
Eurordis (European Organisation for Rare
    Diseases), 305, 306t
euthanasia, amyotrophic lateral sclerosis, 247
evaluation of advocacy, 75
extrinsic motivation, project management, 186
eye-opening, vegetative state, 42

F

Facebook, public relations, 213
facilitators, project management, 182
FACTS & FIGURES in MS, 232
Fagues, P, 124
failure in advocacy, 16–17, 21
    headaches, 341–3
families
    desire to make decisions, 318–19, 320
    end of life decisions, 320–1
family advocacy, 76–8
    amyotrophic lateral sclerosis, 246–7
    dementia, 296–8
FARA (Friedreich's Ataxia Research
    Alliance), 275
FDA *see* Food and Drug Administration (FDA)
Federation of European Neuroscience Societies
    (FENS), 161
finances
    advocacy projects, 64–5
    European Multiple Sclerosis Platform,
        231, 239f
    headaches, 341
    neuropathic pain research, 352
    palliative care, 319
    project management, 181
    science, 71
    see also economics
5Ws and H, 294
flavour carriers, 77

follow-up-treatment
    dementia care, 297
    neuromuscular disorder, 254
Food and Drug Administration (FDA)
    ataxia advocacy, 275
    rare disorder drugs development, 309
Forget me not organisation, 298
Fox, Michael J, 146
FP5, funding, 161t, 162–3
FP6, 161, 161t
    funding, 161t, 162–3
FP7, 162
    funding, 161t, 162–3
FP8-Horizon 2020, European Brain
    Council, 163
FP9, 163–5
Framingham Health Study, stroke, 219
free market economy, Sri Lanka, 57–8
Freud, Sigmund, 34–6
    influence of, 35–6
    revolutionary dream, 34–5
Friedreich Ataxia Parents Group, 275
Friedreich's Ataxia Research Alliance (FARA), 275
Froebel children's education, 38
frontotemporal dementia (FTD), 268–9, 293t
FTD (frontotemporal dementia), 268–9, 293t
Fugh-Berman, A, 56
funding *see* finances

G

gabapentin, neuropathic pain treatment, 348
GAMIAN-Europe (Global Alliance of
    Mental Illness Advocacy Networks
    - Europe), 160
Gandhi, 179
GARD (Genetic and Rare Diseases Information
    Centre), 306t
Gates, Bill, 188
general population, epilepsy knowledge
    lack, 330
Genetic Alliance, 305, 306t
Genetic and Rare Diseases Information Centre
    (GARD), 306t
genetics
    ataxia, 274
    counselling of migrants/refugees, 129
    variability case study, 257–8
genotyping
    Stevens–Johnson syndrome, 257
    toxic epidermal necrolysis, 257
Germany
    ethnicity of migrants, 124
    PSP Germany, 269
    SOS Children's Villages opposition to, 167–8
glioblastomas, 281
glioma
    end-of-life phase, 51
    treatment restriction, 50
Global Action Plan in the Public Health
    Response to Dementia (WHO), 300

Global Alliance of Mental Illness
    Advocacy Networks - Europe
    (GAMIAN-Europe), 160
Global Burden of Disease study
  headaches, 339, 340
  white paper drafting, 142
Global Campaign Against Epilepsy, 330
  Basic Principle and Guidance Instrument for
    Developing, Adopting and Implementing
    Epilepsy Legislation, 333
  Demonstration Projects, 330–1, 334
Global Campaign Against Headache
    (WHO), 343–4
Global Colon Cancer Alliance, 117
Glock, Ralph, 229
Gmeiner, Hermann, 167
goals, project management, 179, 181–6
governments
  advocacy in neuropathic pain, 351–6
  neurology advocacy, 141–4
  role of in health, 83
grassroot advocacy, 8
grasstop advocacy, 8
Great Depression, 38
Gründerzeit, 36
guerilla advocacy, 8
*Guidelines for Ethical Relationship Between
    Physician and Industry* (Royal
    Australasian College of Physicians), 58
Guillain–Barré syndrome, 287

H

Habsburg Empire, history of advocacy, 33
Hanak, Anton, 38
Hansen, Bruno, 161*t*
Hardy, John, 299
harvesting, projects, 366
Haushofer, Johannes, 193
HDlighthouse Families Website, 271
Headache on the Hill (HOH), 342
headaches, 339–46
  cluster headache, 339, 340
  epilepsy *see* epilepsy
  medication-overuse headache, 340
  prevalence, 339
  tension-type *see* tension-type headache
  treatment, 342
healthcare
  costs in epilepsy, 328
  history of, 53
  multidisciplinary care model, 84
  navigating through, 74
  neuropathic pain, 350
  physicians as leaders, 85
  team–nurse relationships, 94
  see also care; medicine
healthcare access
  migrants/refugees, 125
  neuromuscular disorders, 254, 256
  nurses, 93

healthcare provision
  European figures, 155*f*
  nurses, 93
  rare disorders, 304
health fairs, 142–3
health groups, relations to other groups,
    372–3
health, human right as, 61
health literacy, patient activation, 102
health policy, migrants/refugees, 128
health system advocacy, 86
  amyotrophic lateral sclerosis, 249
  neuropathic pain, 351–6
Health Technology Assessment (HTA), 237
Heart and Stroke Foundation (Canada), stroke
    case study, 223
hepatitis
  cancer, 114*b*
  migrants/refugees, 126
Hereditary Disease Foundation, 271
Herzl, Theodor, 33
higher altitude goals, project
    management, 182–3
Hildebrand, Jerzy, 281
hinge factor, 201
Hispanic patients, neuropathic pain, 350
history of advocacy, 33–40
  Habsburg Empire, 33
  Late Enlightenment, 33
  Vienna, 33–4
history of neurology, 69–70
history-taking, 70
HIV infection, migrants/refugees, 126
Horizon 2000, 159
HTA (Health Technology Assessment), 237
human behaviour, advocacy, 61
Human Genome Project, 271
human papilloma virus (HPV) infection,
    cancer, 114*b*
human resources, project management, 181
human rights
  migrants/refugees, 128
  palliative care as, 323
humility, advocacy, 73
Huntington, George, 271
Huntington's disease, 270–1
  assisted dying, 322
hypophysis, 287

I

IBE *see* International Bureau for Epilepsy (IBE)
Ibero-American Stroke Society, 224
IBTA (International Brain Tumour
    Alliance), 116–17
ICD-10 *see* International Classification of
    Disease 10 (ICD-10)
ICD-11 *see* International Classification of
    Disease 11 (ICD-11)
ice-bucket challenge, 195–7
Id, 35

idealism, decline in, 200–1
identification of advocates, 5
IETF (International Essential Tremor Foundation), 269
IFMSA *see* International Federation of Medical Students' Association (IFMSA)
IHA (International Huntington Association), 270–1
IKCC (International Kidney Cancer Coalition), 117
ILAE *see* International League Against Epilepsy (ILAE)
immersion, advocacy, 75–6
IMMPACT (Initiate on Methods, Measurement and Pain Assessment in Clinical Trials), 353
immunization, migrants/refugees, 130
IMRT (intensity modulated radiotherapy), brain tumours, 282–3
incurable disease, case study, 90–2
individuals
　advocacy for, 34–6
　assistance in brain tumours, 285
infections
　cancer, 114*b*
　migrants/refugees, 125–6
information
　advocacy in neurology, 316
　application of advocacy, 105
　brain cancer, 100
　collection from migrants/refugees, 124
　palliative care advocacy, 318
　project management, 181
Initiate on Methods, Measurement and Pain Assessment in Clinical Trials (IMMPACT), 353
Instagram, public relations, 213
Institute of Pain (USA), neuropathic pain prevalence, 347
insurance companies
　counter advocacy, 65
　managed healthcare, 84
　neuropathic pain treatment, 349
intellectual input, advocacy projects, 64
intensity modulated radiotherapy (IMRT), brain tumours, 282–3
internal challenges, SOS Children's Villages, 170–1
internal ratings based (IRB) discussions, 121
internal readiness, advocacy in service providers, 174
international advocacy, 153–8, 193–204
　connections, 202
　lessons learned from "ice bucket challenge," 196–7
　persistence, 202
　prepare for the unexpected, 201
　status quo change, 201–2
　stroke treatment, 194–5
　think locally, act globally, 202

International Brain Tumour Alliance (IBTA), 116–17
International Bureau for Epilepsy (IBE), 330
International Bureau for Epilepsy (IBE), epilepsy advocacy, 331–2, 333
International Classification of Disease 10 (ICD-10), 154
　ICD-11 *vs.*, 156
　non-communicable diseases, 157
　stroke, 194
　topic advisory group, 154
International Classification of Disease 11 (ICD-11), 4, 154, 156
　ICD-10 *vs.*, 156
International Clinical Trials Registry Platform (WHO), 258
International Epilepsy Day, 205
International Essential Tremor Foundation (IETF), 269
International Federation of Medical Students' Association (IFMSA), 198–201
　advocacy training sessions, 199
　case study, 198–200
　learning about advocacy, 200–1
　Youth Pre-World Health assembly, 199
International Huntington Association (IHA), 270–1
International Kidney Cancer Coalition (IKCC), 117
International League Against Epilepsy (ILAE), 142, 330
　epilepsy advocacy, 331–2, 333
international level, palliative care, 323–4
International Organization for Migrants, 128
International Organization of Multiple Sclerosis Nurses (IOMSN), 234
International Parkinson and Movement Disorder Society, 265
International Rare Diseases Research Consortium (IRDiRC), 306*t*
Internet, 207
internists, neuroscience education, 140
The Interpretation of Dreams (Freud), 34–5
interwar years, Vienna, 36–7
intrinsic motivation, project management, 186
IOMSN (International Organization of Multiple Sclerosis Nurses), 234
ipilimumab, 287
IRB (internal ratings based) discussions, 121
IRDiRC (International Rare Diseases Research Consortium), 306*t*
Ireland, Migraine Association of Ireland, 342
isolated autonomy, 44
issue-centred advocacy, 63

J

job retention, multiple sclerosis, 233
Johnson, Beth, 299
Joint Linearization of Mortality and Morbidity (JLMMS), 154, 156

journalists, 207–8
judicial system, neurology advocacy, 143–4

K
Katzman, Robert, 291
kinesis, 26
KISS-rule, 208
knowledge gap, epilepsy care barriers, 329–30
Kogoj, Aleš, 298
Korea, epilepsy Demonstration Projects, 331
Kraus, Karl, 34
Kulturwille, 36

L
language barriers, migrants/refugees health, 129
Late Enlightenment, history of advocacy, 33
Latin America Summit for Stroke, stroke case study, 224
law-making, 62
Lawry, Sylvia, 229, 230*f*
LCE (Lymphoma Coalition Europe), 118
leadership failure
    case study, 197–8
    project failure, 189
leadership training, advocacy in, 64
Lebenswelt, 26
legal rights, migrants/refugees, 123
legislation
    advocacy, 8
    epilepsy advocacy, 333
    migrants/refugees rights, 128
    neurology advocacy, 143
Lehman, J, 98
leprosy, 253
letters to the editor, 210–11
letting come, The Theory U, 29, 29*f*
letting go, The Theory U, 28, 29*f*
Leukaemia Patient Advocates Foundation, 117
levels of advocacy, 8, 14
Levin, Victor, 281
Lewy body dementia, 292, 293*t*
Lewy Body Society, 300
Lifeline Express, 143, 143*f*
life-sustaining treatment, 45–6
    amyotrophic lateral sclerosis, 247
    withdrawal of, 45
Lifting the Burden (LTB) (UK), 343
LMICs *see* low- and middle-income countries (LMICs)
lobbying, advocacy *vs.*, 8
local level, advocacy of, 148*t*
local regional branches, movement disorders, 276
long-term goals
    advocacy, 62–3
    project management, 181–2
long-term impact, advocacy, 66
low- and middle-income countries (LMICs)
    disabled people, 255
    epilepsy, 328

stroke, 127–8
LRRK2 gene, 127
LTB (Lifting the Burden) (UK), 343
Lueger, Karl, 33
Lung Cancer Europe (LuCE), 119
Lymphoma Coalition Europe (LCE), 118
lymphomas, 281

M
Mach, Ernst, 34
Machtwille, 36
macro level, 14
    methods, 75
    palliative care, 323–4
    projects, 366, 372
magnetic resonance imaging (MRI), brain tumours, 282
Mallik, M, 89
management advocacy, 74
MAO-B (monoamine oxidase type B) inhibitors, 267
Marie Curies Triggers for Palliative Care, 317
marijuana, medical, 356
MDA (Muscular Dystrophy Association), 275
MDS (myelodysplastic syndromes), 119
MDS Alliance, 119
media, 373
    distribution list, 208
    information, 209
    neuroscience education, 140
    press releases, 209
    project management, 181
    public relations, 207–8
media kits (press kits), 210
mediation advocacy, 105
Medical Board of Australia, 58
medical decision-making, problems in, 41
medical research, 58
medical students
    idealism, decline in, 200–1
    neuroscience education, 138, 139*f*
Medicare, neuropathic pain, 352
medication-overuse headache, 340
medicine
    definition, 69
    influences on, 71
    mainstream topics, 72
    see also healthcare
Medicins Sans Frontiers, 258
medulla oblongata, brain death, 46
medulloblastomas, 281
Melanoma Patient Network Europe (MPNE), 119
memory, children/teacher education, 140–1
mental education, neuropathic pain advocacy, 351
Mental Health Capacity Act (UK), 318
Mental Health Gap Action Programme (MHGAP) (WHO), 331
mental health service, neuropathic pain, 349

Merleau-Ponty, M, 24
meso level, 8
  methods, 75
  movement disorders, 265
  palliative care, 322–3
  projects, 366, 372
message of advocacy, 63
methods
  advocacy, 74–5
  projects, 64
Meynert, Theodor, 35
MHGAP (Mental Health Gap Action Programme) (WHO), 331
Michael J Fox Foundation (MJFF), 268
micro level, 8
  methods, 75
  projects, 366, 372
Middle East
  Behçet's disease, 126
  consanguinity, 127
migraine, 339
  treatment, 340
Migraine Association of Ireland, 342
Migraine Trust, 342
migrants/refugees, 7, 123–33
  ageing cognitive disorders, 128
  Behçet's disease, 126–7
  consanguinity, 127
  diseases/disorders, 125
  epilepsy, 126
  European health information, 124
  health service access, 125
  infections, 125–6
  information collection, 124
  legal rights, 123
  multiple sclerosis, 126
  national death registers, 124
  neurogenetic diseases, 127–8
  neurology, 125
  non-migrant populations *vs.*, 124–5, 129–30
  originating areas, 123
  socioeconomic status, 125
mild cognitive impairment, participation in research, 49
Millennium Development Goals, 168
mindful communicating, 25–6
mindfulness, 25
minimally conscious state, 43
MJFF (Michael J Fox Foundation), 268
monoamine oxidase type B (MAO-B) inhibitors, 267
Montessori children's education, 38
morality, empowerment, 102–3
motivation, project management, 186–8
motor neuron disease, 50
  see also amyotrophic lateral sclerosis (ALS)
movement disorders, 265–79
  advocacy types, 276
  meso level of action, 265
  unmet advocacy needs, 276–7, 276t

  see also ataxia; atypical parkinsonism; chorea; corticobasal degeneration (CBD); dystonia; essential tremor (ET); Huntington's disease; Parkinson's disease (PD); progressive supranuclear palsy (PSP); tics; Tourette's syndrome
MPE (Myeloma Patient Europe), 117
MPNE (Melanoma Patient Network Europe), 119
MRI (magnetic resonance imaging), brain tumours, 282
MS *see* multiple sclerosis (MS)
MSA (Multiple System Atrophy) Coalition, 269
MS-ATLAs, 232
MS Barometer, 232
MS Cybercafe, 231
MS-ID (Multiple Sclerosis-Information Dividend), 234–6
MSIF (Multiple Sclerosis International Federation), 229
MS-NEED (European MS Nurse Survey), 232
MS-NEED (Multiple Sclerosis-Nurse Empowering Education), 234
MS Nurse Professionals, 234
MTB (multidisciplinary tumour board), 286
Mukand, J A, 97–8
multidisciplinary healthcare
  model of, 84
  nurse care navigator, 93
multidisciplinary tumour board (MTB), 286
multiple sclerosis (MS), 229–41
  data collection, 234–6
  employment, 233
  EU bodies and initiatives, 236–7
  job retention, 233
  migrants/refugees, 126
  nurse advocates, 233–4
  patient advocacy, 233–4
  personality impairment, 47
  treatment restriction, 50
Multiple Sclerosis-Information Dividend (MS-ID), 234–6
Multiple Sclerosis International Federation (MSIF), 229
Multiple Sclerosis-Nurse Empowering Education (MS-NEED), 234
multiple system atrophy, 268
  see also atypical parkinsonism
Multiple System Atrophy (MSA) Coalition, 269
muscular dystrophies, incidence/prevalence, 253
Muscular Dystrophy Association (MDA), 275
Musil, Robert, 34
myasthenia gravis, 287
  incidence/prevalence, 253
Myasthenia Gravis Foundation of America, 308
myelodysplastic syndromes (MDS), 119
Myeloma Patient Europe (MPE), 117
myositis, 287

N

NANO (Neurologic assessment in Neuro-Oncology), 286
National Ataxia Foundation (NAF), 275
National Brain Councils (NBCs), 164–5
national death registers, migrants/refugees, 124
National Health Service (NHS) (UK), 85
National Institutes of Health (NIH)
  ataxia advocacy, 275
  headache advocacy, 342
  Network in Excellence in Neuroscience Clinical Trials, 352
  Rare Disease Clinical Research Network programme, 306
national level, advocacy of, 148*t*
National Multiple Sclerosis Society (US), 229
National Neurology Association (Pakistan), 138, 140
  advocacy in, 147
  legislation advocacy, 143, 144*b*
  patient support groups, 145
  WHO and, 147
National Organization for Rare Disorders (NORD), 275, 305, 306*t*, 308
National Parkinson Foundation, 267
national policies, migrants/refugees health, 129
National Spasmodic Dysphonia Association (NSDA), 272*t*
National Spasmodic Torticollis Association (NSTA), 272*t*
National Tremor Foundation (NTF), 269
Nation Headache Competence Centre (Norway), 342
navigation, application of advocacy, 104
Nazism, 38–9
NCDs *see* non-communicable diseases (NCDs)
need for advocacy, 4–7, 97–9
need recognition, disabled people, 255
negative coping mechanisms, neuropathic pain, 355–6
negative self-advocacy, 6
Netherlands, driving ability and neurological disease, 49
Network in Excellence in Neuroscience Clinical Trials (NeuroNEXT), 352
Neue Mensch, 36
Neurocritical Care Society, 43
  life-sustaining treatment, 45
neurofibromatosis, 256–7
neurological care, neuromuscular disorder, 255
neurological diseases/disorders
  brain cancer, 97–8
  context of, 4
  employment, 144
Neurological Disorders: Public Health Challenges (WHO/WFN), 157
neurological examination, 70
Neurologic assessment in Neuro-Oncology (NANO), 286

neurologists
  advocates as, 72
  primary duty, 53
  self-advocacy, 147, 148*t*
neurology
  additional skills, 71–2
  definition, 41
  development, 70–1
  migrants/refugees, 125
  purpose of advocacy, 62
Neurology Advocacy Awards, European Federation of Neurological Advocacy, 266
Neurology on the Hill, American Academy of Neurology, 143
neurology services, 142
neuromuscular disorders, 253–63
  access to care, 256
  action planning, 259
  advocacy focus, 258–9
  amyotrophic lateral sclerosis *see* amyotrophic lateral sclerosis (ALS)
  barriers to, 254–6
  incidence/prevalence, 253–4
  myasthenia gravis *see* myasthenia gravis
  neurofibromatosis *see* neurofibromatosis
  peripheral neuropathy *see* peripheral neuropathy
  spinal cord injury, case study, 256–7
  Stevens–Johnson syndrome *see* Stevens–Johnson syndrome
  toxic epidermal necrolysis, genotyping, 257
NeuroNEXT (Network in Excellence in Neuroscience Clinical Trials), 352
neuro-oncology, 281–9
  history of, 281–2
  systemic cancer, 285–7
  see also systemic cancer
Neuro-Oncology (journal), 281–2
neuropathic pain, 347–60
  challenges to, 357*t*
  effects of, 348–9
  government advocacy, 351–6
  health system advocacy, 351–6
  new drug development, 348
  patient-level advocacy, 347–9
  patient safety, 354–5
  physician advocates, 349–51
  prevalence, 347
  public education, 355–6
  public–private partnerships, 353
  research, 352–4
  treatment, 348
neuropsychiatry services, access to, 98–9
neuro-psychosocial support, brain cancer, 100
neuro-rehabilitation
  brain cancer, 100
  stroke treatment, 194–5
newspapers, 207

NGOs *see* non-governmental organizations (NGOs)
Nigeria, stroke support, 225
NIH *see* National Institutes of Health (NIH)
NIV (non-invasive ventilation), amyotrophic lateral sclerosis, 247
nivolumab, 287
NNT (number needed to treat), neuropathic pain treatment, 348
NOCEBO, 71
non-communicable diseases (NCDs)
  burden of, 194
  ICD-10, 157
  WHO, 156
non-governmental organizations (NGOs), 146–7, 157, 173
  dementia, 299–300
  international advocacy, 153
  migrants/refugees health, 129
  public relations, 206
  role of in health, 83
non-invasive ventilation (NIV), amyotrophic lateral sclerosis, 247
non-steroidal anti-inflammatory drugs (NSAIDs), diabetic neuropathy, 355
NORD (National Organization for Rare Disorders), 275, 305, 306*t*, 308
Nork Hodepineselskap, 342
North Africa
  Behçet's disease, 126
  consanguinity, 127
  HIV infection, 126
  multiple sclerosis, 126
Norway
  health expenditure, 153
  Nation Headache Competence Centre, 342
  Nork Hodepineselskap, 342
NSAIDs (non-steroidal anti-inflammatory drugs), diabetic neuropathy, 355
NSDA (National Spasmodic Dysphonia Association), 272*t*
NSTA (National Spasmodic Torticollis Association), 272*t*
NTF (National Tremor Foundation), 269
number needed to treat (NNT), neuropathic pain treatment, 348
nurse advocates
  awareness of advocacy, 89
  multiple sclerosis, 233–4
  neuro-oncology, 286
nurse care navigator, 93–4
Nurse PRO training programme, 232
nursing, 89–96
  case study, 90–2
  competencies and skills, 92
  difficulties and conflicts, 94–5
  healthcare access and provision, 93
  patient autonomy, 92
  patient representation, 92–3, 94
  recommendations, 95

O

OMERACT (Outcome Measures in Rheumatoid Arthritis Clinical Trials), 353
oncology wards, case study, 76–7
online resources
  Internet, 207
  press conferences, 213
  project management, 181
  public relations, 209, 212–14
  stroke, 225
Ontario Stroke Study, 223
open charts, patient access, 78
opioids
  abuse epidemic, 354–5
  diabetic neuropathy, 355
  neuropathic pain treatment, 348
  palliative care, 323
orchestration, advocacy, 73
organ donation, 46–7
Organization for Understanding of Cluster Headache (OUCH), 342
originating areas, migrants/refugees, 123
orphan diseases *see* rare disorders
Orphan Drug Act (1983), 308
Orphanet, 306*t*
orthopaedic support, amyotrophic lateral sclerosis, 247–8
OUCH (Organization for Understanding of Cluster Headache), 342
Outcome Measures in Rheumatoid Arthritis Clinical Trials (OMERACT), 353
outcome of advocacy, 65
Out of the Shadows campaign, 330
overmotivation, advocacy dangers, 245
oxycodone, 348

P

PAGs (patient advocacy groups), rare disorders, 305–6, 306*t*, 309
PAHO (Pan American Health Organization), 224
PAIN-CONTRoLS (Patient-Assisted Intervention for Neuropathy: Comparison of Treatment in Real Life Situations), 353
pain, systemic cancer, 286
Pakistan
  healthcare provision, 83
  National Neurology Association (Pakistan) *see* National Neurology Association (Pakistan)
Palatucci programme, 78, 86, 87, 197–8, 294, 351
palliative care, 121, 315–26
  advance care planning, 319–20, 320–1
  advance directive, 319–20
  brain tumours, 283
  care services, 315
  definition, 315
  disease chronicity, 317–18, 322*f*
  early disease progression in, 321

education and, 323–4
financial issues, 319
human right as, 323
international level, 323–4
macro level issues, 323–4
medication, 323
meso level issues, 322–3
patient-related advocacy, 318–21
recognition for, 316–17
social aspects, 319
Pan American Health Organization (PAHO), 224
paralanguage, 26
PARENT Joint Action (cross-border PAtient REgistries iNiTiative), 236
Parent Project Muscular Dystrophy group, 309–10
Parkinsonism, migrants/refugees, 127
Parkinson's disease (PD), 266–7
cognitive impairment, 47
disease chronicity, 317–18
media education, 140
patient associations, 267
personality impairment, 47
research advocates, 267
symptoms, 267
treatment restriction, 50
Parkinson's Disease Foundation (PDF), 267–8
parTisan advocacy, 8
passion, advocacy, 73, 74
paternalism, 44
pathological crying and laughing, amyotrophic lateral sclerosis, 246, 248
Path to Participation (PPP), 233
patient(s)
acknowledge communications, 26
activation, 102–3
autonomy, 70, 92
brain tumour monitoring, 283
cancer-centred care, 114–15
collaboration, 102
dementia, 295–6
education, 136–8, 138b
empowerment, 7, 113–15
group relations, 372–3
identification of needs, 24–8
inquiries to, 21–2
MS relevant outcome data, 238
MS reported outcome data, 238
needs, 21, 22
neuropathic pain safety, 354–5
nurse representation, 94
open chart access, 78
perspectives of, 78
physician interactions, 71
representation by nurses, 92–3
self-documentation example, 27
supportive care needs, 94
tacit knowledge of needs, 24
Patient Advisory Committee (PAC), 113, 115–16, 116–20

patient advocacy, 73, 97–111
multiple sclerosis, 233–4
neuropathic pain, 347–9
organizations, 146
palliative care, 318–21
rare disorders, 305–6, 306t, 309
support groups, 85–6, 145–6, 145b
Patient Advocate Workshops, 266
Patient and Consumer Working Party (PCWP), 233
Patient-Assisted Intervention for Neuropathy: Comparison of Treatment in Real Life Situations (PAIN-CONTRoLS), 353
Patient-Centred Outcomes Research Institute (PCORI), 77–8, 371
movement disorders, 266
neuropathic pain, 353, 354
rare disorder drug development, 309
Patient Protection and Affordable Care Act (2010), 347
PAtient REgistries iNiTiative (PARENT Joint Action), 236
PCORI see Patient-Centred Outcomes Research Institute (PCORI)
PCWP (Patient and Consumer Working Party), 233
European Multiple Sclerosis Platform membership, 233
PD see Parkinson's disease (PD)
PDF (Parkinson's Disease Foundation), 267–8
peer resources, project management, 181
PEG (percutaneous endoscopic gastrostomy) procedure, 248
pembrolizumab, 287
percutaneous endoscopic gastrostomy (PEG) procedure, 248
performing, The Theory U, 30
peripheral nervous system (PNS), cancer, 285
peripheral neuropathy
case study, 256
incidence/prevalence, 253–4
permanent vegetative state, 42
perseverance, advocacy, 74
persistence, international advocacy, 202
persistent vegetative state, 42
personality changes, 47
personalized care, neuropathic pain, 347–8
perspective lists, project management, 182–3
PET (positron emission tomography), brain tumours, 282
Peterson, Ronald, 299
pharmaceutical industry, 53–60
advocacy, 59
European Multiple Sclerosis Platform, 239f
physicians interactions, 54–5
representatives, 54, 55, 56–7
understanding of, 56–7
physical needs, neuromuscular disorder, 255

physical therapy
 brain tumours, 284
 neuropathic pain treatment, 349
physician advocates
 dementia, 298–9
 neuro-oncology, 286
 neuropathic pain, 349–51
 rare disorders, 307
 relations to other groups, 372–3
physician-assisted suicide, 247
physician autonomy, 53–60
 amyotrophic lateral sclerosis, 244
physicians (doctors), 83–7
 advocacy, duty of, 71, 72, 85, 87, 219
 core competencies, 69
 healthcare system leaders as, 85
 managed care role, 84
 patient needs, 25–6
 patient support groups, 85–6
 pharmaceutical industry interactions, 54–5
 pharmaceutical representative visits, 54, 56–7
 roles of, 83–4
 social healthcare system, 85
 training and advocacy, 86–7
PIL (public interest litigations), 144
PLACEBO, 71
planning, dementia advocacy, 294
platforms, public relations, 211, 211t
PNE *see* public neurology education (PNE)
PNS (peripheral nervous system), cancer, 285
Political Action Committee, 143
political crises, migrants/refugees, 124
political thinking, 14
population-based surveys, Global Campaign Against Headache, 343
positive subjects, appreciative inquiry, 28
positron emission tomography (PET), brain tumours, 282
Posner, Jerome, 281
post-ischaemic encephalopathy, cognitive impairment, 47
post-mortem analysis, projects, 366–7
post-traumatic encephalopathy, cognitive impairment, 47
Potts, Daniel, 298
PPP (Path to Participation), 233
PR *see* public relations (PR)
PR Crisis Bible (Cohn), 208
pregabalin, 348
preprocessing, project management, 183–4
presencing, The Theory U, 28, 29, 29f
press conferences, 210
press kits (media kits), 210
primary care physicians, neuroscience education, 140
proactive mindset, project management, 180
problems in understanding
 dementia, 296
 palliative care advocacy, 318
procrastination, project management, 186

productive-age adults, 6
professional advocates, 74, 247–8
professional organizations, healthcare advocacy, 86
prognosis, rare disorders, 304
programme portfolio, SOS Children's Villages, 169, 170f
progressive supranuclear palsy (PSP), 268
 see also movement disorders
project management, 179–91
 advocacy goals, 183–4
 failure of, 188–9
 goals and milestones, 179, 181–6
 higher altitude goals, 182–3
 initiation, 179
 motivation, 186–8
 preprocessing, 183–4
 proactive mindset, 180
 procrastination, 186
 resources, 181
 sound bites, 180–1
 target audience, 180
 to-do lists, 184–6
 working environment, 179–80
projects, 370–2
 content, 371–2
 ending and closing, 364
 harvesting, 366
 learning from, 366
 level of, 372
 methodology in, 64
 ownership of, 7
 post-mortem analysis, 366–7
 resources, 370–1
 results, 363–4, 364b
 tacit knowledge from *see* The Theory U
 to-do lists, 184–5
 tools, 371–2
Prosser, H, 54
pseudoprogression, brain tumours, 283
pseudoresponses, brain tumours, 283
PSP (progressive supranuclear palsy), 268
PSP Association, 269
PSP Australia, 269
PSP Germany, 269
psychoanalysis, 24
psychology, amyotrophic lateral sclerosis, 244–5
publication bias, 77
public education, 75
public health policy
 headache advocacy, 340–1
 movement disorders, 276t
 prevalence, 340
public interest litigations (PIL), 144
public neurology education (PNE), 135–6, 136b
 literature, 138b
public–private partnerships, neuropathic pain advocacy, 353
public relations (PR), 205–15
 advocacy in, 106

advocacy integration, 206
advocacy vs., 205–6
definitions, 206b
instruments of, 208–11, 209b
media relations, 207–8
non-governmental organizations, 206
online, 212–14
platforms, 211, 211t
spokespersons, 211
publishing, 71
purpose of advocacy, 62

Q
quality of life (QoL), amyotrophic lateral sclerosis, 245

R
RACP (Royal Australasian College of Physicians), 58, 59
radiotherapy
  brain tumours, 282–3
  systemic cancer, 285–6
Rare Disease Clinical Research Network programme (RDCRN)
  drug development, 309–10
  National Institutes of Health, 306
rare disorders, 303–13
  definition, 303
  drug development, 308, 309–10
  empowerment and education, 307–8
  medical service provision, 304
  patient advocate groups, 305–6, 306t
  physician advocates, 307
  prevalence, 303
  problems with, 303–5
  prognosis, 304
  treatment lack, 304–5
  unnecessary medical intervention, 303
RD Action, 306t
RDCRN see Rare Disease Clinical Research Network programme (RDCRN)
reactive depression, amyotrophic lateral sclerosis, 244, 248
Reagan, Nancy, 297
real-world boundaries, community advocacy, 107
RECaN (Recognising European Cancer Nursing) project, 116
Recognising European Cancer Nursing (RECaN) project, 116
recognition of needs, disabled people, 255
redirecting, The Theory U, 28, 29, 29f
Reeves, Christopher, 146
referral resource advocacy, 106
refugees see migrants/refugees
regional level of advocacy, 148t
rehabilitation
  brain cancer, 98
  brain tumours, 284–5
Rehabilitation in MS (RIMS), 234

religions, brain death, 46
research
  advance directive, 50
  ethics of, 41
  movement disorders, 276t
  neuropathic pain, 352–4
  Parkinson's disease, 267
  participation in, 49–50
  SOS Children's Villages, 171
residency training programmes, 86–7
resilience, advocacy, 74
resistance to advocacy, 14–15
  case study, 15–16
resources
  project management, 181
  projects, 370–1
resuscitation, brain injury, 44
reviews, to-do lists, 185
revolutionary dream, Freud, 34–5
RIMS (Rehabilitation in MS), 234
Roberts, Julia, 146
Rotary International, 146
Rowling, J K, 146
Royal Australasian College of Physicians (RACP), 58, 59
Rubin, M, 43, 44

S
Sacks, Oliver, 149
SAFE (Stroke Alliance for Europe), 224
Safe Treatment and Opportunities to Prevent Pain Act (STOP), 342
sarcoma, 120
Sarcoma Patient EuroNet (SPAEN), 119–20
scheduling, project failure, 189
Schlesinger, Renate, 35
Schnitzler, Arthur, 34
scholarly practice, advocacy, 74
Schönberg, Arnold, 34
science
  advocacy, 298–9
  consumerism vs., 70
  funding, 71
  headache advocacy, 340
  movement disorder information, 276t
  politics advocacy, 249–50
sedation, head injury, 45
selective serotonin reuptake inhibitors (SSRIs), diabetic neuropathy, 355
self-advocacy
  case study, 5–6
  negative kind, 6
  neurologists, 147, 148t
self-confidence, nurses, 94
self-documentation, 27
self-knowledge, 23
self-management
  brain cancer, 99, 100
  patient activation, 102
self-responsibility, patients, 7

Shapiro, William, 281
shared decision-making model, 44–5
shared decision-making process, 48
short-term objectives of advocacy, 62–3
Shriver, Maria, 297
Singapore, stroke survivors/caregivers/healthcare workers, 225
situational change, international advocacy, 201–2
skills, nurse advocacy, 92
SMART (specific, measurable, assignable, realistic and time-related), 65
　dementia advocacy, 294
　goal setting, 183–4
SNO (Society for Neuro-Oncology), 281
social aspects
　advocacy definition, 8
　amyotrophic lateral sclerosis, 246–50
　palliative care, 319
Social Democrats, Vienna, 37
social healthcare system, 85
social media, 207, 213–14
social networks, dystonia advocacy, 272–3
societal issues
　advocacy in, 62
　cause–effect cycle, 174
Society for Neuro-Oncology (SNO), 281
Society for Neurosciences, 295b
socioeconomic status, migrants/refugees, 125
soft skills, 71
someone else's problem, 48
SOS Children's Villages, 167–76
　advocacy inclusion, 169–70
　data collection, 169
　deinstitutionalization process, 171–2
　development, 167–70
　Eastern Europe, 171–2
　flourishing of, 168
　history, 167–8
　independent research, 171
　internal challenges, 170–1
　international successes, 171–6
　opposition to, 167–8
　programme portfolio, 169, 170f
　stocktaking (2000), 169–70
sound bites, project management, 180–1
South Asia, consanguinity, 127
South Central Library System Advocacy, 295b
South East Asia, health expenditure, 153
SPAEN (Sarcoma Patient EuroNet), 119–20
Specialist Ataxia Centre (London), 275
specialists, 70
speciality care setting, neuromuscular disorder, 254
SPICT (Supportive and Palliative Care Indicators), 317
spinal cord injury, case study, 256–7
spokespersons
　advocacy, 105
　public relations, 211
spontaneous breathing, brain death, 46

sporadic Creutzfeldt–Jakob disease, 296
Sri Lanka
　essential drug policy, 57–9
　free market economy, 57–8
　State Pharmaceutical Cooperation, 57
　stroke advocacy, 226–7
Sri Lanka Freedom Party (SLFP), 57
SSOs (stroke support organizations), 224
SSRIs (selective serotonin reuptake inhibitors), diabetic neuropathy, 355
stakeholders, 75
Stand up For Epilepsy Sports and Epilepsy Project, 334
START-EXTEND IA, 222
State Pharmaceutical Cooperation (SPC) (Sri Lanka), 57
St Christopher's Hospice, 321
Stevens–Johnson syndrome, 257
stigma, epilepsy in migrant communities, 126
STOP (Safe Treatment and Opportunities to Prevent Pain Act), 342
storytelling, 76
stroke, 4, 219–28
　brain injury, 45–6
　case studies, 220–7
　cognitive impairment, 47
　Framingham Health Study, 219
　migrants/refugees, 127–8
　mortality, 219
　online resources, 225
　treatment, 194–5
Stroke Alliance for Europe (SAFE), 224
Stroke Care Act, 144b
StrokeCare.sg, 225
Stroke Network, 224
Stroke Patient Organization, 224
stroke support organizations (SSOs), 224
studies of advocacy, 77–8
sub-Saharan Africa
　health expenditure, 153
　HIV infection, 126
　stroke, 128
sudden unexplained death in epilepsy (SUDEP), 328
SUDEP (sudden unexplained death in epilepsy), 328
Superego, 35
Supportive and Palliative Care Indicators (SPICT), 317
supportive care needs
　brain tumours, 283
　patients, 94
surgical resection, brain tumours, 282
surrogate decision-makers, 44
survival rates, brain cancer, 98
suspending, The Theory U, 28, 29f
Sustainable Development Goals (2015–2030) (UN), 173–4, 175f
Sweden, driving ability and neurological disease, 49

sympathy, advocacy, 73
symptomatic care, amyotrophic lateral sclerosis, 249
synergy, 14
systemic cancer, 285–7

T

TA (Tourette's Action), 274
tacit knowledge
   advocacy projects to *see* The Theory U
   needs of, 23–4
   patient needs of, 24
TAG (topic advisory group), ICD-10, 154
TAN (Tremor Action Network), 269
Tandler, Julius, 36–9, 37
target audience, project management, 180
TB (tuberculosis), migrants/refugees, 125
teachers, neurology education, 140–1
team numbers, advocacy in neurology, 316
teamwork, 14
tension-type headache, 339
   prevalence, 340
terminology/nomenclature, 160
theoretical background, 23–4
The Theory U, 28–30, 29*f*
tics, 273–4
time to decide, palliative care advocacy, 318
tobacco use, cancer, 114*b*
to-do lists, project management, 184–6
tools, projects, 371–2
top-down advocacy, 8
topic advisory group (TAG), ICD-10, 154
Tourette Association of America, 274
Tourette's Action (TA), 274
Tourette's syndrome, 273–4
toxic epidermal necrolysis, genotyping, 257
Toyotaization, 70
training in advocacy, 78
   physicians, 86–7
traumatic brain injury, dementia, 292
treatment
   ethical restrictions, 50–1
   identification of gaps, 164
   inequalities in multiple sclerosis, 235
Treatment of Painful DPN guidelines, American Academy of Neurology, 350
Tremor Action Network (TAN), 269
Tremor Research Group (TRG), 269
TRG (Tremor Research Group), 269
tricyclic antidepressants, diabetic neuropathy, 355
triggers, palliative care, 317
tuberculosis (TB), migrants/refugees, 125
tumour-directed treatment, 50
twinning, epilepsy advocacy, 334
Twitter, 213

U

underprivileged population, 6
unexpected, prepare for, 201
UNICEF, 258
United Kingdom (UK)
   assisted dying, 322
   care coordination, 93
   headache advocacy, 342
   Specialist Ataxia Centre (London), 275
United Nations (UN)
   alternative care for children guidelines, 172–3
   Convention on the Rights of the Child, 171
   health as a human right, 61
   Sustainable Development Goals (2015–2030), 173–4, 175*f*
United States (US)
   American Academy of Neurology (AAN) *see* American Academy of Neurology (AAN)
   American Headache Society, 342
   American Heart Association, 224
   American Library Association Advocacy Institute, 295*b*
   American Medical Association (AMA), 307
   American Stroke Association, 224
   Americans with Disabilities Act, 258
   care coordination, 93
   headache advocacy, 341, 342
   Ibero-American Stroke Society, 224
   Latin America Summit for Stroke, 224
   managed healthcare, 84
   Myasthenia Gravis Foundation of America, 308
   National Multiple Sclerosis Society, 229
   Neurology on the Hill, 143
   Pan American Health Organization (PAHO), 224
   rare disorders prevalence, 303
   Tourette Association of America, 274
   Wyoming Parkinson's Disease Community, 266
unnecessary medical intervention, rare disorders, 303
urban signature, 37
Utermohlen, William, 300

V

vaccination, migrants/refugees, 130
value of treatment (VOT) for brain disorders in Europe, 163
vascular dementia, 292
vegetative state, 42
Vienna
   elderly care home, 15–16
   history of advocacy, 33–4
   interwar years, 36–7
   Social Democrats, 37
The Vienna System, 37–8
virtual advocacy, 271
virtual boundaries, community advocacy, 107
virtual press conferences, public relations, 213
visionary, project management, 182
The Voice of 12,000 People (EURORDIS), 304
VOT (value of treatment) for brain disorders in Europe, 163

W

Walley, T, 54
war, advocacy of, 61–2
Wazana, Ashley, 54
websites, 212
Western Europe, health expenditure, 153
Western Health (Melbourne, Australia), stroke case study, 220–2
Western Ontario and McMaster Universities Arthritis Index (WOMAC), 353
WFN *see* World Federation of Neurology (WFN)
WHA *see* World Health Assembly (WHA)
whistle-blowing, 74
white papers, neurology advocacy, 141–2, 141*b*
WHO *see* World Health Organization (WHO)
Wickramasinghe, S A, 57
Williams, Robin, 146
Will, Robert, 298
Wilson, Charles, 281
Wittgenstein, Ludwig, 34
WOMAC (Western Ontario and McMaster Universities Arthritis Index), 353
women's rights, migrants/refugees, 129, 130
working environment, project management, 179–80
World Alzheimer's Day, 205
World Alzheimer's Month, 205
World Bank
  health expenditure estimates, 153
  World Report on Disability, 255–6
World Brain Atlas (WHO), 86
World Brain Day, 86, 205
World Congress of Neurology, training days, 86
World Federation of Neurology (WFN), 86
  Atlas: Country Resources for Neurological Disorders, 156–7
  dementia recommendations, 157
  epilepsy advocacy, 332, 333
  international advocacy, 153
  Neurological Disorders: Public Health Challenges, 157
  neuromuscular disorder, 254
  palliative care, 323
  white paper drafting, 142
World Federation of Neuro-Oncology Societies, 282
World Health Assembly (WHA)
  dementia recommendations, 157
  epilepsy advocacy, 332
  WHO, 199
World Health Organization (WHO)
  advocacy dementia, 295*b*
  Atlas of Epilepsy Care, 328, 330
  dementia recognition, 300
  dementia recommendations, 157
  epilepsy advocacy, 330, 333
  Global Action Plan in the Public Health Response to Dementia, 300
  Global Campaign Against Headache, 343–4
  headache education, 339
  healthcare provision figures, 154
  International Clinical Trials Registry Platform, 258
  Mental Health Gap Action Programme, 331
  migrants/refugees health, 128
  National Neurology Association and, 147
  Neurological Disorders: Public Health Challenges, 157
  neuromuscular disorder, 254
  non-communicable diseases, 156
  palliative care definition, 315
  patient-centred care, 115
  rare disorders, 308
  role of, 83
  stroke, importance of, 224
  white paper drafting, 142
  World Brain Atlas, 86
  World Health Assembly, 199
  World Report on Disability, 255–6
World Parkinson's Day, 205
World Press Trends (2016), 207
World Report on Disability (WHO/World Bank), 255–6
World Stoke Association (WSO), 86
World Stroke Association (WSA), 226–7
  ICD-11 consultation, 156
World Stroke Campaign, 219
World Stroke Day, 205, 224
  China 2015, 226
  Sri Lanka 2009, 226
Written Declaration of Epilepsy, European Parliament, 332
WSA *see* World Stroke Association (WSA)
WSO (World Stoke Association), 86
Wyoming Parkinson's Disease Community, 266

Y

Year of the Brain (YOTB 2014), European Brain Council, 164–5
Youth Pre-World Health assembly, International Federation of Medical Students' Association, 199
YouTube, public relations, 213

The manufacturer's authorised representative in the EU for product safety is
Oxford University Press España S.A. of el Parque Empresarial San Fernando de
Henares, Avenida de Castilla, 2 – 28830 Madrid (www.oup.es/en or product.
safety@oup.com). OUP España S.A. also acts as importer into Spain of products
made by the manufacturer.

www.ingramcontent.com/pod-product-compliance
Ingram Content Group UK Ltd.
Pitfield, Milton Keynes, MK11 3LW, UK
UKHW022230230426
12048UKWH00016BA/1165